PROGRESS IN SYSTEMIC LUPUS ERYTHEMATOSUS RESEARCH

PROGRESS IN SYSTEMIC LUPUS ERYTHEMATOSUS RESEARCH

TOMAS I. SEWARD
EDITOR

Nova Biomedical Books
New York

For permission to use material from this book please contact us:
Telephone 631-231-7269; Fax 631-231-8175
Web Site: http://www.novapublishers.com

LIBRARY OF CONGRESS CATALOGING-IN-PUBLICATION DATA

Progress in systemic lupus erythematosus research / TomasI. Seward (editor).
p. ; cm.
Includes bibliographical references and index.
ISBN-13: 978-1-60021-861-3 (hardcover)
ISBN-10: 1-60021-861-X (hardcover)
1. Systemic lupus erythematosus. I. Seward, tpmas I.
[DNLM: 1. Lupus Erythematosus, Systemic. WR 152 P964 2008]
RC924.d.L85P76 2008
616.7'7--dc22

2007030893

Published by Nova Science Publishers, Inc. ✦ New York

Contents

Preface		**vii**
Expert Commentary	Therapeutic Plasmapheresis in the Treatment of Complicated Systemic Lupus Erythematosus *Claudia Stefanutti, Fabio Mazza and Valeria Riccieri*	
Expert Commentary	Pregnancy, a Challenge in Patients with Systemic Lupus Erythematosus *Javier A. Cavallasca and Maria del Rosario Maliandi*	**9**
Short Communications	Influence of Exercise on the Peripheral Circulation in Patients with Systemic Lupus Erythematosus and Systemic Sclerosis *Etsuko Maeshima and Kanako Furukawa*	**17**
Chapter 1	New Frontiers in the Research of Cardiovascular Disease Associated with Systemic Lupus Erythematosus *Laura Gonzalez-Lopez, J. I. Gamez-Nava and Arnulfo Nava*	**29**
Chapter 2	Comorbidity in Systemic Lupus Erythematosus: Aspects of Cardiovascular Disease, Osteoporosis and Infections *Irene E. M. Bultink, Ben A. C. Dijkmans and Alexandre E. Voskuyl*	**77**
Chapter 3	Severe Tissue Trauma Triggers Lupus Autoimmune Disease *Khairul Anam, Mihret Amare, Shruti Naik, Kathleen A. Szabo and Thomas A. Davis*	**105**
Chapter 4	Immunotherapy with Ig-Derived Peptides in SLE: Current Status and Directions *Antonio La Cava and Bevra H. Hahn*	**131**

Chapter 5	Autoantibodies as Prognostic or Diagnostic Markers of Psychiatric Manifestations in SLE *Paola Margutti, Federica Delunardo, Tania Colasanti, Ettore Piro and Elena Ortona*	155
Chapter 6	High-Dose Immunosuppression with Autologous Stem Cell Transplantation in Severe Refractory Systemic Lupus Erythematosus *Igor A. Lisukov, Vera V. Sergeevicheva, Svetlana A. Sizikova, Alexander D. Kulagin, Irina V. Kruchkova, Andrey V. Gilevich, Alexey E. Sizikov, Ludmila P. Konenkova, Elena R. Chernykh, Olga Y. Leplina and Vladimir A. Kozlov*	**177**
Chapter 7	MR Spectroscopy, Diffusion and Diffusion Tensor Imaging in Systemic Lupus Erythematosus *Pia C. Sundgren, Patricia Cagnoli and William McCune*	**193**
Chapter 8	Personalized Medicine for Systemic Lupus Erythematosus: A New Challenge for the Near Future *Ana M. Bertoli and Luis M. Vilá*	**211**
Chapter 9	Therapeutic Potential of HMG-CoA Reductase Inhibitors (Statins) in Systemic Lupus Erythematosus *Przemyslaw J. Kotyla and Bogna Sliwinska-Kotyla*	**227**
Index		**245**

PREFACE

This new book is devoted to leading-edge research developments in lupus which is a condition of chronic inflammation caused by an autoimmune disease. Autoimmune diseases are illnesses that occur when the body's tissues are attacked by its own immune system. The immune system is a complex system within the body that is designed to fight infectious agents, for example, bacteria, and other foreign invaders. One of the mechanisms that the immune system uses to fight infections is the production of antibodies. Patients with lupus produce abnormal antibodies in their blood that target tissues within their own body rather than foreign infectious agents. Because the antibodies and accompanying cells of inflammation can involve tissues anywhere in the body, lupus has the potential to affect a variety of areas of the body. Sometimes lupus can cause disease of the skin, heart, lungs, kidneys, joints, and/or nervous system. When only the skin is involved, the condition is called discoid lupus. When internal organs are involved, the condition is called systemic lupus erythematosus (SLE).

Chapter 1 - Cardiovascular disease is a major cause of mortality in patients with systemic lupus erythematosus (SLE). Around 52% of the autopsies performed in SLE in our centre have shown cardiac involvement and most of these disorders were not diagnosed pre-mortem [1].

Current topics for research are accelerated atherosclerosis, pulmonary hypertension, development of valvular disease and new other forms of cardiac involvement. Most of the patients deceased by cardiovascular disease have an accelerated atherosclerosis. Some authors reported a substantial increase in risk of fatal vascular event in women with SLE compared with matched controls. New methods such as electron-beam computed tomography have demonstrated a highly prevalence of coronary disorder even in asymptomatic patients. Additionally, high resolution carotid ultrasonography has shown a high prevalence of carotid lesions. Both cellular and molecular mechanisms of the accelerated atherosclerosis are complex and not entirely explained by the traditional cardiovascular risk factors, therefore, the research targets on nontraditional factors.

Pulmonary hypertension is relevant by its morbidity and mortality. Previously considered as rare entity; new non-invasive studies have detected patients with earlier involvement; our group have reported a prevalence of 18% in a series of 204 patients assessed by Doppler echocardiography. A follow-up study in our cohort observed an increase of 4 times greater of risk for cardiac failure in patients with asymptomatic pulmonary pressure >40 mmHg. Strategies for the treatment of pulmonary hypertension include immunosuppressive therapy, prostanoids, phosphodiesterase inhibitors or endothelin receptor antagonists. Most of the current information related with the response to these treatments proceeds from short-term studies with a wide variability in the outcome measures making necessary additional research in this area.

There is also a renovate interest in the valvular disease, recent studies show association between antiphospholipid antibodies and mitral valve nodules or mitral regurgitation, the potential effects of these antibodies on the endothelial activation require to be evaluated.

Cardiac dysfunction is another important area for research; several studies have shown a high prevalence of left ventricular diastolic dysfunction. In the authors series this manifestation is present in around 63%. Nevertheless, to date no follow-up studies have been done to evaluate the importance of diastolic dysfunction on the morbidity or mortality.

In summary cardiovascular disease in systemic lupus represents a very exciting area for research being necessary to increase the number of long-term prospective cohorts and well-designed controlled trials in order to improve the clinical care of the patients with this involvement.

Chapter 2 - Over the last decades, the survival of patients with systemic lupus erythematosus (SLE) has improved dramatically. Having improved treatment for active lupus disease, the challenge is now to understand and prevent the long-term complications of the disease, which may be due to the disease itself or the therapies used. To date, long-term complications of SLE are now considered to be important, including cardiovascular disease, osteoporosis and infections.

Cardiovascular disease in patients with SLE, including coronary artery disease, ischemic cerebrovascular disease, and peripheral vascular disease, is the result of premature atherosclerosis. Besides the traditional risk factors (like hypertension, hypercholesterolaemia and smoking), renal insufficiency, raised homocysteine levels, and the presence of anti-phospholipid, antibodies have been recognized as additional risk factors for cardiovascular disease in SLE. Recent studies have demonstrated that the nitric oxide pathway and its endogenous inhibitor asymmetric dimethylarginine may also be involved in the pathogenesis of cardiovascular organ damage in SLE. The metabolic syndrome and insulin resistance in SLE patients are current topics of research in this field.

Several studies have demonstrated a high prevalence of low bone mineral density in patients with SLE, especially in females. In the last few years, more attention is paid to osteoporotic fractures, one of the items of the organ damage index for SLE, and likely the most preventable form of musculoskeletal organ damage in SLE patients. Recent studies have demonstrated an increased frequency of symptomatic vertebral and nonvertebral fractures in patients with SLE. Moreover, a high prevalence of mostly asymptomatic vertebral fractures in patients with SLE was detected. These vertebral fractures were associated with previous use of intravenous methylprednisolone. The importance of identifying vertebral fractures in SLE patients is illustrated by the observed association between prevalent vertebral fractures and reduced quality of life as well as an increased risk of future vertebral and nonvertebral fractures in the general population.

Infection imposes a serious burden on patients with SLE. In case series, infectious complications were found in 25% to 45% of SLE patients, and infection as primary cause of death has been demonstrated in up to 50% of SLE patients. Defects of immune defence and treatment with corticosteroids and other immunosuppressive agents are supposed to play a role in the pathogenesis of infections in SLE. Recently, research has focused on the role of the lectin pathway of complement activation in the occurrence of infections in SLE.

In this review the results of recent studies on cardiovascular disease, osteoporosis and infectious complications in SLE will be discussed.

Chapter 3 - Systemic lupus erythematosus (SLE) is a chronic, complex autoimmune disease characterized by high levels of non-organ-specific, self-reactive antibody production leading to immune complex formation. The etiology of this autoimmune disease remains elusive. The disease results in multiple health problems including increased infection, renal and skin disorders, neurological complications, osteoporosis, rheumatoid arthritis, osteoarthritis, and fibromylagias. Tissue damage associated with severe injury can result in profound immune dysfunction that involves suppressive cell types and a cascade of inflammatory and tissue reparative mediators. Mice from MRL strains have been used as models to study SLE pathogenesis. Wild type MRL/MpJ mice exhibit SLE autoimmune disorders but symptoms are manifested much later in life (70-90 weeks) compared to MRL/MpJ-*Fas*^{lpr} mice (17-22 weeks) which possess a lymphoproliferative mutation. Based on our preliminary findings, the authors hypothesize that following traumatic tissue injury, the activation of specific cell types, cytokines and other mediators involved in wound healing and repair processes may be critical in triggering lupus-like disease. The authors investigated the role of a severe (15% total body surface area) full-thickness cutaneous burn on the early onset of lupus-like autoimmune disease in young adult, lupus prone wild type MRL/MpJ mice, and control BALB/c mice. MRL/MpJ mice develop autoimmune disease 4-15 weeks post injury, manifested by skin lesions, vasculitis, epidermal ulcers, cellular infiltration, splenomegaly, lymphadenopathy, hypergammaglobulinemia, elevated autoantibodies, and renal pathologies including proteinuria, glomerulonephritis, and immune complex deposition. Post-injury survival rate of injured MRL/MpJ mice is significantly reduced due to autoimmune related complications. In contrast, neither uninjured MRL/MpJ mice nor burned BALB/c displayed signs of autoimmunity or premature death. The authors analyzed mRNA expression of numerous cytokines at the wound margins in the skin at days 1-7 post injury. The authors results do not reveal an early or clear Th1 or Th2 cytokine expression pattern during the early wound repair process but demonstrate a correlation between the pathogenic effects of dysregulated interleukin-beta (IL-1β), interleukin-6 (IL-6), tumor necrosis factor alpha (TNF-α) and prostaglandin-E2 (PGE2) synthesis and the early onset of lupus-like disease. Interestingly, the authors found that normal skin isografts transplanted onto the dorsum of MRL/MpJ mice with healed wounds (30- 40 days post burn injury) are rejected within 7 days after transplantation. In contrast, skin grafts transplanted onto uninjured age-matched MRL/MpJ achieved long-term survival. Collectively, these findings suggest that traumatic injury exacerbates inflammatory skin disease and the early onset of severe multi-organ SLE pathogenesis.

Chapter 4 - Understanding the mechanisms that control autoimmune reactivity is an essential step to improve management of autoimmune diseases including systemic lupus erythematosus (SLE). In SLE, the interaction between hyperactive T cells and B cells causes dysregulated production of autoantibodies that by themselves or in immune complexes fix to tissue and cause organ damage. The immune cell subsets that take part in this process have come under intense scrutiny in the past few years, and new information has been acquired on how they interact to induce and/or modulate disease. This information has also led to the development of autoantibody-derived peptide therapies that can effectively influence murine SLE. This chapter describes the rationale, current experimental evidence, preclinical models, and future directions for the use of autoantigen- and Ig-derived peptides in SLE. Considering that autoantibodies in lupus patients have amino acid sequences similar to those of murine antibodies, and at similar locations, it is likely that some of those strategies will be potentially useful in the therapy of human SLE.

Chapter 5 - In the course of Systemic Lupus Erythematosus (SLE), a variety of psychiatric disturbances are reported, including mood disorders (depressive symptoms), psychosis and anxiety. The reported prevalence of psychiatric disorders in SLE varies widely, ranging from 17% to 75%, but the diagnosis of these syndromes is difficult and depends on the exclusion of complications due to an iatrogenic effect of drugs, to metabolic abnormalities or to infections. Moreover, the diagnosis requires a careful psychiatric evaluation to exclude merely reactive psychological disturbances.

It has been suggested that several autoantibody specificities play a role in the pathogenesis of neuropsychiatric SLE. Potential pathogenic relevance has been attributed to, among others, antineuronal, antiphospholipid, antiganglioside, anti-DNA, anti-ribosomal P protein and anti-endothelial cell antibodies. However, particularly regarding psychiatric syndromes, conflicting results have been reported on the association between serum autoantibodies and symptoms.

The diagnostic and/or prognostic role of autoantibodies associated to psychiatric disorders in SLE is discussed.

Chapter 6 - Carry out a prolonged studies to elucidate the role of high dose immunosupression therapy (HDIST) with autologous hematopoietic stem cells transplantation (SCT) in the treatment of severe and refractory autoimmune disease. In this study the authors analyzed single center experience of HDIST followed by SCT for refractory SLE.

The 13 patients with SLE, who had disease progression despite previously treatment with pulse Cy intravenous, prednisolone (standard doses and pulse therapy), oral Cy, azathioprine or metotrexate, were enrolled in the clinic of our Institution from 1998 to 2007. All patients were seriously ill, with SLE disease activity indices (SLEDAI) of 6-30, including cases with central nervous system lupus, lung vasculitis, carditis, nephritis with nephrotic syndrome and cytopenia. Autologous haemopoietic stem cells were collected from bone marrow (n=4) or mobilized from peripheral blood with Cy (3g/m2/once) and granulocyte colony-stimulating factor (G-CSF) (n=9). Pretransplant conditioning regimens included BEAM ± ATG (n=2), Melphalan 140 mg/m^2 + Etoposid 1600 mg/m^2 (n=2), Cy 200 mg/kg ± ATG (n=2) and Melphalan 120 mg/m^2 (n=1), Cy 140 mg/kg (n=6). Transplanted CD34+ MNC were more then 2x106/kg. Median time to an absolute neutrophil count (ANC) greater than 0,5x10^9 /l and platelet count greater than 50x10^9/l was 11 and 15 days, respectively. Three patients died on days 11, 22 and 63 due to transplant-related complications. All of the patients who died due to transplant-related complications had long history of the corticosteroids treatment, multiple and severe episodes of infections pre-SCT and received more then one anticytoststic drugs or ATG as conditioning regimen. All of the alive transplanted patients, who recovered hematopoiesis, showed improvement in disease activity: 8 (CR) and 2 (PR). The median follow up is now 14 month. One patient died due to lung vasculitis progression after 8 years after SCT. We conclude that HDIST followed by SCT for refractory SLE is feasible, effective and achievement of prolonged, corticosteroid-free remissions is a reality.

Chapter 7 - Although clinical assessment is the cornerstone of SLE and NPSLE diagnosis; it can be difficult to make and is frequently presumptive. MR findings play an important role in supporting a clinical diagnosis and findings include volume loss, focal white matter hyperintensity, diffusion abnormalities due to ischemic injuries, evidence of prior hemorrhage or infarct, and meningeal enhancement. Nevertheless, several previous studies have shown that conventional pre-and post-contrast enhanced brain MR appear normal in approximately one third of both symptomatic and asymptomatic NPSLE patients and even more frequently in SLE patients. It has been suggested that other modalities such as MR spectroscopy (MRS), diffusion weighted imaging (DWI) and diffusion tensor imaging (DTI) could be additional tools in the evaluation and monitoring of SLE and NPSLE patients. This chapter will describe these new MRI techniques, recent research results and trends, and discuss if these techniques may add any valuable information that may further elucidate the pathogenesis of NPSLE. These techniques may possibly aid in diagnosing and differentiating NPSLE from other diseases with similar acute clinical symptoms as well as in monitoring disease progression.

Chapter 8 - Systemic lupus erythematosus (SLE) is a chronic disease with higher morbidity and mortality when compared to the general population. Disease outcome varies among patients, in part, because they do not respond the same to a given treatment modality. There is, therefore, a clear need for drug treatments to be selected according to the characteristics of an individual patient, in order to improve efficacy and reduce the number and severity of adverse drug reactions. Personalized medicine means the prescription of specific therapeutics best suited for an individual. This novel treatment approach should be regarded as an ongoing progression of healthcare which is advancing with genomic tools. Although still a translational challenge into the practice of rheumatologists, data for immunosuppressive drugs (mainly coming from transplant patients) is now available and waiting to be introduced in the field of autoimmune diseases such as SLE. Examples of that are genetic studies of drug metabolizing systems that can affect the efficacy, pharmacokinetic and tolerability profile of drugs such as azathioprine, cyclosporin A, mycophenolate mofetil, cyclophosphamide and glucocorticoids, among others. Although quite attractive, implementation of pharmacogenomics may not be so simple. Ideally the genetic trait should be accomplished with a well characterized patient from the socio-demographic, cultural and ethnic background as well as co-morbidities and drug exposure history, variables known as being modifier factors for drug efficacy and tolerability. Major efforts should also be made to systematically evaluate the patient; in this sense, validated outcome measures of disease activity, accumulated damage and health-related quality of life could be very valuable to quantify drug response. Worldwide integrated genomic information should also be an unequivocal subject for the future. Although quite attractive, personalized medicine is not without some drawbacks; cost, infrastructure and worldwide networking are not minor issues to overcome. Finally, personalized medicine must be strongly interpreted from the ethics perspective and regulated by the law.

Chapter 9 - Systemic lupus erythematosus is a connective tissue disorder of unknown origin and a relatively bad prognosis. In the last fifty years the big progress in the treatment of the condition has been made, resulting in the improvement of prognosis and prolongation of the life span. Nowadays we are prepare enough to manage the acute form of the disease, treat acute vasculitis lupus nephritis, decrease inflammation. As the result of extension of the life span the lupus face has been changed. Today a premature atherosclerosis is considered the main risk factor for increased mortality among lupus patients. The premature development of atherosclerosis is a well known clinical phenomena since the work of Urowitz and colleagues who described the term bimodal peak of mortality and attributed the second peak of mortality to premature development of atherosclerosis and its fatal complications. For almost two decades the mechanism of the atherosclerosis in lupus had not been explained satisfactory. In the early nineties of the last century Ross suggested that atherosclerotic process is an inflammation in its nature. Now atherosclerosis is considered a chronic inflammatory condition of the vessel wall. In the recent years many immunological mechanisms in the development and progression of the atherosclerotic lesions have been recognized. Since the atherosclerosis and atherosclerosis in lupus patients share the same pattern of inflammation it would be reasonable to treat the patients with a drug that cools the inflammation on one side and halts progression of atherosclerosis on the other.

Statins, inhibitors of HMG-CoA reductase, a key enzyme in the pathway of cholesterol synthesis have been commonly used in the therapy of ischemic coronary events and the control of hypercholesterolemia. In last years evidence was accumulated suggesting that action of statins go far beyond lipid lowering properties and may affect function of immune system cells. An array of anti-inflammatory effects has now been identified, including reduced production of pro-inflammatory cytokines, chemokines and adhesion molecules; reduced expression of inducible major histocompatibility complex (MHC) class II molecules by antigen presenting cells (APC); lowering of C-reactive protein levels and reduced production of reactive oxygen species. The effect that is separated from lipid lowering properties is sometimes called pleiotropic action of statins. The beneficial effect is often seen before the normalization of lipid profile suggesting that action of statins comprises at least two mechanism – cholesterol synthesis inhibition and direct effect on arterial wall and endothelium.

Such pleiotropic effect may benefit patients with autoimmune rheumatic diseases, including lupus.

The repertoire of drugs used in the treatment of systemic autoimmune disorders is characterized by unfavorable influence on lipid profile in patients treated, thus may perpetuate the development of atherosclerosis evoked by the inflammatory process itself.

In this regard statins may act on two main fields; being a concomitant therapy for autoimmune disorders and normalize the lipid profile abnormalities in patients with connective tissue disorders.

This overview assesses the evidence for using statins in patients with systemic lupus erythematosus.

In: Progress in Systemic Lupus Erythematosus Research
Editor: Tomas I. Seward, pp. 1-8
ISBN 978-1-60021-861-3

Expert Commentary

THERAPEUTIC PLASMAPHERESIS IN THE TREATMENT OF COMPLICATED SYSTEMIC LUPUS ERYTHEMATOSUS

Claudia Stefanutti*, Fabio Mazza and Valeria Riccieri
Department of Clinical and Medical Therapy – Plasmapheresis Unit and Rheumatology Laboratory – University "La Sapienza"of Rome 'Umberto I' Hospital. Rome, Italy

ABSTRACT

Systemic Lupus Erythematosus (SLE), can be complicated by nephritis and various forms of vasculitis. The treatment is aimed at reducing the autoimmune reaction, responsible for vascular damage, and is usually done with immunosuppressive agents. The therapeutic approach for immune complex-mediated vasculitis, as with most systemic autoimmune diseases, is aimed at reducing the pathological immune complexes and autoantibodies. However, conventional drug treatment is not always successful and has a high side-effects potential, especially during long-term therapy. It is also well-known that is not always effective to avoid the development of complications. Such severe cases need definitely of innovative therapeutic approaches, because of their poor prognosis. Indications for the use of therapeutic plasmapheresis in SLE have undergone several modifications since the first treatment in 1974. Once thought to be a promising treatment for selected aspects of SLE, conventional apheresis has been limited as a co-therapeutic adjunct in managing the disorder. Conventional plasmapheresis techniques such as plasma-exchange have considerable disadvantages. The non-selective removal of plasma constituents and the necessary substitution with foreign plasma or human albumin

* Corresponding Author: Stefanutti Claudia, M.D., Ph.D., Professor of Internal Medicine. Specialties: Emergency Surgery; Liver and Metabolic Diseases. Head of Plasmapheresis Unit. Clinical and Medical Therapy Department. University of Rome "La Sapienza". Policlinico "Umberto I". Viale del Policlinico 155, 00161 Rome. Italy (EU). Tel. +390649970578 ; Fax. +39064440290 ; +390649970141 ; Email: plasmaferesi@tin.it; c.incas@flashnet.it

is associated with a certain range of possible side-effects (anaphylactoid reactions, infections). More recently, a new technique called Immunoadsorption Apheresis (IA) was introduced. IA is different from traditional plasmapheresis in that the plasma is filtered through dextran sulphate membranes and then reinfused. A clinical evaluation of the effect of conventional plasmapheresis and IA, with the additional pharmacological therapy in the management of patients affected by SLE, who are non responsive to drugs was performed in our Unit. The outcome of the above mentioned clinical study confirmed the opportunity of a combined therapeutic approach using pharmacological and non pharmacological treatment of Lupus Nephritis. The double association treatment might be potentially extended to other complications of the disease, such as vasculitis. It is reasonable to infere that the acceptable clinical result obtained, appears to be most probably related to the use of a combined therapeutic strategy, rather than to one treatment only. The above reported experience should be clearly confirmed by increasing the clinical sample. A case-controlled, randomized study should be the target of further investigations. On the other side prominent, conflicting ethical considerations, such as the controversial role and complexity of the so called sham-apheresis, as 'placebo', should be taken into account. The therapeutic potential of IA in combination with immunosuppressive drugs should be furtherly investigated not only in SLE, but also in other autoimmune diseases, with circulating pathological immune complexes. Immunoadsorption treatment using dextran sulfate membranes showed to be effective in the removal of anti-DNA antibodies, that are closely associated with pathogenicity in SLE, improving progressively the renal function. In conclusion, it is argued that syncronised therapy is useful at least in inducing a faster remission in patients with proliferative lupus nephritis, non responsive to the immunosupressive agents alone.

INTRODUCTION

Autoimmune diseases are of considerable medical and economic importance since the age- and sex- adjusted prevalance rate as in the first half of the 90's was approximately 1.22 per 1000 (US white population), and can sometimes follow a complicated course. Within the frame of autoimmune diseases, Systemic Lupus Erythematous (SLE) is recognized to be undoubtedly a serious disease with involvement of several organ(s) and systems. The goal of treatment is to relieve symptoms and protect organs by decreasing inflammation and/or the level of autoimmune activity. Patients with mild symptoms may need only intermittent courses of antiinflammatory treatment. Those with involvement of internal organ(s) may require high doses of corticosteroids in combination with other drugs that suppress the immune system. Nonsteroidal antiinflammatory drugs (NSAIDs) are generally used in attempt of reducing inflammation and pain in muscles, joints, and other tissues. Corticosteroids are more effective than NSAIDs in reducing inflammation and restoring function when the disease is active. Hydroxychloroquine is an antimalarial agent that demonstrated to be particularly effective for patients with fatigue, skin, and joint disease. Immunosuppressive medications (methotrexate, azathioprine, cyclophosphamide) are used for treating patients with more severe manifestations of SLE with involvement of internal organ(s). Patients with SLE can develop different combinations of symptoms and organ involvement developing severe complications such as nephritis, peripheral neuropathy, and various form of vasculitis. The immunosuppressive pharmacological treatment is the first line intervention of the above mentioned complications. However, it is relatively common to observe the failure of the pharmacological approach in terms of avoiding even severe complications in SLE. Furthermore, particularly on long-term course, the conventional treatment based on immunosuppressive drugs may be complicated by the occurrence of mild to severe side effects. In patients with severe neurological or renal disease, therapeutic plasmapheresis (plasma-exchange) (PE) was used to remove antibodies and other immune substances from the blood to suppress immunity. Plasmapheresis has also been used to remove cryoglobulins that can lead to vasculitis, after precipitation. It is widely recognized that therapeutic apheresis might be a useful tool in the therapeutic management of certain rheumatic diseases when their clinical evolution includes life-threatening complications not responding to the conventional immunosuppressive treatment alone. Apheresis 'per se' cannot exclude the pharmacological treatment that should be associated in a combined therapeutic strategy designed in order to allow the best possible approach to attain a favourable clinical outcome. The dextran sulfate cellulose column immunoadsorption system (Selesorb® Kaneka Corporation, Osaka, Japan) (IA), can selectively remove circulating anti-DNA antibody, anti-cardiolipin antibody, and immune complex from the bloodstream. "In vitro" experimental study on plasma of patients with SLE showed that Selesorb® has high adsorbent capacity of anti-DNA antibody, anti-cardiolipin, and immune complexes, but not for total proteins, albumin, immunoglobulins, and complement. Rather than the unselective removal of plasma, adsorption procedures allows the selective or specific removal of immunoglobulins and circulating immune complexes, which seems to be a more reasonable and pathogen-removal oriented approach. In SLE in which antibodies and immune complexes play significant roles, corticosteroids and other immunosuppressive drugs have been used to suppress antibody production to favourably interfere with disease activity. A common clinical experience confirmed that immunosuppressive drugs such as methotrexate azathioprine and cyclophosphamide, and/or PE, may be beneficial in the above mentioned illness. However, controlled studies to assess definitely their efficacy are not available. The primary advantage of IA to plasmapheresis is that fluid substitution is not necessary and thus, the risk of allergic reactions and potential transmission of infections is definitely reduced. However, the potential disadvantage inherent in more specific elimination might be insufficient in removing the pathological substances underlying the disease. In autoimmune diseases, the columns used are mostly those with adsorbers with different binding capacities for immunoglobulins and/or circulating immune complexes. In this pivotal study, we report our clinical experience on patients with SLE, with an immunoadsorption apheresis technique, where immunoglobulins and immune complexes were selectively removed from the plasma by columns containing dextransulfate on cellulose (Selesorb®).

METHODS

Immunoadsorption Plasmapheresis: (Selesorb®)

Selesorb® (Kaneka Corp., Osaka, Japan) is a chemical affinity technique able at removing anti-double-stranded DNA antibodies (anti-dsDNA), selectively from the blood of patients with immune disorders and it is based on immunoadsorption with a dextran sulphate cellulose column (figure 1, 2). The process is thought to work via cross-reactivity of anti-dsDNA with dextran sulphate, which is negatively charged (polyanion). A Kaneka MA-01 (Kaneka Corp., Osaka, Japan) system was used as plasma separator. The total volume of plasma to be processed through the columns was determined from the titer of anti-DNA antibody, and body weight. A plasma volume of 45 ml/kg or from 2.5-3.5 l was processed, and the treatment interval ranged from two to three days. The disease activity was also taken into account as defined by the recurrence or remission of symptoms related to the complication responsible for the extracorporeal treatment of the patient.

Patients

We treated a total of 6 patients, 5 females and 1 male, (mean age: 39.5 years) with SLE, submitted to therapeutic plasmapheresis using Selesorb® immunoadsorption system (Table 1). Informed consent was obtained from all patients. The majority of the above mentioned patients showed at least one severe complication related to the pre-existing immunological disorder, not responding to the conventional medical approach. The mean blood volume processed per session, was of approximately 3000 ml.

Results

Patients affected by SLE improved after treatment with IA. Vasculitis was completely recovered in one patient although nephritis symptoms were substantially unchanged. The complete remission of nephritis was observed in the other five patients (table 1). The mean serum creatinine values in patients with SLE before and after IA apheresis are reported in table 2. The progressive significant decline of proteinuria after 1-year treatment with apheresis in one patient belonging to the above mentioned group is reported in figure 3. The progressive decrease of blood nitrogen and creatinine levels in a second patient along with a relatively significant faster reduction of proteinuria was obtained after no.12 sessions of IA apheresis (figures 4, 5, 6). Plasma total protein and albumin levels, before and after immunoadsorption apheresis, did not show statistically significant variations. There were no short-term or long-term changes of clinical importance in electrolytes, hepatic and renal function tests, albumin and coagulation parameters. In conclusion, 5 patients out 6 showed an overall improvement. It is to be underlined, that the patients enrolled in this study were definitely identified as to be *very poor* or *none-responders* to the pharmacological treatment, prior to be submitted to the combined treatment with therapeutic apheresis.

Discussion

Autoimmune diseases include a broad and heterogeneous group of diseases characterized by inflammation and damage to the blood vessels, thought to be induced by an autoimmune response. Vasculitis may occur alone or in combination with other diseases, and may be confined to one organ or involve several organ systems. Individual disease range from the mild to the severe. Symptoms vary widely, even within the same disease. Although there is no definite cure for SLE, for the vast majority of people with the disease, effective treatment can reduce the most painful symptoms, and decrease inflammation processes. Medications often are prescribed for people with SLE, depending on which organ(s) are involved, and the severity of involvement. Commonly prescribed medications include: nonsteroidal anti-inflammatory drugs, such as aspirin and ibuprofen, usually recommended for muscle and joint pain, and arthritis. Acetaminophen and corticosteroids, are used to reduce inflammation and suppress activity of the immune system. Antimalarials are prescribed for skin and joint symptoms. In general, it may take a long-time before these drugs demonstrate a beneficial effect. Immunomodulating pharmacological agents suppress activity of the immune system and biologic drugs block the production of specific antibodies, like those against DNA, or act by suppressing the synthesis of antibodies through other mechanisms. We know from the literature that Azathioprine reduced all cause mortality but did not improve renal outcomes. Cyclophosphamide reduced the risk of increasing serum creatinine but not the mortality. Induction with cyclophosphamide and steroids, as far as it is known, is probably the best acceptable therapy, particularly because of the benefit found in terms of preservation of renal function. Until now the therapeutic approach of cyclophosphamide-steroids is probably the best pharmacological treatment to be associated to PE. Plasmapheresis, is also performed for severe symptoms. Although there are no controlled studies, uncontrolled observations suggest that this therapy may obtain a reduction in the plasma creatinine concentration in 55 to 87 percent of patients. Renal function can be improved or at least stabilized with the above described therapeutic approach, although death from active vasculitis remains a major clinical event. A reasonable plasmapheresis prescription is to exchange one plasma volume three times weekly for two to three weeks. However, in 1992, a randomized, controlled trial of Lewis EJ et al. comparing a standard-therapy regimen of prednisone and cyclophosphamide with a regimen of standard therapy plus plasmapheresis in 86 patients with severe lupus nephritis in 14 medical centers failed to improve the clinical outcome in patients with SLE and severe nephritis, as compared with the standard regimen alone. Photopheresis, gamma globulin, interferon, and plasmapheresis are all more recent treatment options which mechanisms of action are not completely understood, but have been reported as to be at least effective in slowing or interrupting the progression of the disease. They may not be a cure, but have put patients in a state of remission, without the side effects of depressing the immune system. Absolute recognized SLE indications of plasmapheresis include hyperviscosity, cryoglobulinemia, pulmonary hemorrhage and Thrombotic Thrombocytopenic Purpura. However, it may also be useful in cyclophosphamide-resistant, serious, organ-threatening disease. Refinements in apheresis technology may expand the indications. In most cases, our patients trated with IA obtained relief of symptoms and complications has been obtained. However, the therapeutic potential of IA in combination with immunosuppressive drugs shuld be investigated further not only in SLE, but also in other autoimmune diseases, with circulating pathological immune complexes. In this study immunoadsorption showed to be able at removing with high efficiency a great amount of immunoglobulins from the bloodstream. Notwithstanding, it is to be underlined that conventional PE removes antibodies and other plasmatic factors to about 50 to 75%, although the evidence of therapeutic effects is mainly derived from case observation, uncontrolled case series, and prospective controlled trials have been rarely performed even with conventional plasmapheresis. Even other biochemical parameters related to inflammation and local organ involvement such as creatinine and creatinkinase concentrations were reduced on average. As far as the role of IA in the treatment of autoimmune diseases is concerned, the reasonable question could be: when is to be suggested? In our opinion, in severe, aggressive forms, poorly sensitive to the usual pharmacological approach (poor- none- responder patients). In patients who cannot be submitted to the conventional treatment because of intolerance and high incidence of side effects or adverse reactions. We guess that a careful selection of candidates is mandatory. In this clinical pivotal study no adverse reactions or complications were noted. So far, standardized recommendations regarding frequency, intensity and duration of treatment, and combining immunosuppressive treatment cannot be given. This preliminary clinical experience showed that the use of a "combined" therapeutic approach is probably a better model strategy in the management of patient affected by immunological disorders non responsive to conventional therapy. The therapeutic contribution of IA in combination with immunosuppressive drugs in the treatment of refractory SLE needs deeper investigations, increase in the number of subjects to be studied, a case-control randomized design, and the evaluation of a long-term follow-up. To our knowledge trials like above using most refined apheretical techinique such as IA apheresis are lacking. In our opinion this is an area that needs futher investigation, comparison to existing therapeutic regimens, and in particula, well-designed studies on the proposed combined approach: innovative selective apheresis and immunosuppressive drugs.

References

[1] Suzuki K, Hara M, Harigai M, et al.Continuous removal of anti-DNA antibody, using a new extracorporeal immunoadsorption system, in patients with systemic lupus erythematosus. *Arthritis and Rheumatism* 1991; 34(12): 1546-52.

[2] Hashimoto H, Tsuda H, Kanai Y, et al. Selective removal of anti-DNA and anticardiolipin antibodies by adsorbent plasmapheresis using dextran sulfate columns in patients with systemic lupus erythematosus. *J. Rheumatol.* 1991; 18:545-51.

[3] Lewis EJ, Hunsicker LG, Lan SP, Rohde RD, Lachin JM. A controlled trial of plasmapheresis therapy in severe lupus nephritis. The Lupus Nephritis Collaborative Study Group. N Engl J Med 1992; 326(21): 1373-79.

[4] Ishizuka T, Suzuki K, Hara M, et al. Successful use of immunoadsorption therapy to treat diffuse proliferative glomerulonephritis in a patient with systemic lupus erythematosus. *Japanese Journal of Rheumatology* 1993; 4(3): 175-182.

[5] Matsuki Y, Suzuki K, Kawakami M, et al. High-avidity anti-DNA antibody removal from the serum of systemic lupus erythematosus patients by adsorption using dextran sulfate cellulose columns. *Journal of Clinical Apheresis* 1996; 11: 30-35.

[6] Funauchi M, Ikoma S, Enomoto H, et al. High-Affinity anti-DNA antibody parallels clinical course of immunoadsorption therapy for systemic lupus erythematosus. *Internal Medicine* 1996; 35(5): 367-72.

[7] Jones JV, Cumming RH, Bucknall RC, et al. Plasmapheresis in the management of systemic lupus erythematosus? *Lancet* 1996; i: 709-711).

[8] Funauchi M, Ikoma S, Imada A, Kanamaru A.Combination of Immunoadsorption Therapy and High-dose Methylprednisolone in Patients with Lupus Nephritis; Possible Indications in Patients with Early Stage. *J. Clin. Lab. Immunol.* 1997; 49: 47-57.

[9] Funauchi M, Imada A, Horiuschi A, et al. Effect of immunoadsorption therapy in systemic lupus erythematosus. *Jpn. J. Apheresis* 1997; 16(1): 192-3.

[10] Matsuki Y, Suzuki K, Kawakami M, Ishizuka T, Hidaka T, Nakamura H. Adsorption of anaphylatoxins from the plasma of systemic lupus erythematosus patients using dextran sulfate cellulose columns. *J. Clin. Apheresis*. 1998; 13(3):108-13.

[11] Kutsuki H, Takata S, Yamamoto K, Tani N. Therapeutic selective adsorption of anti-DNA antibody using dextran sulfate cellulose column (Selesorb) for the treatment of systemic lupus erythematosus. Ther Apher 1998; 2(1):18-24. Review.

[12] Schneider KM: Plasmapheresis and immunoadsorption: different techniques and their current role in medical therapy. *Kidney Int. Suppl.* 1998; 64:S61-5. Review.

[13] Nakamura Y, Yoshida K, Itoh S, et al. Immunoadsorption plasmapheresis as a treatment for pregnancy complicated by systemic lupus erythematosus with positive antiphospholipid antibodies. *American Journal of Reproductive Immunology* 1999; 41: 307-11.

[14] Uramoto KM, Michet CJ Jr, Thumboo J, Sunku J, O'Fallon WM, Gabriel SE.Trends in the incidence and mortality of systemic lupus erythematosus, 1950-1992. *Arthritis Rheum.* 1999;42(1):46-50.

[15] Hidaka T, Suzuki K, Matsuki Y, Takamizawa-Matsumoto M, Kataharada K, Ishizuka T, Kawakami M, Nakamura H, Yabuki T, Kutsuki H: Evaluation of adsorption selectivity dextran sulfate bound cellulose beads for the removal of anti-DNA antibodies. *Ther. Apher.* 1999; 3(1):75-80.

[16] Korbet SM, Lewis EJ, Schwartz MM, Reichlin M, Evans J, Rohde RD. Factors predictive of outcome in sever lupus nephritis. Lupus nephritis collaborative study group. *Am. J. Kidney* 2000; 35(5): 904-14.

[17] Braun N, Bosch T: Immunoadsorption, current status and future developments. *Expert Opin. Investig. Drugs* 2000; 9(9): 2017-38.

[18] Suzuki K: The role of immunoadsorption using dextran-sulfate cellulose columns in the treatment of systemic lupus erythematosus. *Ther. Apher.* 2000; 4(3): 239-43.

[19] Wallace DJ. Apheresis for lupus erythematosus: state of the art. *Lupus* 2001; 10(3):193-6. Review.

[20] Nakaji S: Current topics on immunoadsorption therapy. *Ther. Apher.* 2001; 5(4):301-5.

[21] Kamijo Y, Kaneko Y, Ichikawa T, Kobayashi N, Koyama T, Kakegawa T, Kamijo H, Kono K, Minami S, Tanaka N, Arakura H, Hirata M, Higuchi M, Kiyosawa K, Hora K. A case of nephrotic syndrome due to lupus nephritis which was controlled with low-density lipoprotein apheresis. *Ther. Apher.* 2002; 6(6):459-62.

[22] Avenhaus B, Avenhaus W, Schneider M, Domschke W, Gaubitz M. Development of an in vitro miniature model to simulate immunoadsorption in patients with systemic lupus erythematosus. *J. Clin. Apheresis* 2002;17(4):183-9.

[23] Blake JS, Butani L. Rapidly progressive lupus glomerulonephritis and concomitant microangiopathy in an adolescent. *Lupus* 2002;11(8):533-5.

[24] Danieli MG, Palmieri C, Salvi A, Refe MC, Strusi AS, Danieli G. Synchronised therapy and high-dose cyclophosphamide in proliferative lupus nephritis. *J. Clin. Apheresis* 2002;17(2):72-7.

[25] Braun N, Junger M, Klein R, Gutenberger S, Guagnin M, Risler T. Dextran sulfate (Selesorb) plasma apheresis improves vascular changes in systemic lupus erythematosus. *Ther. Apher.* 2002; 6(6):471-7.

[26] Cagnoli L; Italian Society of Nephrology.Instructions and implementations for percutaneous renal biopsy. Guidelines for the therapy of glomerular nephropaties. *G. Ital. Nefrol.* 2003; 20 Suppl 24: S3-47.

[27] Doria A, Rondinone R. Cosa è il lupus. In: *Il lupus: la malattia dai mille volti*. Milan: GPAnet, 2004: 21-38.

[28] Kaoru Sugimoto, Ken Yamaji, Kwang-Seok Yang, Yoshinori Kanai, Hiroshi Tsuda, Hiroshi Hashimoto Immunoadsorption Plasmapheresis Using a Phenylalanine Column as an Effective Treatment for Lupus Nephritis Therapeutic Apheresis and Dialysis 2006; 10 (2), 187–192.

[29] Stefanutti C Stefanutti C, Di Giacomo S, Mareri M, Ceccarelli F, and Valesini G. Cyclophosphamide and Immunoadsorption Apheresis Treatment of Lupus Nephritis Nonresponsive to Drugs Therapy *Alone Biodrugs* 2005; 19 (2):129-133.

[30] Micheloud D, Nuño L, Rodríguez-Mahou et al. MEfficacy and safety of Etanercept, high-dose intravenous gammaglobulin and plasmapheresis combined therapy for lupus diffuse proliferative nephritis complicating pregnancy. *Lupus* Volume 15, Number 12, December 2006, pp. 881-885(5).

In: Progress in Systemic Lupus Erythematosus Research
Editor: Tomas I. Seward, pp. 9-15
ISBN 978-1-60021-861-3

Expert Commentary

PREGNANCY, A CHALLENGE IN PATIENTS WITH SYSTEMIC LUPUS ERYTHEMATOSUS

Javier A. Cavallasca and Maria del Rosario Maliandi
Division of Rheumatology, Hospital de Clinicas "Jose de San Martin",
School of Medicine, University of Buenos Aires, Buenos Aires, Argentina

INTRODUCTION

Systemic lupus erythematosus (SLE) is a multi-system autoimmune disease that typically affects women of childbearing age. The peaks incidence of SLE occurs between the ages of 15 and 40 years, with an estimated female to male incidence of 9:1. Most studies analyzing the relationship between SLE and pregnancy, observed an increased of fetal and maternal risks, notably when pregnancy occurs in active SLE. Also the frequent association between SLE and antiphospholipid syndrome (APS) represent another risk situation for this patients and the product of conception.

FERTILITY

Fertility in SLE patients is not impaired in the absence of severe disease, end stage renal disease and cytotoxic medications. The main risk factor for premature ovarian failure is the use of cyclophosphamide, and is closely related to age and total dose received. The use of azathioprine, cyclosporine and methotrexate is not associated with ovarian failure.

INFLUENCE OF PREGNANCY ON SLE

Normal pregnancy is associated with palmar and facial erythema that can mimic a lupus rash , difusse arthralgias and joint efussions which may be confused with lupus arthritis, hair loss, mild anemia because of hemodilution and thrombocitopenia.

Whether lupus flares are more frequent during pregnancy remains controversial. While some authors hold that pregnancy is not a cause of disease exacerbations, other researchers have found exacerbations in 74% of cases. This may be due to the differences in study populations, the number of patients included in the series, methodological differences in the study design, the existence or lack of a control group, and the definition of flare that is being used.

Flares can be present during all trimesters and in the puerperium period, generally they involve minor organ manifestations (e.g. cutaneous), however major organs manifestations (e.g renal flares) can occur.

According to the services of Rheumatology and Obstetrics of the Hospital de Clínicas José de San Martin, University of Buenos Aires, which includes 72 pregnancies in 61 SLE patients followed between 1986 and 2004 , fourteen disease exacerbations were identified (19%). The majority of flares were mild, skin was the most common manifestation (27%) and there were five cases of renal exacerbations (7%).The third trimester was the one with most exacerbations and during puerperium they were observed in three patients (4%).

Flare rates have consistently been highest in patients with poorly controlled SLE, particularly these with lupus nephritis (LN), renal failure and hypertension.

Therefore patient should be advised to become pregnant when the disease is inactive, and for at least 6 months if they have history of renal involvement.

INFLUENCE OF SLE ON PREGNANCY: *OBSTETRIC AND FETAL OUTCOME*

Historically lupus pregnancy was associated with a high rate of obstetric and fetal complications. These include spontaneous abortion, late miscarriage, intrauterine growth retardation, preterm delivery and prematurity. With the widespread use of careful monitoring and treatment schedules of these patients many improvements in both fetal and maternal pregnancy outcomes have occurred, with an overall fetal loss as high as 50% in unplanned pregnancies versus 13% in planned pregnancies. In our series there were 61 live births, 85%, (one twin birth), six stillbirth (8%) and 5 spontaneous abortions (7%).

Reported incidences for preterm delivery have ranged between 17-49% in recent studies, and lupus activity, hypertension and corticosteroid use are the strong predictors of preterm birth. In our experience forty six percent of 72 pregnancies ended in preterm deliveries. Significantly more women in the preterm delivery group were taking $\geq$ 10 mg/day of prednisone compared to the term delivery group.

Lupus and Hypertensive Pregnancy Complications

Lupus pregnancy is associated with an increased risk of pre-eclampsia of 13-32%, especially in the setting of lupus nephritis. Pre-eclampsia and eclampsia can mimic lupus with both presenting as edema, thrombocytopenia, hyperuricemia, anemia, hypertension, proteinuria, hematuria and seizures in eclampsia.

Pre-eclampsia is often difficult to distinguish from active LN. Investigations of serum complements C3, anti DNA antibodies and urinary sediment can help to differenciate between both diseases. We have seen in our study, gestational hypertension in 15 pregnancies (21%) and preeclampsia in 8 pregnancies (11%). No eclampsia or HELLP syndrome (hemolysis, elevated liver enzymes, low platelets) occurred.

Lupus Nephritis (LN)

On the other hand, the activity of LN at conception greatly impacted on fetal losses which ranged between 25-57% in women with active LN versus 8-12.5% in those with stable renal disease. In our report patients whose disease manifested as nephritis had live births in 70% of pregnancies, however, no association with abortions or stillbirths was seen.

Antiphospholipid Syndrome (APS)

The APS confers increased risks of abortions, fetal intrauterine growth retardation and death, thrombosis in the mother and severely early onset of preeclampsia. Two studies have reported that if an APL positive lupus patient left untreated, would only have a live birth rate of 20%, but with the use of low dose aspirin, the live birth rate increased to 42-44%, and with combined low dose low molecular weight heparin(LMWH) live birth rates doubled to 71-80%. In our series, 85% of pregnancies in patients with APS resulted in live newborns, 4 of which (30%) also had low birth weight.

Neonatal Lupus Erythematosus

All lupus patient contemplating pregnancy should have an anti-Ro/SSA, anti-La/SSB status determined, these antibodies are present in 30-50% of SLE patients. They cross the placenta and cause neonatal lupus in 1% of babies born to these mothers, and subsequent children have a 25% risk. The majority of the affected babies suffer a transient and often mild lupoid rash lasting 3-6 months, but the most severe complication is congenital heart block(CHB), which is diagnosed by fetal bradycardia at 16-23 weeks of gestation , with a mortality of 20% in the neonatal period.

The first fetal echocardiogram should be obtained at 16 weeks of gestation and then weekly for high risk infants (prior fetus with CHB) or every 2 weeks in lower risk settings.

In our study, there was only one infant with CHB in an anti-Ro/SSA positive mother. Although intrauterine dexamethasone was administered, the infant did not survive.

Drugs in Pregnancy and Breastfeeding

SLE in women in their reproductive years may need drugs treatment during pregnancy , puerperium and in the breastfeeding period , to control maternal disease and to ensure successful pregnancy outcome.

Because only drugs considered safe can be studied in pregnant or lacting women, the number of controlled studies is small, and only information on the safety of drugs during these periods is derived from experimental and precilinical studies.

Non Steroidal Antinflammatory Drugs (NSAID)

Cox-1 and Cox-2 are involved in ovulation and implantation. Several case reports and small series have described transient infertility after treatment with non-aspirin NSAID, such as indomethacin, diclofenac, piroxicam and naproxen, also some studies in animals and humans have shown that these drugs can inhibit the rupture of the luteinized follicle.

Non selective Cox inhibitors are not teratogenic and can be continued during the first and second trimesters, but all NSAID (except aspirin add less than 100 mg/day) after gestational week 20 th can cause constriction of the ductus arteriosus and impair fetal renal function. They should be withdrawn at gestational week 32.

In relation to low dose aspirin (LDA) there is no consensus on when to stop it before delivery. Some advice cessation of the treatment one week before a planned delivery with epidural anesthesia. Other experts do not stop LDA in patients with APS.

Most NSAID are excreted in very small quantities into breast milk. The American Academy of Pediatrics considers ibuprofen, indomethacin, diclofenac, piroxicam, naproxen, mefenamic acid, tolmetin, and flufenamic acid to be compatible with breastfeeding.

At present there are no reliable data on selective Cox-2 inhibitors.

Costicosteroids

11-β hydroxi steroid dehydrogenase in the placenta converts cortisol and costicosterone to inactive forms. On the other hand fluorinated corticosteroids (betamethasone and dexamethasone), are less well metabolized by the placenta. High dose (> 30 mg/day) glucocorticoid therapy is associated with major maternal complications including hyperglicemia, diabetes mellitus and hypertension.

Stress doses of hydrocortisone at delivery are recommended in patients on corticosteroids long term therapy.

Breast feeding is allowed with moderate doses of corticosteroids.

ANTIMALARIAL DRUGS

Chloroquine and hidroxichloroquine cross the placenta with no significant difference in the mean concentration in maternal and cord blood.

Different articles did not find an increase in congenital malformations or cardiac conduction disturbances in children exposed antenatally to these drugs.

The suppression of this drugs may produce a SLE flare so, when indicated continue antimalarials during pregnancy and lactation.

Methotrexate

Methotrexate is contraindicated during pregnancy and in the breastfeeding period . It must be withdrawn three months before a planned pregnancy.

Cyclophosphamide (CYC)

CYC is gonadotoxic in both women and men. Cryopreservation of sperm and sperm banking is the method of choice in men, preservation of gonadal function in women is best done with a gonadotrophin-releasing hormone agonist.

This drug is contraindicated during pregnancy and the breast feeding period. As MTX, it must be withdrawn three months before a planned pregnancy.

Azathioprine (AZA)

It does not adversely affect the fertility of both women and men. It can be used during pregnancy at daily dose not exceeding 2 mg/kg/day.

Nursing is not recommended by the American Academy of Pediatrics.

Cyclosporin A (Cs A)

It can be used in pregnancy at the lowest effective dose, with close control of maternal blood pressure and renal function during therapy. Breastfeeding is not recommended.

Mycophenolate Mofetil (MMF)

MMF is contraindicated during pregnancy. The drug should be stopped at least 5 six weeks before a planned pregnancy. Breastfeeding is not allowed.

Leflunomide

Leflunomide is contraindicated during pregnancy and breastfeeding. Discontinue 2 years prior to conception. Consider the use of cholestiramine to enhance elimination from the body until plasma levels of leflunomide are undetectable.

Tacrolimus

It may be maintained during pregnancy at the lowest possible dose. Nursing is possible.

Intravenous Immunoglobulin

It can be used in pregnancy and in the breastfeeding period.

Conclusion

Pregnancy in a lupus patient continues to be a major challenge for the physician and it should be considered as a high – risk situation. However, if it is planned when the disease is stable and under close supervision by a multidisciplinary team, we could expected for the mother and her baby a good outcome.

References

Clowse ME, Magder LS, Witter F, Petri M. The impact of increased lupus activity on obstetric outcomes. *Arthritis Rheum*. 2005 ;52:514-21.

Lockshin MD. Pregnancy does not cause systemic lupus erythematosus to worsen. *Arthritis Rheum*. 1989;32:665-70.

Nossent HC, Swaak TJ. Systemic lupus erythematosus. VI. Analysis of the interrelationship with pregnancy. *J. Rheumatol.* 1990; 17:771-6.

Khamashta MA, Hughes GR. Pregnancy in systemic lupus erythematosus. *Curr. Opin. Rheumatol.* 1996 ;8:424-9.

Cervera R, Font J, Carmona F, et al. Pregnancy outcome in systemic lupus erythematosus: good news for the new millennium. *Autoimmun Rev*. 2002;1:354-9.

Kutteh WH. Antiphospholipid antibody-associated recurrent pregnancy loss: treatment with heparin and low-dose aspirin is superior to low-dose aspirin alone. *Am. J. Obstet. Gynecol.* 1996 ;174:1584-9.

Rai R, Cohen H, Dave M, Regan L. Randomised controlled trial of aspirin and aspirin plus heparin in pregnantwomen with recurrent miscarriage associated with phospholipid antibodies (or antiphospholipid antibodies) *BMJ.* 1997 ;314:253-7.

Norella C T Kong. Pregnancy of a lupus patient- a challenge to the nephrologist. *Nephrol. Dial Transplant* 2006;21:268-272.

Moroni G, Ponticelli C. The risk of pregnancy in patients with lupus nephritis. *J. Nephrol.* 2003 ;16:161-7.

Meyer O. Making pregnancy safer for patients with lupus. *Joint Bone Spine*. 2004 ;71:178-82.

Dhar JP, Sokol RJ. Lupus and pregnancy: complex yet manageable. *Clin. Med. Res.* 2006;4:310-21.

Ostensen M, Khamashta M, Lockshin M,et al. Anti-inflammatory and immunosuppressive drugs and reproduction. *Arthritis Res. Ther*. 2006;8:209-.

In: Progress in Systemic Lupus Erythematosus Research
Editor: Tomas I. Seward, pp. 17-27
ISBN 978-1-60021-861-3

Short Communications

INFLUENCE OF EXERCISE ON THE PERIPHERAL CIRCULATION IN PATIENTS WITH SYSTEMIC LUPUS ERYTHEMATOSUS AND SYSTEMIC SCLEROSIS

Etsuko Maeshima [*] ***and Kanako Furukawa*** [**]
[*]Department of Health and Sport Management,
Osaka University of Health and Sport Sciences, Japan
[**]Third Department of Internal Medicine,
Wakayama Medical University
811-1 Wakayama-city, Wakayama, 641-0012 Japan

ABSTRACT

We evaluated the influence of exercise on the peripheral circulation in patients with systemic lupus erytematosus (SLE) and systemic sclerosis (SSc). Six patients with SLE (SLE group), 10 patients with SSc (SSc group), and 11 members of their families or medical staff (control group) were studied. After listening to a 1-hour lecture while seated, the subjects performed stretching exercise. The blood pressure, pulse rate, and skin temperature were measured prior to exercise and after 10 minutes of rest following the exercise session. The skin temperature at the fingertip was used as an index of the peripheral circulation. There were no significant changes of blood pressure and pulse rate after exercise in any of the 3 groups. Although there was no significant change of skin temperature after exercise in the SLE group, the post-exercise skin temperature was significantly lower than the pre-exercise temperature in the SSc group, ($P<0.05$). Moreover, the post-exercise skin temperature of the SSc group was significantly lower than that of the other two groups. Exercise is likely to cause exacerbation of peripheral

[*] 1-1 Asashirodai, Kumatori-cho, Sennan-gun, Osaka 590-0496, Japan. e-mail:etsukom@ouhs.ac.jp. Fax: +81-724-53-8818. Tel:+81-724-53-8845

circulatory disturbance in SSc, even when patients perform low-intensity exercise. Therefore, it is necessary to monitor the peripheral circulation by measuring the skin temperature when patients with such diseases perform exercise.

Keywords: systemic lupus erythematosus, systemic sclerosis, exercise, peripheral circulation.

INTRUDUCTION

The beneficial effects of exercise include a decrease of sympathetic nervous tone, dilation of the peripheral blood vessels, increased dermal blood flow, and mental relaxation, as well as improvement of lifestyle-related diseases [1]. Recently, more and more people in Japan have begun to incorporate exercise into their daily lives for health maintenance and promotion, as well as for the prevention of various diseases. It is expected that patients with autoimmune diseases may benefit from daily exercise in terms of improvement of their peripheral circulation, and exercise may also help to alleviate problems caused by their medications, such as hypertension, diabetes, and osteoporosis. There have been reports that exercise is beneficial for lupus fatigue [2-4] and that it improves the aerobic capacity, quality of life (QOL), and depression in patients with systemic lupus erythematosus (SLE) [5]. In patients with systemic sclerosis (SSc), it is thought that exercise capacity is a useful index of pulmonary function [6-8]. However, the effect of exercise on the peripheral circulation of such patients have not yet been examined. Accordingly, we investigated whether exercise improved the peripheral circulation of patients with SLE or SSc.

SUBJECTS

Among patients with autoimmune diseases who underwent consultations for patients with intractable diseases at a health center in Wakayama Prefecture, 16 patients (3 men and 13 women) were studied. They did not have Raynaud's phenomenon, cyanosis, ulcers, or finger defects at the time of the consultation, and they were all willing to cooperate with the investigation. In addition, 11 members of their families and some of the medical staff (4 men and 7 women) were studied as a control group, making a total of 27 subjects. The autoimmune disease was SLE [9] in 6 patients (SLE group) and SSc [10] in 10 patients (SSc group). All of the patients were well-controlled and were being treated as outpatients.

METHODS

After listening to a 1-hour lecture while seated, the subjects performed stretching exercise involved moving the upper or lower extremities while seated for 30 minutes. The blood pressure, pulse rate, and skin temperature were measured before exercise and after 10 minutes of rest following the completion of exercise. The blood pressure and pulse rate were measured in the right arm (brachial artery) using an automated sphygmomanometer (Terumo Electronic Sphygmomanometer, Terumo Corporation, Japan, Tokyo). The skin temperature was employed as an index of the peripheral circulation, and was measured at the palmar aspect of the tips of the right and left index fingers using an instantaneous dermatherm (Scalar Corporation, Tokyo). A "decreased skin temperature" was defined as a decrease of skin temperature on either the right or left side by 0.5 degrees or more, while an "increased skin temperature" was defined as an increase by 0.5 degrees or more. The patients also evaluated their own symptoms (pain, paresis, and cold sensation of the hands, fingers, and feet) on a three-point scale ("improved," "unchanged," or "aggravated"), and filled in questionnaires.

The lecture was held at the health care center for patients treated at institutions both inside and outside Wakayama Prefecture, so a detailed medical history or information about current medications was not obtained.

Results were subjected to statistical analysis using the Wilcoxon signed-rank test, the Kruskal-Wallis test, and the chi-square test.

RESULTS

1. Age

The age of the patients ranged between 32 and 82 years (48.5 ± 18.4 years) in the SLE group, 46 and 76 years (63.2 ± 9.4 years) in the SSc group , and 30 and 74 years (53.2 ± 15.8 years) in the control group, with no significant differences among the three groups.

2. Blood Pressure

Systolic Pressure

The pre-exercise systolic blood pressure ranged from 90 to 156 mmHg (115.7 ± 24.8 mmHg) in the SLE group, 110 to 156 mmHg (130.1 ± 17.5 mmHg) in the SSc group, and 99 to 150 mmHg (124.9 ± 15.0 mmHg) in the control group, showing no significant differences among the three groups.

The post-exercise systolic pressure ranged from 100 to 154 mmHg (120.7 ± 22.8 mmHg) in the SLE group, 104 to 176 mmHg (132.0 ± 25.5 mmHg) in the SSc group, and 105 to 186 mmHg (131.2 ± 23.1 mmHg) in the control group, again showing no significant differences. There was also no significant change of systolic pressure after exercise in any of the groups (Figure 1).

Diastolic Pressure

The pre-exercise diastolic blood pressure of the SLE, SSc, and control groups ranged from 62 to 88 mmHg (75.2 ± 10.1 mmHg), 58 to 91 mmHg (74.4 ± 12.8 mmHg), and 65 to 87 mmHg (75.1 ± 6.8 mmHg), respectively, with no significant differences among the three groups. The post-exercise diastolic pressure ranged from 64 to 98 mmHg (76.2 ± 14.2

mmHg), 58 to 101 mmHg (77.1 ± 15.0 mmHg), and 58 to 94 mmHg (78.4 ± 9.8 mmHg), respectively, and there were also no significant differences among the groups. Furthermore, there was no significant change of blood pressure after exercise in any group (Figure 2).

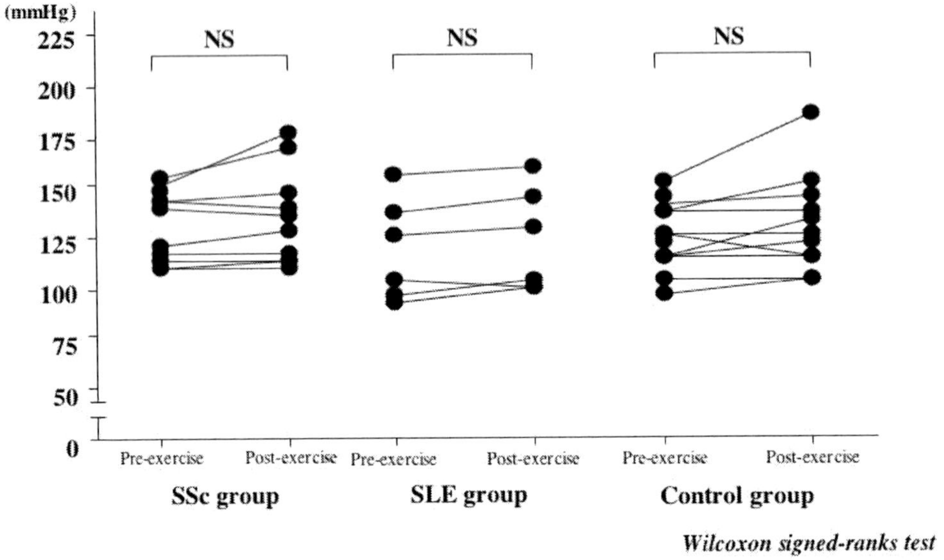

Figure 1. Systolic blood pressure. There were no significant changes after exercise in any group.

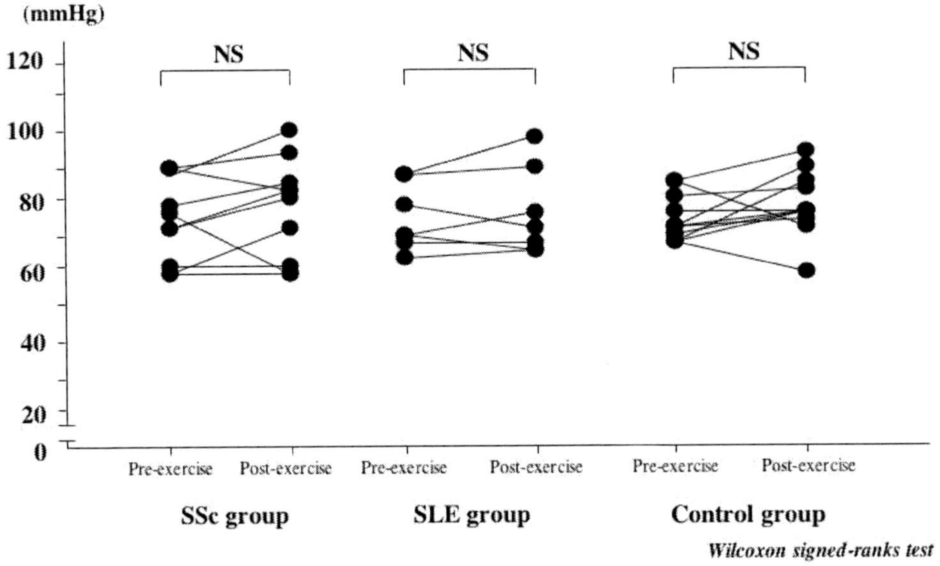

Figure 2. Diastolic blood pressure. There were no significant changes after exercise in any group.

3. Pulse Rate

The pre-exercise pulse rate of the SLE, the SSc, and the control groups ranged from 57 to 88 bpm (74.3 ± 11.9 bpm), 60 to 85 bpm (70.5 ± 9.5 bpm), and 43 to 109 bpm (74.0 ± 17.8 bpm), respectively, with no significant differences among the three groups. Post-exercise pulse rates ranged from 54 to 79 bpm (71.7 ± 10.0 bpm), 65 to 87 bpm (73.7 ± 6.8 bpm), and 50 to 120 bpm (74.5 ± 19.8 bpm), respectively, again showing no significant differences. There was also no significant change of the pulse rate with exercise in any of the groups (Figure 3).

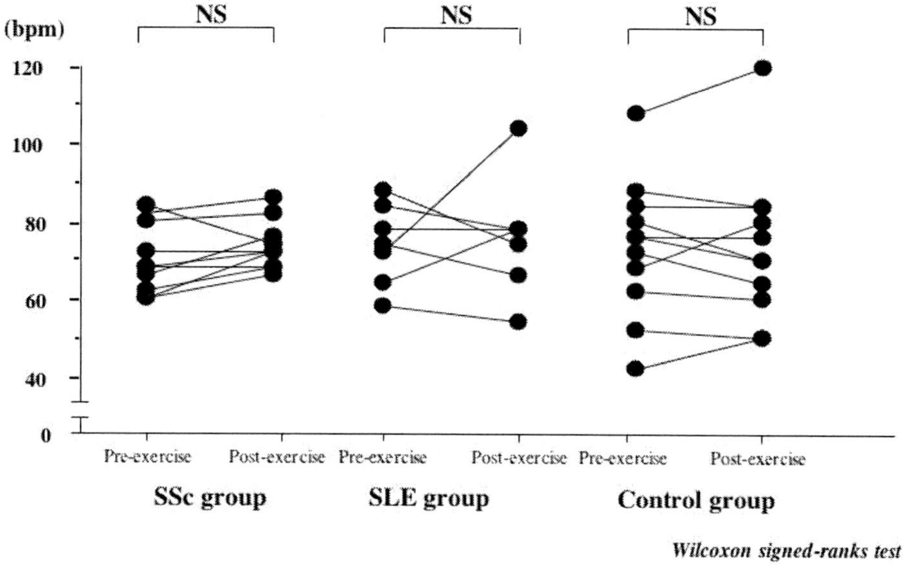

Figure 3. Pulse rates. There were no significant changes after exercise in any group.

4. Skin Temperature

Right Index Finger

The pre-exercise skin temperature of the right index finger ranged from 25.9 to 32.9°C (31.4 ± 2.7°C), 22.1 to 32.1°C (28.9 ± 4.0°C), and 22.8 to 34.6°C (30.7 ± 3.9°C) in the SLE, SSc, and control groups, respectively, with no significant differences among the groups. The post-exercise skin temperature ranged from 26.7 to 34.9°C (32.1 ± 2.9°C), 21.8 to 33.4°C (27.8 ± 4.4°C), and 22.9 to 34.7°C (31.8 ± 3.4°C), respectively, showing differences among the three groups. There was a significant difference between the SLE group and the SSc group (P<0.05), as well as between the SSc group and the control group (P<0.05) (Figure.4).

Left Index Finger

The pre-exercise skin temperature of the left index finger ranged from 24.9 to 33.4°C (31.1 ± 3.2°C), 21.1 to 32.0°C (28.2 ± 3.8°C), and 23.1 to 34.6°C (30.5 ± 4.2°C) in the SLE, SSc, and control groups, respectively, showing no significant differences.

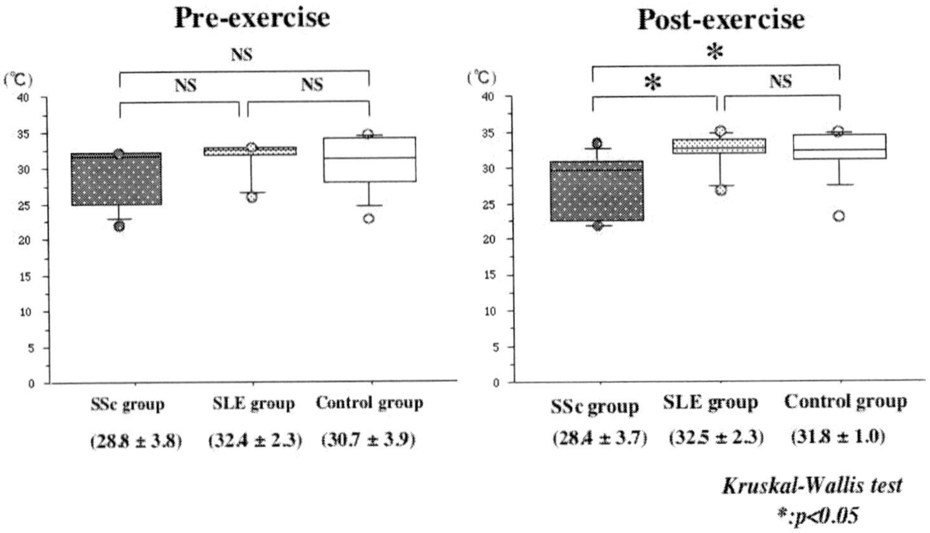

Figure 4. Pre-exercise and post-exercise skin temperature of the right index finger. The pre-exercise skin temperature showed no significant differences among the three groups. However, the post-exercise skin temperature showed variation among the groups. There was a significant difference between the SSc group and the SLE group ($P<0.05$), as well as between the SSc group and the control group ($P<0.05$).

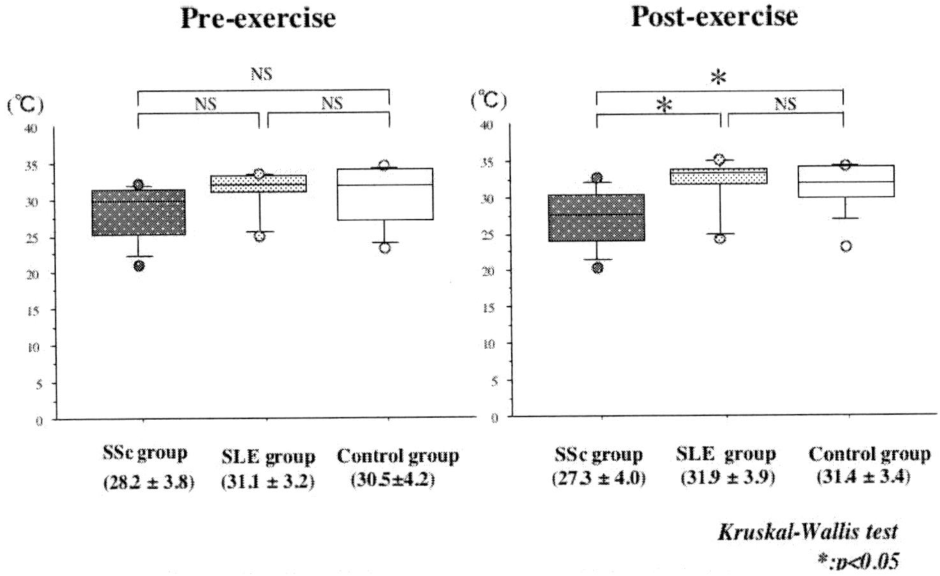

Figure 5. Pre-exercise and post-exercise skin temperature of the left index finger. The pre-exercise skin temperature showed no significant differences among the three groups. However, the post-exercise skin temperature showed variation among the groups ($P<0.05$). There was a significant difference between the SSc group and the SLE group ($P<0.05$), as well as between the SSc group and the control group ($P<0.05$).

Post-exercise skin temperature ranged from 24.2 to 35.0°C (31.9 ± 3.9°C), 20.2 to 32.6°C (27.3 ± 4.0°C), and 22.9 to 34.2°C (31.4 ± 3.4°C), respectively, showing variation among the three groups. There was a significant difference between the SLE group and the SSc group (*P*<0.05), as well as between the SSc group and the control group (*P*<0.05) (Figure. 5).

When the skin temperature of each group was compared between before and after exercise, there were no significant changes in the SLE group or the control group. In the SSc group, however, the post-exercise skin temperature of the right finger showed a significant decrease compared with the pre-exercise value (*P*<0.05) (Figure. 6A, B).

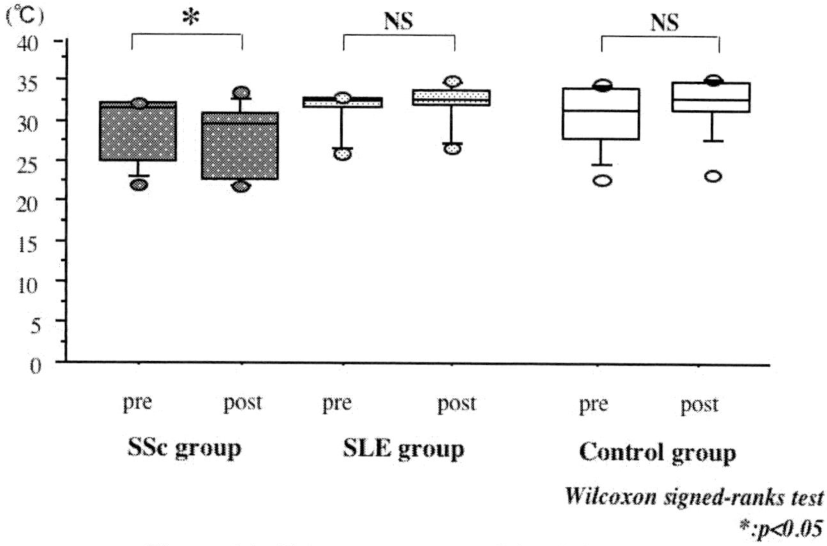

Figure 6A. Skin temperature of the right finger.

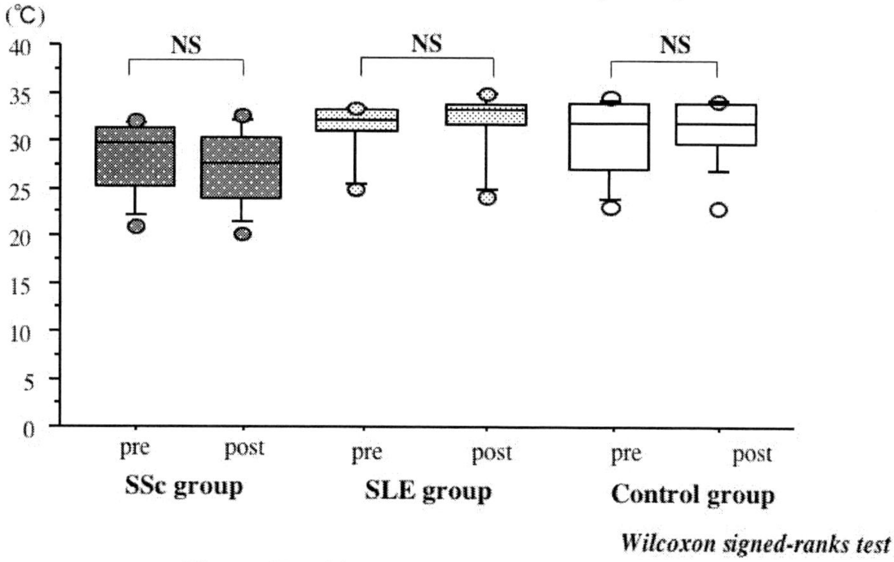

Figure 6B. Skin temperature of the left finger.

Figure 6A, 6B. Comparison of the skin temperature before and after the exercise in each group. There were no significant changes in the SLE and control groups, but the SSc group had a significantly lower post-exercise skin temperature of the right finger compared with the pre-exercise value (*P*<0.05).

5. Post-Exercise Interview

Among the 6 patients in the SLE group, one patient stated that his/her symptoms (pain, pareisis, or cold sensation) were "aggravated" (the skin temperature increased). On the other hand, 5 patients reported that their symptoms were "unchanged" or "improved" (3 of them had an increased skin temperature and 2 (33.3%) had a decreased skin temperature). In the SSc group, 2 patients answered that their symptoms were "aggravated," and both of them had a decrease of skin temperature with exercise. On the other hand, although 8 patients answered that their symptoms were "unchanged" or "improved," only 1 of them had an increase of skin temperature and 6 (60.0%) of them had a decrease of temperature. In the control group, all of the subjects answered that their symptoms were either "unchanged" or "improved." Among them, 7 subjects had an increase of skin temperature and 4 had a decrease. There were no significant differences among the three groups (Table 1).

Table 1. Subjective symptoms and the skin temperature

	Subjective symptoms	Decreased skin temperature	Increased skin temperature	unchanged
SSc group (n=10)	"improved" or "unchanged	6 cases (60%)	1 case (10%)	1 case (10%)
	"aggravated"	2 cases (20%)	0 case (0%)	0 case (0%)
SLE group (n=6)	"improved" or "unchanged	2 cases (33.3%)	3 cases (50%)	0 case (0%)
	"aggravated"	1 case (9.1%)	1 case (9.1%)	0 case (0%)
Control group (n=11)	"improved" or "unchanged	4 cases (36.4%)	7 case (63.6%)	0 case (0%)
	"aggravated"	0 case (0%)	0 case (0%)	0 case (0%)

Discussion

Peripheral Circulation

There have been some previous reports about the effects of exercise in patients with autoimmune diseases. The effect of bicycle ergometer aerobic exercise for eight weeks was assessed in 23 SLE patients, showing that exercise did not exacerbate their disease and that it actually improved their aerobic capacity and fatigue [2]. Ramsey-Goldman et al. divided 10 SLE patients into two groups, which were an aerobic exercise group and a range of motion/muscle strengthening group, and examined the influence and safety of these different kinds of exercise on fatigue and functional status [3]. Neither type of exercise exacerbated disease activity, while both improved fatigue, functional status, cardiovascular fitness, and muscle strength, as well as increasing bone turnover. Tench et al. also reported the use of appropriately graded aerobic exercise for the management of fatigue in SLE patients [4]. These authors concluded that exercise was effective for improvement of fatigue, depression, and aerobic capacity, but the influence of exercise on the peripheral circulation was not examined. It has also been reported that exercise is useful for evaluation of lung function in SSc [6-8], but the influence on the peripheral circulation has not been examined in SSc patients either.

No significant changes of the blood pressure and pulse rate were observed after exercise was performed in this study, and there were also no significant differences among the groups. Thus, this study assessed low-intensity exercise that did not affect the blood pressure and pulse rate. However, the digital skin temperature (used as an index of peripheral circulation) decreased significantly after exercise in the SSc group. Skin temperature is regulated by contraction and dilation of the cutaneous blood vessels. An increment cutaneous blood flow increases the skin temperature and a decline of blood flow decreases the skin temperature. During exercise, the cutaneous vessels dilate and cutaneous blood flow increases, which causes the skin temperature to rise [1]. In this study, the skin temperature after exercise was significantly lower in the SSc group than in the other two groups, and the skin temperature after exercise lower than the temperature before exercise. On the other hand, there were no significant changes of the skin temperature after exercise in the SLE and control groups.

Paroxysmal vasospasm of the fingers, or Raynaud's phenomenon, is a frequent abnormality in patients with SSc, mixed connective tissue disease, and SLE. Raynaud's represents dysregulation of the neuroendothelial control of vascular tone and it is essentially an exaggerated vasospastic response to cold or emotion. The prevalence of Raynaud's phenomenon in SLE takes the middle range between the rate of 95% found in patients with scleroderma and the level of 3% seen in those with rheumatoid arthritis [11]. Raynaud's phenomenon is nonspecific and may be present for years before the development of other changes due to SLE, SSc, or dermatomyositis. Such vasospasm is regarded as the main cause of the disturbance of peripheral circulation in many autoimmune diseases, including SLE [11]. However, patients with SSc not only have abnormal vascular function (vasospasm), but also develop changes of vessel structure and the nervous system, an imbalance between vasodilation and vasoconstriction, abnormal platelet function, and abnormal erythrocyte deformation [12-14]. Generally, vasospasm due to Raynaud's phenomenon rarely leads to permanent damage, although small ulcers on the fingers can occur following prolonged and frequent attacks. However, disturbance of the digital circulation is more prominent in SSc compared with other autoimmune diseases, and ulcers at the tips of the digits are included in the criteria defining this disease. Thus, it seems that peripheral circulatory disturbance is more severe in SSc compared with other autoimmune diseases.

When recommending exercise for patients with SSc, we should emphasize that it is important to undergo assessment of the peripheral pulses or skin temperature measurement.

Interview Findings

The results of the interviews showed no significant differences among the three groups. In the SLE group, 2 patients answered that their symptoms were "unchanged" or "improved, although their skin temperature decreased. Even in the SSs group, in which the pre-exercise skin temperature was significantly lower than that of the other groups and the post-exercise temperature was even lower, approximately 80% of the patients answered that their symptoms were "improved" or "unchanged." This shows the difficulty of evaluating a decrease of skin temperature during or after exercise only on the basis of patients' symptoms. The reason for the discrepancy between the changes of symptoms and the actual skin temperature is unclear. It is possible that activity had a beneficial influence such as a refreshing feeling, which may make it difficult for patients to notice the deterioration of their peripheral circulation. The refreshing effect of exercise or decreased transmission of pain is often discussed in association with β-endorphin, which is secreted by the pituitary gland and immunocompetent cells [15,16]. However, previous reports indicate that exercise above a certain intensity threshold is required to promote the secretion of β-endorphin, and it is unlikely that secretion of this hormone was increased by the low-intensity exercise performed in our study.

Among patients whose skin temperature decreases after exercise, it can be one of the risk factors for exaceerbation of digital ulcers or necrosis. Therefore, when patients with peripheral circulatory disturbance perform exercise, it is necessary to monitor the status of their peripheral circulation by skin temperature measurement.

Conclusion

During low-intensity exercise, there were no significant differences of blood pressure and pulse rate between patients with autoimmune disease and the healthy control group. A decrease of peripheral blood flow was not observed in the SLE patients. However, SSc patients were likely to show deterioration of peripheral circulation even with low-intensity exercise. Therefore, it is necessary to monitor the peripheral circulation by assessing the peripheral pulses or skin temperature when patients with such diseases perform exercise.

References

[1] Karacabey K. (2005). Effect of regular exercise on health and diseases. *Neuroendocrinol. Lett.*, 26, 617-623.

[2] Robb-Nicholson LC, Daltroy L, Eaton H, Gall V, Wright E, Hartley LH, Schur PH, LiangMH. (1989). Effects of aerobic conditioning in lupus fatigue: a pilot study. *Br. J. Rheumatol.*, 28, 500-505.

[3] Ramsey-Goldman R, Schilling EM, Dunlop D, Langman C, Greenland P, Thomas RJ, Chang RW. (2000). A pilot study on the effects of exercise in patients with systemic lupus erythmatosus. *Arthritis Care Res*, 13, 262-369.

[4] Tench CM, McCarthy J, McCurdie I, White PD, D'Cruz DP. (2003). Fatigue in systemic lupus erythematosus: a randomized controlled trail of exercise. *Rheumatology*, 42, 1050-1054.

[5] De Carvalho MRP, Sato EI, Tebexreni AS, Heidecher RTC, Schenkman S, Neto TLB. (2005). Effects of supervised cardiovascular training program on exercise tolerance, aerobic capacity, and quality of life in patients with systemic lupus erythematosus. *Arthritis Rheum*, 53, 838-844.

[6] Alkotob ML, Soltani P, Sheatt MA, Katsetos MC, Rothfield N, Hager WD, Foley RJ, Silverman DI. (2006). Reduced exercise capacity and stress-induced pulmonary hypertension in patients with scleroderma. *Chest*, 30, 176-181.

[7] Villalba WO, Sampaio-Barros PD, Pereira MC, Cerqueria EM, Leme CA Jr, Marques-Neto JF, Paschoal IA. (2007). Six-minute walk test for the evaluation of pulmonary disease severity in scleroderma patients. *Chest*, 131, 217-222.

[8] Buch MH, Denton CP, Furst DE, Guillevin L, Rubin LI, Wells AU, Matucci-Cernic M, Riemekasten G, Emery P, Chadha-Boreham H, Charef P, Roux S, Black CM, Seibold JR. (2007). Submaximal exercise testing in the assessment of interstitial lung disease secondary to systemic sclerosis: reproducibility and correlations of the 6-min walk test. *Ann. Rheum. Dis.*, 66, 169-173.

[9] Tan EM, Cohen AS, Fries JF, Masi AT, McShane DJ, Rothfield NF, Schaller JG, Talal N, Winchester RJ. (1982). The 1982 revised criteria for the classification of systemic lupus erythematosus. *Arthritis Rheum.*, 25, 1271-1277.

[10] Clements PJ, Lachenbruch PA, Seibold JR, Zee B, Steen VD, Brennan P, Silman AJ, Allegar N, Varga J, Massa M. (1993). Skin thickness score in systemic sclerosis: an assessment of interobserver variability in 3 independent studies. *J. Rheumatol.*, 20, 1892-1896.

[11] Wallace DJ. (1997). Clinical and laboratory features in systemic lupus erythematosus: Cutaneouse and cutaneovasucular manifestation of systemic lupus erythematosus. In: Wallace DJ, Hahn HB (Eds.), *Dubois' Lupus Erythematosus* (5th edition, pp.693-721). Baltimore, Maryland: William and Wilkins.

[12] Generini S, Kahaleh B, Matucci-Cerinic M, Pignone A, Lombardi A, Ohtsuka T. (1996). Raynaud's phenomenon and systemic sclerosis. *Ann. Ital. Med. Int.*, 11, 125-131.

[13] Herrick AL. (2005). Pathogenesis of Raynaud's phenomenon. *Rheumatology*, 44, 587-596.

[14] Seibold JR. (2005). Connective tissue disease, scleroderma, and inflammatory myopathies: Scleroderma. In: Harris Jr ED, Budd R, Genovese MC, Firestein GS, Asrgent JS, Sledge GB (Eds.), *Kelley's Textbook of Rheumatology* (7th edition, pp.1279-1308). Philadelphia, Pennsylvania: Elsevier Saunders.

[15] Goldfarb AH, Jamurtas AZ. Beta-endorphin response to exercise. *Sports Med.* 1997; 24: 8-16.

[16] Heinz H, Kornelia H, Gramsch C, Katz N, Hempelmann G, Teschemacher H. Beta-endorphin (1-31) in the plasma of male volunteers undergoing physical exercise. *Psychoneuroendocrinology* 2000; 25: 551-562.

In: Progress in Systemic Lupus Erythematosus Research ISBN 978-1-60021-861-3
Editor: Tomas I. Seward, pp. 29-75

Chapter 1

NEW FRONTIERS IN THE RESEARCH OF CARDIOVASCULAR DISEASE ASSOCIATED WITH SYSTEMIC LUPUS ERYTHEMATOSUS

Laura Gonzalez-Lopez,* J. I. Gamez-Nava,** and Arnulfo Nava**

*Department of Internal Medicine - Rheumatology,
Hospital General Regional 110
Prolongacion Circunvalacion-Oblatos 2208,
Guadalajara, Jalisco, México, 44340. Prostgraduate Program of Public Health Sciences
Centro Universitario Ciencias de la Salud Universidad de Guadalajara
**Division of Musculoskeletal and Autoinmune Diseases,
Clinical Epidemiology Research Unit
Hospital de Especialidades del Centro Medico Nacional de Occidente
Belisario Domínguez 1000, Guadalajara,
Jalisco, México, 44320

ABSTRACT

Cardiovascular disease is a major cause of mortality in patients with systemic lupus erythematosus (SLE). Around 52% of the autopsies performed in SLE in our centre have shown cardiac involvement and most of these disorders were not diagnosed pre-mortem [1].

Current topics for research are accelerated atherosclerosis, pulmonary hypertension, development of valvular disease and new other forms of cardiac involvement. Most of the patients deceased by cardiovascular disease have an accelerated atherosclerosis. Some authors reported a substantial increase in risk of fatal vascular event in women

* Correspondence to: L. Gonzalez-Lopez, Salto del Agua 2192, Col. Jardines del Country. Guadalajara, Jalisco, Mexico, 44210. Email: lauragl@mail.udg.mx; jaimemrom@prodigy.net.mx. Telephone/ Fax: +52-33-38-54-13-69.

with SLE compared with matched controls. New methods such as electron-beam computed tomography have demonstrated a highly prevalence of coronary disorder even in asymptomatic patients. Additionally, high resolution carotid ultrasonography has shown a high prevalence of carotid lesions. Both cellular and molecular mechanisms of the accelerated atherosclerosis are complex and not entirely explained by the traditional cardiovascular risk factors, therefore, the research targets on nontraditional factors.

Pulmonary hypertension is relevant by its morbidity and mortality. Previously considered as rare entity; new non-invasive studies have detected patients with earlier involvement; our group have reported a prevalence of 18% in a series of 204 patients assessed by Doppler echocardiography. A follow-up study in our cohort observed an increase of 4 times greater of risk for cardiac failure in patients with asymptomatic pulmonary pressure >40 mmHg. Strategies for the treatment of pulmonary hypertension include immunosuppressive therapy, prostanoids, phosphodiesterase inhibitors or endothelin receptor antagonists. Most of the current information related with the response to these treatments proceeds from short-term studies with a wide variability in the outcome measures making necessary additional research in this area.

There is also a renovate interest in the valvular disease, recent studies show association between antiphospholipid antibodies and mitral valve nodules or mitral regurgitation, the potential effects of these antibodies on the endothelial activation require to be evaluated.

Cardiac dysfunction is another important area for research; several studies have shown a high prevalence of left ventricular diastolic dysfunction. In our own series this manifestation is present in around 63%. Nevertheless, to date no follow-up studies have been done to evaluate the importance of diastolic dysfunction on the morbidity or mortality.

In summary cardiovascular disease in systemic lupus represents a very exciting area for research being necessary to increase the number of long-term prospective cohorts and well-designed controlled trials in order to improve the clinical care of the patients with this involvement.

Cardiovascular disease is a major cause of mortality in patients with systemic lupus erythematosus (SLE). Several studies have found increase in cardiovascular involvement in autopsies. Around 52% of the autopsies performed in SLE in our centre show cardiac involvement and most of these disorders were not diagnosed pre-mortem [1].

Current topics for research are accelerated atherosclerosis, pulmonary hypertension, development of valvular disease and new other forms of cardiac involvement. All the cardiac structures can be involved in the heart including pericardium endocardium, myocardium, valves and conduction tissue. Also are involved the arteries including both pulmonary as coronaries.

PERICARDITIS

Pericarditis is one of the most well documented cardiac involvements in SLE and is included among the manifestations described in the ARA/ACR classification criteria. Pericarditis has been demonstrated by echocardiography between 11-54% of the patients with

SLE [2]. This manifestation can be asymptomatic or with severe symptoms and even life-threatening, severe complications as cardiac tamponade, constrictive pericarditis and purulent pericarditis are fortunately rare. Effusions are associated with disease activity. The diagnosis of pericarditis or pericardial effusion frequently is unsuspected or the symptoms are only mild and transitory. Figure 1 shows a case of pericarditis observed in an autopsy from a patient with SLE in our centre. Note the thickening of the pericardium and the mild inflammatory infiltrate.

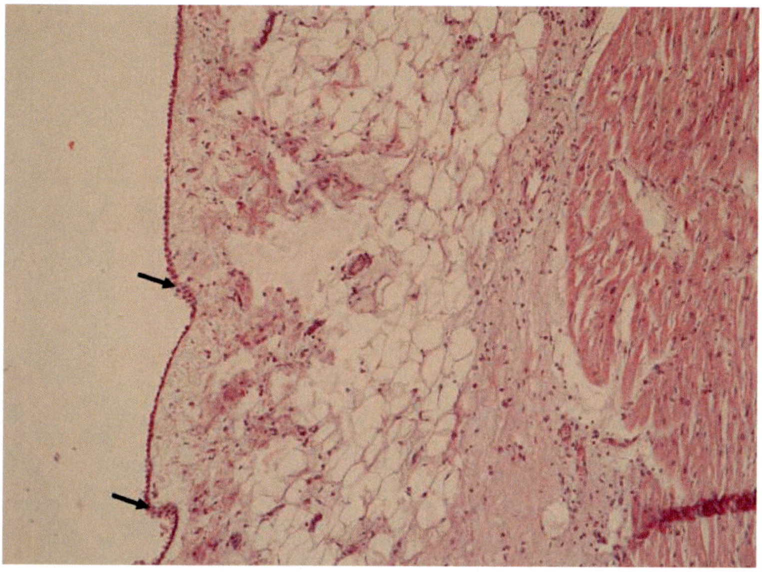

Figure 1. Shows a case of lupus pericarditis observed in autopsy from our hospital. The presence of thickening of pericardial and hyperplasia of the mesothelial cells can be observed (black arrow). A mild to moderate inflammatory infiltrate is present. Hematoxylin-Eosin staining 40 x. (Photo courtesy Dr. Maria R. Flores-Marquez, Department of Pathology, CMO IMSS, Guadalajara, Mexico).

From a study in China from 310 patients retrospectively evaluated only 18 had pericarditis or pericardial effusion reported in their charts clinical, from these the main signs for suspicion were precordial pain in 7 (39%), dyspnea in 11 (61%), pericardial rub in only one patient, typical abnormalities in the ECG were found in 7 (39%), and cardiomegaly on the chest radiograph in 8 (44%), although in 17 (94%) the pericarditis was documented by the echocardiography [3]. The treatment for pericarditis and/or pericardial effusion depends of the severity of the involvement. For mild cases usually the treatment with nonsteroidal anti-inflammatory drugs and corticosteroids (prednisone 0.5 mg / kg / day or equivalent) are sufficient [2]. In severe cases such as tamponade or associated myocarditis this complication must be managed with the patient hospitalized. Some patients have a good response with intravenous bolus of methylprednisolone (1 g daily for three days) [2, 3]. Cardiac tamponade is developed when fluid accumulation in the pericardial space raise the pressure surrounding the heart impairing the cardiac filling, resulting in elevated venous pressure and impaired cardiac output leading to shock. This constitutes an emergency that can be fatal if not treated opportune and appropriateness. Echocardiography is the best method for the diagnosis of tamponade showing a diastolic collapse of the free wall of the right atrium and/or the right ventricle, the collapse is exaggerated during expiration because the right heart filling is reduced [4]. There is a lack of controlled studies evaluating immunosuppressive drugs in severe pericardial involvement. The "corner stone" of the treatment for cardiac tamponade is drainage of the pericardial effusion. Medical treatment is usually ineffective and only constitute an adjuvant therapy while is available the pericardial drainage [4]. The use of inotropic agents to treat the shock caused by cardiac tamponade is usually ineffective and the mechanical ventilation without pericardial drainage may produce a sudden drop in blood pressure with impairment of cardiac filling [4].

Algorithm for the treatment of pericarditis in SLE

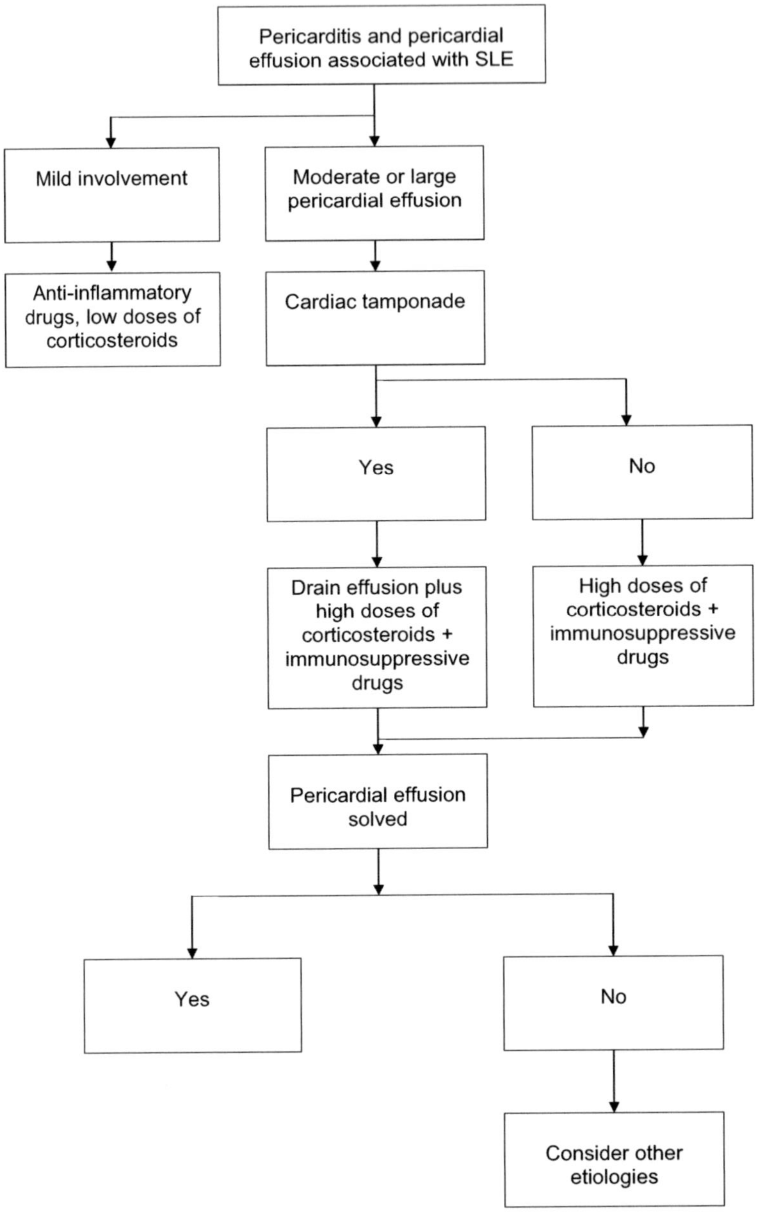

MYOCARDITIS

Several studies have reported that myocarditis is an infrequent finding in lupus. A recent report describes a small series of 11 patients diagnosed with acute myocarditis associated with lupus [5]. The following symptoms were present at the time of the admission: dyspnea 10/11, fever 6/11, orthopnea 5/11, paroxysmal nocturnal dyspnea 4/11, chest pain 4/11, leg swelling 3/11 and palpitations 2/11 [5]. The clinical signs are unspecific showing basal crackles on chest auscultation 8/11, raised jugular venous pressure 6/11, tachycardia 6/11, gallop rhythm 5/11, peripheral oedema 4/11, new murmur 3/11, or irregular pulse rate 1/11. Some series have found association between myocarditis with positive anti-dsDNA antibody or low C3 or C4 levels [5]. Acute myocarditis usually is associated with other organ involvement including nephropathy, lymphopaenia, leukopaenia, thrombocytopenia or anaemia [5]. Only one-third of the patients have elevated creatine kinase. Lupus anticoagulant or anticardiolipin antibodies are not useful markers for myocarditis in SLE [5].

Histological findings of myocarditis include small foci of fibrinoid necrosis with infiltrates of plasma cells, lymphocytes and foci of myocardial fibrosis [2]. Immunocomplexes and complement deposits can be found in the myocardium and their blood vessels [2]. Figure 2 and 3 shows a case of myocarditis by SLE observed in autopsy in our hospital. Figure 2 shows a 40X image showing foci of inflammation composed by lymphocytes with some macrophage and plasmatic cells. Figure 3 shows a 60x image showing associated fibrinoid necrosis associated with the inflammatory cells.

Noninvasive myocardial imaging techniques for myocarditis include echocardiography, nuclear imaging with gallium or indium labeled antimyosin antibodies and magnetic resonance imaging [6].

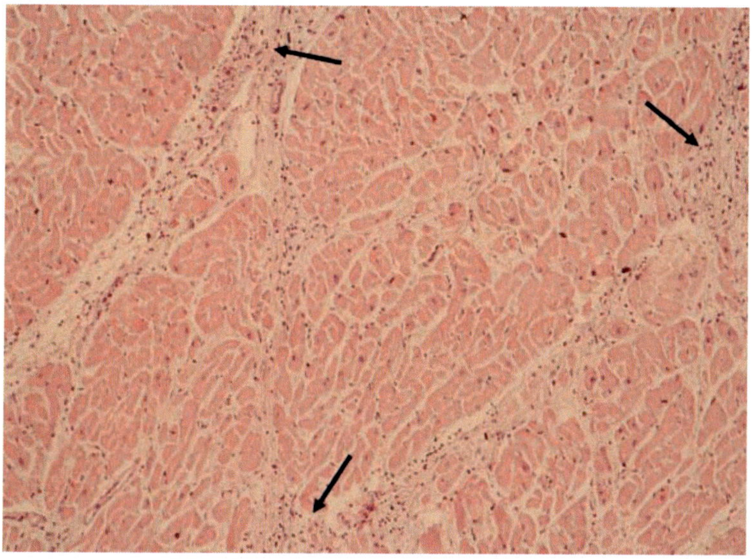

Figure 2. Shows a case of lupus myocarditis observed in an autopsy from our centre. Note the presence of inflammatory infiltrates in the myocardium (black arrows). Hematoxylin-Eosin staining 40 x. (Photo courtesy Dr. Maria R. Flores-Marquez, Department of Pathology, CMO IMSS, Guadalajara, Mexico).

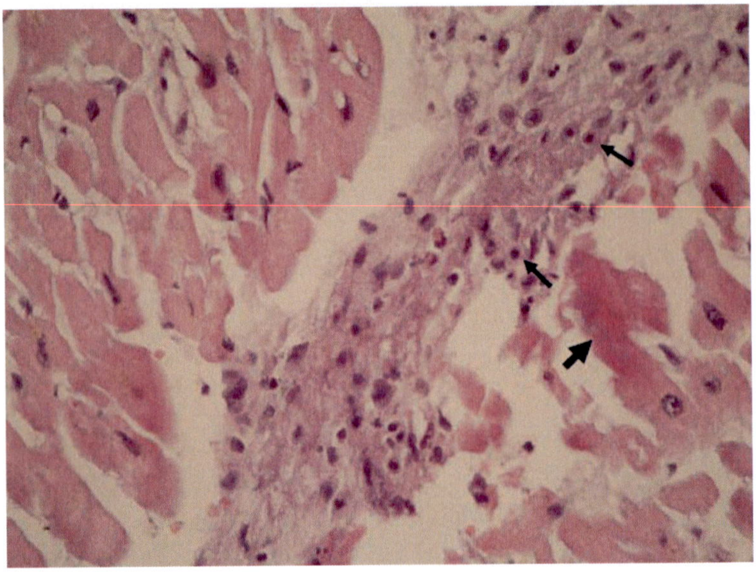

Figure 3. Details of the inflammatory infiltrate observed in myocarditis. Note the predominance of mononuclear cells (thin arrows). Also note the necrosis of some myocardial fibers (wide arrow). Hematoxylin-Eosin staining 60 x. (Photo courtesy Dr. Maria R. Flores-Marquez, Department of Pathology, CMO IMSS, Guadalajara, Mexico).

Echocardiography in Myocarditis

Echocardiography is the method most amply used in the clinics for support the diagnosis of myocarditis. Findings in the echocardiography include left and/or right ventricular dysfunction, segmental wall motion abnormalities (such as hypokinetic, akinetic or diskinetic wall) [7]. These findings in the echocardiography are not conclusive, and other confirmatory techniques should be used when possible. Echocardiography can be used as a method to evaluate the response to the therapy; most of the abnormalities in acute myocarditis improve or even may disappear. Recent techniques such as tissue Doppler imaging and myocardial velocity measurements are useful to evaluate the changes in function of the therapy.

Scintography

Scintography studies have recovered renovated interest in myocarditis specially indium monoclonal antibody fragments that are directed against myosin. These autoantibodies bind to cardiac myocytes that have exposed myosin to extracellular fluid space. Therefore, these autoantibodies are markers of myocyte necrosis, and reflect the extent of this necrosis. This method differs from the traditional use of gallium that detects only myocardial inflammation [6]. Some authors have evaluated the performance of the antimyosin antibodies in patients with suspected myocarditis. In a series of patients who were evaluated by endomyocardial biopsy and their histopathologic results were used "as gold standard". The antimyosin antibodies showed a high sensitivity (91-100%) and high negative predictive value (93-

100%), but very low specificity (31-44%) or positive predictive value (28-33%) [8]. Therefore, the antimyosin imaging can be considered as useful test for exclusion of myocarditis in case of negative results but is not very useful to confirm myocarditis in case of positive findings and further confirmatory procedures should be performed.

Magnetic Resonance

Contrast-enhanced magnetic resonance is another useful technique used for the diagnosis of myocardial inflammation [6]. Myocarditis is associated with myocyte injury tissue edema and cellular swelling. Therefore, the assessment of T1 and T2 relaxation times are useful for detection of myocarditis, as well as, the following of this complication [9]. MRI can help to difference patients with myocardial infarction from those with myocarditis [10]. Patients with myocardial infarction have a segmental early subendocardial defect with a delayed high enhancement predominantly anteroseptal. Instead, patients with myocarditis have no early defect and they present focal or diffuse nonsegmental, nonsubendocardial delayed enhancement predominantly in an inferolateral location [10]. In a recent study were compared 6 patients with active SLE (2 of them with myocarditis) versus 5 patients inactive and 5 healthy volunteers with the aim to determine differences in myocardial T2 relaxivity in MRI [11]. Active SLE patients, independently of myocardial involvement or not had significantly higher T2 relaxation times compared with inactive SLE and controls. Also, 3/6 active patients (two of them with myocarditis) had abnormal focal areas of increased signal intensity and wall hypokinesis [11]. Focal areas of contrast intake were detected in these patients. This intriguing report concludes that active SLE patients had high myocardial T2 relaxation times, even without a myocardial involvement. Further studies need to be performed to evaluate the role of MRI using endomyocardial biopsy as gold standard in patients with suspicion of myocarditis associated to SLE.

Endomyocardial Biopsy

Endomyocardial biopsy is an invasive method that confirms the presence of myocarditis, although may cause severe complications, therefore their utilization is limited. Some indications of the endomyocardial biopsy have been proposed [12] including: the exclusion of common etiologies of dilated cardiomyopathy, subacute or acute symptoms of heart failure refractory to standard treatment, worsening of ejection fraction refractory to therapy, development of arrhytmias affecting the hemodinamics specially progressive heart block or ventricular tachycardia, heart failure with concurrent rash fever or peripheral eosinophilia or suspicion for giant cell myocarditis [12]. Small series of patients have been evaluated with endomyocardial biopsy in SLE. Sakaguchi et al, evaluated 14 endomyocardial biopsies in lupus where the main finding is fibrosis, whereas, only 4/11 patients showed moderate cell interstitial infiltration [13]. Immunofluorescence of these biopsies shows immunoglobulin G, and fibrinogen deposits in the membrane of myocytes and interstitium.

Figure 4. Shows a substitution of the myocardial fibers by fibrosis (Masson staining). This image can be observed in cases of chronic inflammation by increase in the collagen synthesis.

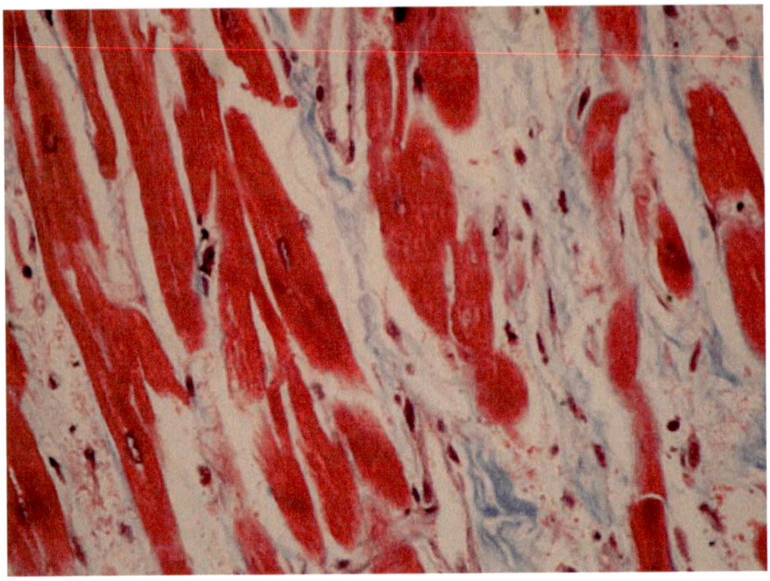

Figure 4. Masson staining showing extensive fibrosis between the myocardial fibers (blue color) observed in response to chronic inflammation of the myocardium. (Photo courtesy Dr. Maria R. Flores-Marquez, Department of Pathology, IMSS, Guadalajara, Mexico).

Treatment of Myocarditis

All the patients with myocarditis by SLE should be hospitalized and followed with supportive care in a similar way to other forms of myocarditis [14]. These supportive measures include diuretics to decrease ventricular filling pressures, and angiotensin converting-enzyme inhibitors to diminish vascular resistance. Some patients may require most potent vasodilators such as sodium nitroprusside. Digoxin should be used with extreme precaution because can increase proinflammatory cytokines. Inotropic agents or use of a ventricular assist device can be required for some patients; sometimes can be required antiarrhythmic agents in case of atrial or ventricular arrhythmias. Due to acute myocarditis constitute a severe manifestation of disease activity in SLE this should be treated with corticosteroids and immunosuppressive drugs, although most of the evidence of the effect of this drugs in SLE is obtained from case-series. Currently, there are not controlled trials to evaluate the efficacy of immunosuppressive drugs in myocarditis by SLE. In a case-series of 11 patients with myocarditis (5), all received high dose of systemic corticosteroids including prednisone, hydrocortisone or in more severe cases intravenous methylprednisolone. Most of the half of them [7/11], were treated with intravenous cyclophosphamide associated with corticosteroids, although two of them deceased after the first infusion of cyclophosphamide secondary to infections [5].

Atherosclerosis in SLE

Most of the patients with SLE who have deceased by cardiovascular disease had an accelerated atherosclerosis. Atherosclerosis can be considered a chronic inflammatory condition on the vessel wall characterized by lipids (cholesteryl esters mainly) accumulated within the macrophages (foam cells) and smooth muscle cells in the intimal layer [15]. The lesions progress into atherosclerotic plaques composed by extracellular matrix component smooth muscle cells, macrophages, connective tissues, lymphocytes and a fibrous cap over a pool of extracellular lipid [15]. Current theories indicate that in atherosclerosis coexist an active inflammation and an autoimmune process [15, 16].

Premature or accelerated atherosclerosis in SLE was initially described in 36 autopsies performed by Bulkley and Roberts in 1975 [17]. In 1976 Urowitz et al, reported a bimodal mortality pattern in SLE, calling the attention to the consequences of atherosclerosis particularly to the high incidence of myocardial infarction as a major cause of death in those patients with longer disease duration [18]. Many groups have confirmed the high frequency of accelerated atherosclerosis in SLE. The two main consequences of atherosclerosis are coronary and cerebrovascular disease. Some authors have reported a cumulative prevalence of coronary artery disease in SLE of 6 to 10%, although subclinical disease may occurs in 35 to 40% of the patients [19].

Traditional risk factors explain only partially the high frequency of atherosclerotic complications. Recently, a number of "new" risk factors for the development of atherosclerosis in SLE have been proposed. These include autoantibodies such as anti-*B*2 glycoprotein I, antiphospholipid antibodies, anti-oxidized LDL (anti-Ox-LDL), and anti-heat shock protein 60/65 (anti-HSPs). Currently, is also revalorized the role of some traditional risk factors such as homocysteine and C-reactive protein (CRP). Finally, some studies have investigated the role of cytokines, factors that participate in cell-to-cell interactions, and some infections in the genesis of atherosclerosis. The table 1 describes the risk factors associated with accelerated atherosclerosis.

Table 1. Risk factors for atherosclerosis in SLE

Traditional risk factors	Nontraditional risk factors
(a) Dyslipidemia	Antiphospholipid antibodies (aPLs)
(b) Hypertension	Anti-oxidized low-density lipoproteins (anti-OxLDL)
(c) Inflammation (CRP)	Anti heat shock proteins (anti-HSPs)
(d) High levels of homocysteine	Proinflammatory Cytokines
(e) Smoking	Infections
(f) Utilization of corticosteroids	
(g) Lifestyle	
(h) Disease activity	

Traditional Risk Factors

The traditional risk factors for development of atherosclerosis have been extensively studied in SLE. New clues have been found about the mechanisms and effects of these risk factors for SLE patients.

Dyslipidemia in SLE

Although dyslipidemia is highly prevalent in SLE and their role on the atherogenesis seems to be one of the most studied, some authors have shown evidence that this risk factor is not frequently assessed in the ordinary clinical practice. Al-Herz et al, observed in a retrospective charts review that serum lipid profiles were measured only in 37 from 60 patients (62%) in a lupus clinic and in 19 from 123 (15%) patients obtained from private practice [20]. In 56 patients where the lipid profile was obtained, 31 (55%) of them had dyslipidemia underlying the importance of to assess this risk factor in the lupus clinics.

There has been described a typical pattern of dyslipidemia in SLE that is characterized by low high-density lipoprotein (HDL), raised triglycerides (TGs), and mild or no elevation of low-density-lipoprotein, with a raising of lipoprotein (a) (Lp(a)) [21, 22]. There is a close relationship between disease activity and dyslipidemia in these patients [23]. Some mechanisms are supposed to participate in the association between dislypidemia and disease activity. There is considered that an impairment in the activity of lipoprotein lipase (enzyme responsible for the catabolism of chylomicrons), is responsible for the elevated levels of triglyceride found in SLE. One study detected in 47% from 105 patients with SLE autoantibodies directed against lipoprotein lipase with capacity for inhibition of this enzyme [24].

Hypertension and Smoking

Elevated high blood pressure is highly prevalent in SLE. Recent studies showed that this risk factor has a prevalence that ranges from 12 to almost 30% of the patients [25, 26]. Both, smoking as systemic hypertension constitute two well documented risk factors for coronary and cerebrovascular disease. Both factors increase the levels of tissue factor (formerly known as thromboplastin), that is a key initiator of the coagulation cascade that leads to fibrin formation [27]. Tissue factor is involved in the pathogenesis of atherosclerosis by promoting thrombus formation and to induce migration and proliferation of vascular smooth muscle cells [27]. Smoking has multiple other effects on the atherogenesis producing vascular inflammation and abnormalities in the oxidative stress. Different studies have shown that smokers have higher leucocytes counts in blood, increase in C-reactive protein (CRP), interleukin-6 and higher serum levels of soluble intercellular adhesion molecules [28]. Smoking may increase the expression of metalloproteinases and plasmin. Metalloproteinases are expressed in the atherosclerotic plaques where may contribute to instability of the plaque and the rupture stimulating neovascularization via generation of angiogenic peptides [28]. In patients with SLE, smoking has been found consistently as a major risk factor for atherosclerosis and cardiovascular events. In a recent study Urowitz reported in an extensive number of patients surged from a cohort that smoking was one of the major factors associated with atherosclerotic vascular events in SLE [29]. In a multiethnic cohort of patients with SLE performed in the United States smoking also was found as one of the strongest predictors for vascular events, together with elevated levels of CRP and antiphospholipid antibodies [30]. These data suggest the need to discourage smoking in patients with SLE and to inform the patients the increase of risk for a vascular event in case of persistence of this behavior.

Homocysteine in SLE

Homocysteine is an aminoacid containing sulfur produced during the metabolism of methionine with multiple effects on the vascular endothelium. High levels of homocysteine are prothrombic, increased collagen production and decrease the availability of nitric oxide. Elevated homocysteine has been proposed as cerebrovascular and cardiovascular risk factor in SLE. One of the earliest observations about the possible role of homocysteine in the atherosclerosis of SLE was made in a prospective cohort study by Petri et al [31]. They observed a prevalence of plasmatic hyperhomocysteinaemia (>14.1 mumol /l) in 15% of their patients. After adjusting by other traditional risk factors hyperhomocysteinaemia increased the risk for stroke (OR=2.44, 95%CI 1.04-5.75, p=0.04) and arterial thrombotic events (OR=3.9, 95%CI 0.97-12.54, p=0.05). Further studies have confirmed the association between elevated levels of homocysteine and thrombosis [32, 33]. However, these findings are not consistently reported [34].

Homocysteine levels can be decreased by the utilization of folic acid and vitamin B supplementation. Statins used for treatment of hyperlipidemia can also decrease the hyperhomocysteinaemia. Nevertheless, although homocysteine is a potentially modifiable factor for cardiovascular events in SLE, currently there is a lack of controlled trials to evaluate the effect of a normalization of the levels of homocysteine on the rate of cardiovascular events in SLE. These trials are required to define if hyperhomocysteinemia is truly a risk factor that requires be treated or constitutes only an epiphenomenon of the systemic inflammation in SLE.

Corticosteroids

Corticosteroids are associated with increase of risk factors for atherosclerosis including the redistribution of body fat, modifications in blood pressure, and effects on the plasmatic glucose. The alterations on the lipid profiles are related with the doses of corticosteroids. More than one decade ago, MacGregor et al observed that prednisone dose lower than 10 mg/ daily did not affect the lipid profile, whereas, higher dose can increase the levels of triglycerides and some apolipoprotein [35]. Other authors have subsequently confirmed this strong association of lipid levels and corticosteroids [36].

Although, the role that play the corticosteroids in the accelerated atherosclerosis in SLE is not simple. Intriguingly, the corticosteroids may also improve the "protective factors" for atherogenesis. Corticosteroids can suppress the inflammation and some of their components that are related with atherosclerosis. These facts explain in part some of the controversial findings reported in the literature. Roman et al. [37] observed that those patients with carotid atherosclerosis had received a lower total cumulative dose of corticosteroids compared with patients without carotid plaques. Corticosteroids therefore, have a complex role in the pathogenesis of atherosclerosis; strategies to decrease the doses using other drugs such as antimalarials can contribute to improve the rates of accelerated atherosclerosis in SLE.

Inflammation

Atherosclerosis has an important inflammatory component, examination of plaques of atherosclerosis shows infiltration of T cell lymphocytes and macrophages observed mainly in early stages. Several substances facilitate the infiltration by inflammatory cells including the monocyte chemotactic protein-1 (MCP-1), and different adhesion molecules. Inflammatory mechanisms contribute to instability and rupture of plaques. Interferon (IFN) has been found in the area surrounding atherosclerotic plaques. IFN contribute to the instability of a plaque and rupture, through to reduce collagen synthesis in conjunction with increase in the synthesis of matrix metalloproteinases leading to destabilization of the plaque, fissuring it and provoking the rupture [38, 39].

High levels of C-reactive protein (CRP), detected by high-sensitivity immunoassay are considered strong predictors for coronary artery disease. CRP is synthesized in the liver in response to different cytokines including interleukin-6. Studies in vitro have shown that CRP activates the complement system, induces the production of MCP-1, increase the expression of cellular adhesion molecules (CAM), stimulate the monocyte production of tissue factor and are mediators in the macrophage uptake of LDL [40]. High levels of CRP also produce an endothelial dysfunction mediated through their effects in to suppress vascular endothelial cell expression and the activity of endothelial nitric oxide synthase [40]. This endothelial dysfunction is considered nowadays an important component of the initiation of atherogenesis. CRP has other important actions implicated on the atherogenesis including promote a procoagulant state mediated by their effects in inducing of plasminogen activator inhibitor-1, and increase the erythrocyte adhesiveness and subsequent aggregation [40].

TNF-α and IL-1

Different studies have been observed evidence of the participation of TNF-α and IL-1 in the atherosclerotic plaques. Both cytokines have a number of effects on the atherogenesis including to stimulate the smooth muscle proliferation, induce local inflammation in blood vessels, activation of macrophages, promote expression of cell adhesion molecules and induce secretion of matrix metalloproteinases [41]. Both IL-1 and TNF-α, are powerful inhibitors of lipoprotein lipase leading to increase the levels of triglycerides. TNF-α also exerts other metabolic effects related with atherosclerosis including redistribution of adipose tissue and impairment in the insulin sensitivity [41]. Some authors have described in women with SLE and history of cardiovascular disease an increase in plasmatic levels of TNF-α and soluble receptors of TNF1 and TNF2 compared with those patients without cardiovascular disease [42]. Patients with cardiovascular disease also had a positive correlation between levels of TNF-α and cholesterol or triglycerides [42].

Autoantibodies

a) Anti-Oxidized Low Density Lipoproteins (Anti-Oxldl Antibodies)

After the migration from the blood circulation to the subendothelial layer of the artery, the low-density proteins (LDL) particles suffer an oxidative modification which is atherogenic. These oxidized LDL promote proliferation of smooth muscle of the arteries, activate monocyte-macrophages, increase the foam cell formation, leukocyte recruitment and interfere with endothelium mediated relaxation [43-45].

The oxidation of LDL transform these lipoproteins in antigenic. Autoantibodies reacting with oxidized LDL have been found in the atherosclerotic plaques. In animal models, the titers of antibodies against oxidized LDL (anti-Ox-LDL) correlates with the progression of atherosclerosis and in humans, the presence of anti-Ox-LDL is independent risk factor for progression of carotid plaques [15].

b) Antiphospholipid Antibodies

Beta 2-glycoprotein I, is a molecule located on the surface of endothelial cells, in subendothelial regions and the intimal of the arteries. Antibodies directed against to *Beta* 2-glycoprotein I (anti-*B*2-GPI) have been associated with the development of atherosclerosis. *B*2-GPI can bind Ox-LDL resulting in the complexe denominated *B*2-GPI-Ox-LDL, a very stable complex that may accelerate the process of atherosclerosis [43]. Antibodies directed against this complexe increases LDL uptake by macrophages contributing to the foam cell formation. Anti-*B*2-GPI also binds endothelial cells inducing the expression of adhesion cell molecules increasing the adhesion of monocytes to the endothelium [46]. Interestingly, further evidence in several studies considered functional differences in the classes of immunoglobulin that are compound of the antibodies anti-*B*2-Ox-LDL. Whereas, IgG autoantibodies directed against B2-GPI-ox-LDL are atherogenic, the IgM anti-ox-LDL seems to be protective [46, 47].

Anticardiolipin antibodies have a controversial association with cardiovascular events. In a study performed in middle-age-men, the frequency of anticardiolipin antibodies was greater in those patients who developed myocardial infarction or death associated to cardiac event compared with patients who did not developed cardiac disease [48]. However, a more recent study failed to find a positive association between high titres of antibodies anticardiolipin antibodies, anti-Ox-LDL and myocardial infarction [49]. In patients with SLE the presence of antiphospholipid antibodies is associated with coronary disease. In a prospective cohort of 166 patients with SLE after the adjustment by other important risk factors, the presence of lupus anticoagulant increase the probability to develop ischemic coronary disease and stroke

[50]. Other cohort studies have also confirmed the increase in risk for coronary artery disease in SLE patients with antiphospholipid antibodies [51, 52].

Anti-Heat Shock Proteins

Heat shock proteins (HSPs) have been found in atherosclerotic plaques and there is some evidence regarding an association between plaque inflammation and higher levels of antibodies directed against these HSPs [53]. The role of this anti-HSP in atherosclerotic lesions can be explained as an effect in response to the injured endothelium that expresses HSPs, or instead, be a cross-reaction originally directed against some microorganisms that infected the arterial walls where HSPs may be expressed as response to these infections. In support of the second hypothesis, experimental models have observed that the rabbit vascular cells infected by Chlamydia pneumoniae (infection that has been linked to atherosclerosis), express the HSP-60 leading to mitogenic effects with increase in the number of vascular smooth muscle cells that is a step in the development of atheroma [54]. Anti-HSPs 65/60 are experimentally involved in endothelial cytotoxicity [55]. Higher titres of anti-HSP65 have been associated with advanced carotid atherosclerotic lesions and an increase in the risk for 5-year mortality [56]. Anti-HSP65 antibodies have been also associated with coronary calcification assessed by electron-beam computed tomography [57].

Infections

Chlamydia Pneumoniae is an infectious agent associated with the development atherosclerosis. Lipopolysaccharides of this microorganism are associated with increase in the levels of C-reactive protein, and HSP-60 both involved in the development of atherosclerosis and the inflammation of the vascular bed. Molecular evidence of Chlamydia infection has been found in some patients with SLE and coronary artery calcification evaluated by electron beam computed tomography [58]. Although, many confounding factors can be implied in these findings and other studies should be performed to confirm this possible association. Therefore, in the case of be confirmed the role of infections in atherosclerosis further therapeutic strategies should be evaluate to treat these infections to reduce the risk of coronary disease in SLE.

Cohort Studies and Risk Factors for Atherosclerosis

A number of cohort studies have recently evaluated the effect of different risk factors on the development of vascular events. These studies are important because may proportionate important clues for evaluation of causal associations. In the lupus cohort of Toronto University from 1,087 patients included the frequency of atherosclerotic vascular events was 10.9% [29]. A number of factors were associated with cardiovascular events particularly was interesting the observed association with neuropsychiatric involvement [29]. LUMINA, is a multiethnic cohort performed in United States. In this cohort 546 patients were assessed for risk factors associated with the subsequent development of vascular events including myocardial infarction or angina, stroke and peripheral arterial involvement. The frequency of vascular events was 6.2%, being more frequently observed the cerebrovascular involvement (18 events), followed by cardiovascular (13 events) and peripheral vascular (5 events). The risk factors associated with vascular events were older age, current smoking, longer follow-up time, elevated serum levels of C-reactive protein and antiphospholipid antibodies (30). In the Hopkins Lupus Cohort, 380 patients with SLE were followed in order to assess the development of atherosclerosis and/or coronary artery disease. Patients with lupic anticoagulant developed a higher frequency of myocardial infarction (22%), but antiphospholipid antibodies were not associated with subclinical atherosclerosis including carotid plaques or coronary calcification [51].

Whereas, an important number of cohort studies have been developed to assess atherosclerosis in adults patients with SLE. The information proceeding from follow-up studies in pediatric population is limited. The incidence and risk factors for atherosclerosis in pediatric patients are not well known. In a recent prospective cohort, 139 children were followed in order to determine the role of active disease and therapy on the abnormalities of lipid levels [59]. A reduction in the prednisone dose during the follow-up was associated with decrement in the levels of cholesterol and triglycerides, whereas, those patients with proteinuria developed increase in cholesterol, triglycerides and LDL levels [59].

Diagnostic Methods in Atherosclerosis

The approaches to study atherosclerosis can be classified in two different forms: Those that the outcomes rely on clinical events (or primary endpoints) including myocardial infarction, stroke or death caused by atherosclerotic complications, being these events presented late in the disease. The second approach is based in to study surrogate measures that detect atherosclerosis earlier, where the impact of preventive strategies can modify the natural course of the disease. Therefore, for this second approach the useful of noninvasive techniques for the detection of atherosclerosis even in asymptomatic patients can be utilized in order to establish opportune therapeutic measures. Overall, the assessment of atherosclerosis may involve noninvasive techniques (B-mode ultrasound or electron beam computed tomography), semi-invasive techniques or invasive techniques (coronary angiography).

Coronary Angiography

Coronary angiography is the gold standard technique to assess the severity of stenosis of coronary arteries caused by atherosclerosis. Angiitis of the coronary vessels, thrombosis caused by hypercoagulable states, and coronary spasm that are entities to be considered in SLE, can also be assessed by coronary angiography [60]. Figure 5 shows a partial obstruction of the coronary artery caused by atheroma in the coronary angiography.

An "old concept" in coronary disease, is that in order to produce a myocardial infarction is required a significant occlusion of the coronary artery usually higher than 50%. However, more recent evidence suggests that the rupture of an atherosclerotic plaque can produce myocardial infarction even without significant coronary stenosis. Vulnerable atherosclerotic plaques that are associated with mortality have been studied in their histopathology.

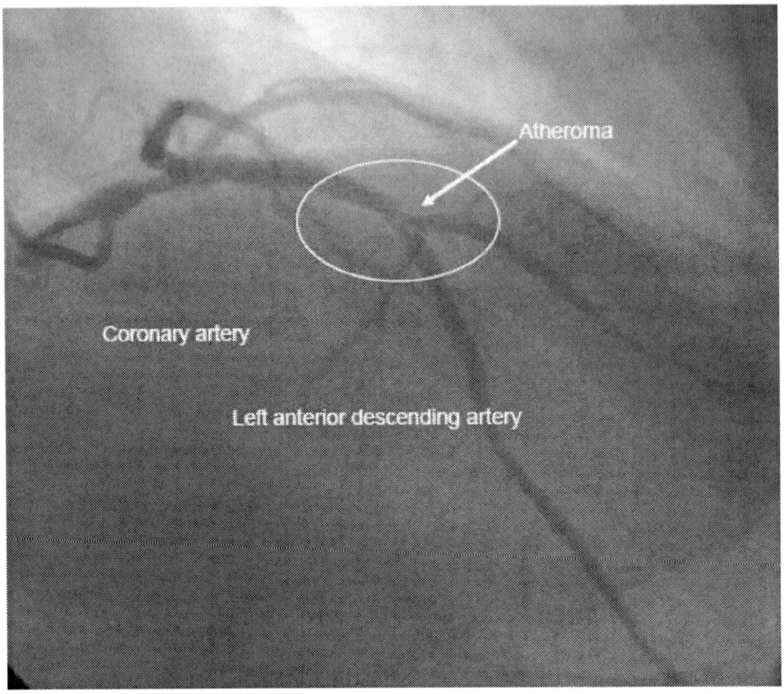

Figure 5. Coronary angiography showing the presence of atheroma that produces an incomplete obstruction of the vascular lumen in a patient with systemic lupus erythematosus.

In general around 60% of the plaques susceptible of rupture have a thrombogenic core of lipids, macrophages, T cells, neovascular formation and calcium deposits. Presumably the ruptures of these types of plaque are caused by the macrophages digestion and the apoptosis of smooth muscle cells induced by cytokines. Whereas, in another 30-40% of patients without coronary stenosis there are coronary thromboses overlie plaques with significant luminal inflammation [61]. In SLE patients inflammatory cells infiltrate may be considered a major marker of plaque vulnerability even independently of plaque structure or stenosis. Therefore, major efforts need to be done in order to determine by other techniques the coronary involvement without the limitations of coronary angiography.

Intracoronary Ultrasonography

This technique can be useful to identify atheroma in arteries with normal angiography providing insights into the extent and distribution of atherosclerotic plaque and evaluating both the vessel wall and plaque morphology [62].

Intracoronary ultrasound is useful to evaluate the plaque core. A calcified plaque is echoreflective, whereas, a fibrous plaque is hyperechoic and a plaque with a lipid-rich core is hypoechoic. The reliability of this technique is higher to distinguish calcifications in the plaques or fibrous plaques but decreases significantly to distinguish lipid-rich plaques. Since the epidemiological point of view, this technique is limited by their invasiveness and their complications. To date, there are no published reports evaluating the role of this technique in lupus patients.

Electron Beam Computed Tomography and Helical Computed Tomography

The evaluation of coronaries by electron beam computed tomography and helical computed tomography constitute two related techniques to evaluate calcification in coronary arteries using computed tomography. Pathological studies have shown a good correlation between the severity of calcification in atherosclerotic plaques and the severity and extend of coronary heart disease [63]. Under this basis, the assessment of coronary calcification constitutes a valuable surrogate measure to detect early atherosclerosis. Currently, there is some studies assessing the prevalence of coronary calcification in SLE assessed by electron beam computed tomography. In an interesting study, the performance of the Framingham risk score for increased cardiovascular risk was evaluated in asymptomatic women with SLE. These patients were also evaluated by electron beam computed tomography in order to detect coronary atherosclerosis [64]. There were no statistical differences in the Framingham scores between patients with SLE and controls, although; the prevalence of coronary calcification was significantly higher in SLE (19.4% versus controls 6.2%, $p=0.02$). This study shows two important aspects: the prevalence of asymptomatic coronary disease is high in SLE and the performance of Framingham risk score to predict coronary calcifications in SLE is low and can underestimate the true risk for coronary disease. Another recent study evaluated the variables associated with coronary artery calcification by electron beam computed tomography in SLE. Higher age, homocysteine concentrations and disease duration were associated with coronary artery calcification [65]. The association between hyperhomocysteinaemia and coronary artery calcification is relevant because is a modifiable risk factor and future studies should evaluate the effectiveness of therapies used to decrease this and other risk factors in order to reduce the incidence of coronary calcifications. Future studies with electron beam computed tomography of the coronary arteries also should demonstrate their utility as predictors of hard outcomes in SLE patients.

Magnetic Resonance Coronary Angiography (MRCA) and Positron Emission Tomography

MRCA can provide a 3 dimensional of the coronary arteries being useful to detect large stenoses. Although, small stenoses can be not detected constituting an important limitation in terms of its utility for the prevention of coronary disease complications. Positron emission tomography (PET) can be used to evaluate coronary flow and flow reserve. The main disadvantage is its inability to detect coronary stenosis lower 50%. Some authors found in patients with hypercholesterolemia show that myocardial blood flow can be improved after lipid lowering therapy suggesting a promissory role in the research of results of lipid-lowering therapy [66]. So far the evaluation of these strategies in SLE requires additional studies.

B-Mode Ultrasound

B-mode ultrasound constitutes a noninvasive technique for the visualization of intima-media thickness (IMT) in the lumen of the carotid, aortic or femoral arteries [67]. Carotid IMT measurement correlates adequately with coronary atherosclerosis and is an independent risk factor for coronary heart disease in general population. Patients with SLE have a higher prevalence of carotid plaques shown by this technique compared with controls [68].

A potential of this technique is to monitor the changes in IMT in response to therapy. Strategy that requires be evaluated in future studies of prevention for coronary heart disease in SLE.

Myocardial Perfusion Scintigraphy

Some recent series have showed that a high proportion of patients with SLE had abnormalities in scintigraphy. One study found a prevalence of 28% of abnormalities evaluated with scintigraphy with single photon computed tomography with technetium 99-sestamibi. None of these patients had angina or antecedents suggestive of coronary involvement. Factors associated with abnormalities in the scintigraphy in this study were associated with diabetes mellitus, lower levels of HDL or concurrent vasculitis [69]. Issues regarding to specificity and predictive values of this technique in SLE should be solved in future researches.

Coronary Flow Reserve Evaluated by Doppler

Coronary flow reserve (CFR) measurement is used to assess epicardial coronary stenoses. CFR also, can be utilized to examine the integrity of microvascular circulation. Transthoracic Doppler echocardiography is a useful technique to measure the blood flow velocity. This technique is reliable to measure the blood flow velocity in the distal and middle segment of left anterior descending coronary artery, circumflex coronary artery and right coronary artery. Currently, the use of contrast enhancement combined second harmonic-imaging technique increased the feasibility of the transthoracic Doppler echocardiography [70]. The clinical applications of the transthoracic Doppler to assess CFR include: functional assessment of coronary stenosis, to detect severe stenoses, assessment of the wall motion, evaluate the impairment of microvascular circulation. Doppler echocardiography to assess CFR also can be used to refer a patient for a therapeutic procedure (such as percutaneous transluminal coronary angioplasty), to monitor coronary restenosis or assessment of a reperfused myocardial infarction. The utility of this method in SLE to predict patients who will develop coronary artery disease require to be evaluated by prospective cohorts.

Treatment of Atherosclerosis in SLE

The treatment for accelerated atherosclerosis in SLE can be classified as a) preventive (oriented to modify in asymptomatic patients the risks for a hard outcome such as myocardial infarction or death), focused to decrease the progression and complications in a patient with a previous cardiovascular event (such patients who already developed angina or myocardial infarction) that is also known as "secondary prevention".

The preventive treatment of atherosclerosis requires the early recognition of a patient in risk. Risk factors such as smoking, obesity, diabetes mellitus, or physical inactivity should be treated. Bruce et al reported that a significant proportion of their patients with SLE who developed acute coronary events had a previous inadequate management of some potentially reversible risk factors particularly hypercholesterolemia, smoking and obesity [71]. A more recent study of this group reported that only 285 of their patients with hypercholesterolemia were treated with lipid lowering treatment [72]. These two studies underline the importance to treat adequately the risk factors for atherosclerosis in SLE. Patients with abnormalities in the studies that show atherosclerosis including electron beam computed tomography or B-mode ultrasound of the carotid should be considered candidate for preventive treatment in order to decrease the risk of a hard outcome such as myocardial infarction or stroke.

Antimalarial Drugs in Atherosclerosis

Several reports have found a significant benefit of antimalarial drugs in decrease the levels of cholesterol [73-75]. Together with their effects in cholesterol, antimalarial drugs exerts effects in increase the levels of HDL and decrease levels of LDL. Recently, it has been demonstrated an increase in the clearance of LDL cholesterol in patients with SLE who receive chloroquine [76]. Antimalarial drugs should be considered in patients with SLE that have abnormalities in their lipid profile, as a strategy to prevent atherosclerotic complications. These drugs can be useful for reduce the abnormalities in the lipid profile in patients who receive prednisone [77]. However, there is a lack of studies evaluating the effect of these drugs using subrogate measures of atherosclerosis such as B-mode ultrasound or electron beam computed tomography. This constitutes an interesting are for further research in atherosclerosis.

Statins in SLE

Statins inhibit 3-hydroxy-3methylglutaryl coenzyme A (HMG-CoA) reductase. The drug has effects decreasing the levels of lipids and affecting immune responses having a pleiotropic pharmacological activity. Statins decrease the levels of C-reactive protein [78], decrease the levels of some proinflammatory cytokines such as interleukin-6 and TNF-α [79]. Statins has immunomodulatory properties reducing the inflammatory component of the atherosclerotic plaque [80]. Statins should be used with careful in SLE: is well established the effect of these drugs on lipid metabolism, although statins may increase the B cell reactivity by enhancing the Th2 immune response [80]. Statins have been associated with lupus like syndrome and develop of antinuclear antibodies in patients without rheumatic disorders with this treatment [80]. On the opposite side of these findings, in animal models of lupus, statins may have benefits. Atorvastatin for example administered in murine models of SLE reduce titres of anti-dsDNA antibodies, decrease the deposit of immunoglobulin on the glomeruli, and decrease the proteinuria and azotemia [80]. Therefore, is important a deeper evaluation of the effects of statins in patients with SLE. Unfortunately, there are some barriers to evaluate statins in controlled clinical trials in patients with SLE. A recent paper was unable to perform a randomized controlled trial of pravastatin in SLE caused by the lack of participation, and high rates of dropouts [81]. These authors informed subsequently a decrement in the total cholesterol and LDL observed in the group of patients who received pravastatin compared with those who did not receive the drug, although the utilization of corticosteroids decreases the effectiveness of the statin [82]. Patients with SLE usually receive a multiplicity of medications that increase the risk of side-effects and the willingness of the patients to receive new drugs. Patients who are nonparticipants have more concerns about their health status, the medication used in the trial and the possible inclusion in the placebo group compared with those who accept their participation [83]. Trials evaluating preventive strategies should take into account the possible high rates of no-participation of these patients. A double-blind multicenter trial is required in order to raise a sufficient sample of patients to evaluate the effect of statins in SLE and give a relevant information to support the clinical decision making.

Aspirin Therapy

The lack of evidence from controlled trial about the benefits of aspirin in the prevention of myocardial infarction in SLE is intriguing, because aspirin is an old-drug with recognized benefits to decrease the rates of coronary disorders in other populations. An important number of randomized controlled trials have shown that low-dose aspirin decrease the risk for myocardial infarction in men of the general population. However, a randomized trial was unable to demonstrate benefits in healthy postmenopausal women in order to decrease the rates of nonfatal myocardial infarction or death from cardiovascular causes [84]. In SLE there is a lack of controlled studies to evaluate if aspirin decrease or not the risk for myocardial infarction. This is an important issue that requires to be evaluated in controlled trials, because these patients constitute a high-risk group for cardiovascular events by the factors enunciated previously. Although, other factors should be considered, among these factors is quite relevant that a high proportion of patients with SLE are concurrently treated with nonsteroidal anti-inflammatory drugs (NSAIDs). There is evidence in the literature that the concomitant regular utilization of NSAIDs interferes with the benefits of low-dose aspirin in the prevention of myocardial infarction [85]. This finding is particularly important in patients with SLE that are chronic consumers of NSAIDs and further studies should be performed to solve if aspirin can be protective in SLE even with the concomitant administration of NSAIDs.

Angiotensin-Converting–Enzyme Inhibitors

Angiotensin converting-enzyme inhibitors (ACEI) are frequently used to treat the hypertension in SLE patients, although, to date there are no controlled studies have been performed to evaluate their role on the reduction of the cardiovascular mortality in these patients. The evidence of the literature on other populations shows that ACEI reduces the rates of death from cardiovascular causes, myocardial infarction and stroke in high-risk patients for the development of coronary heart disease including among these diabetes mellitus [86, 87]. But there is no information regarding the long term effects on the protection of coronary heart disease in SLE with the use of these drugs. Therefore, although the evidence in other populations point-out to additional benefits with these drugs in atherosclerosis, is currently required to evaluate the effect of ACEI inhibitors on the primary and secondary prevention of atherosclerotic complications in SLE.

General Measures Used for Atherosclerosis

Because of the evidence that moderate and high doses of corticosteroids contribute to the development of coronary heart disease in patients with SLE, it is recommended the utilization of these drugs at the lowest dosage guided by the severity of the disease activity, and reducing these doses when possible. An adequate evaluation of the disease activity is mandatory to take appropriate measures regarding to the corticosteroid dosage. Because the evidence described above also denote that corticosteroid can be also protective if they are used adequately in patients with chronic inflammation.

Treatment of Atherosclerotic Complications

In 2004 Ward reviewed in a state hospitalization database the outcomes of all the hospitalizations for myocardial infarctions and strokes in patients with SLE and compared them with the outcomes in controls without SLE [88]. No significant differences were observed between SLE and controls in the following outcomes: risk of in-hospital mortality or congestive failure, although men with SLE had longer length of stay compared with controls [88]. A number of case-reports have been published describing the results of percutaneous transluminal coronary angioplasty and coronary stent in SLE, although; there is a lack of information of follow-up studies to evaluate the rates of coronary restenosis in these patients. Being an interesting issue to be evaluated in future cohort studies because the restenosis could be expected be higher in these patients due to the high number of coronary risk factors that they present.

Conclusions in the Management of Risk Factors for Atherosclerosis

In an excellent paper Bruce summarize some of the recommendations to treat the risk factors of atherosclerosis [89]. The strategy recommended is to select targets that should be achieved by individual patients. These targets should be take into account the main risk factors for coronary heart disease such as blood pressure, levels of lipids, other comorbid diseases (such as diabetes mellitus or obesity), smoking, etc. Patients with SLE can be beneficiated with aspirin if they have additional risk factors such as a previous event of coronary heart disease, or presence of antiphospholipid antibodies. ACE inhibitors are recommended for patients with heart failure, diabetes mellitus or left ventricular hypertrophy [89]. Currently, there is adequate evidence to recommend antimalarial drugs in those patients with an abnormal lipid profile, although the data for take a position about statins is waiting for controlled studies. Strategies in order to decrease homocysteine levels in SLE are still without be evaluated by controlled trials and therefore is uncertain their benefit in SLE.

Pulmonary Hypertension

Definition

Pulmonary arterial hypertension (PAH) is an elevation of the pulmonary vascular pressure caused by an increase in pulmonary arterial with or without increase in the venous pressure. Hemodynamically, PAH can be defined as an increase of the pulmonary artery pressure at resting greater than 25 mm Hg at rest or greater than 30 mm Hg during exercise measured invasively with a pulmonary artery catheter. Although, other definitions are based in a measure systolic pulmonary artery pressure greater than 30 mm Hg [90].

The prevalence of pulmonary hypertension in SLE depends of the method employed for the assessment. In the clinical context PAH can be identified in various scenarios: a) during a directed assessment for the pulmonary pressure in a symptomatic patient, b) during the screening of patients at risk or c) be discovered incidentally during the evaluation of an asymptomatic patient.

Prevalence Studies

Prevalence of PAH reported in SLE depends of the design of the study and the method used for the diagnosis. PAH in SLE was considered previously as a very rare entity and with very high-mortality at the short term of follow-up, this because that in earlier studies PAH was diagnosed almost exclusively during a cardiac catheterization performed in patients with severe symptomatology. Similar findings are found in studies based in diagnostic obtained from clinical charts where PAH seems to be observed infrequently in SLE. A more recent retrospective study found only 46 patients with PAH from a lupus cohort of 786 patients [91]. Nevertheless, one of the main disadvantages of this study is the lack of a systematic assessment to exclude PAH in the remaining 740 other patients [91], limiting the validity of their conclusions.

Nowadays, the utilization of non-invasive methods particularly the Doppler echocardiography has allowed the early detection in asymptomatic population. In patients evaluated by Doppler echocardiography the prevalence of PAH in SLE goes from 11% to 43% [92-94]. In a prospective study we systematically assessed 204 outpatients with SLE from two rheumatology clinics using Color-Doppler echocardiography technique, obtaining a prevalence of PAH of 18% (defining PAH as a finding of systolic pulmonary artery pressure >30mmHg) [95]. However, there are important concerns about the specificity of Doppler compared with catheterism and the reproducibility of the Doppler studies when they are evaluated sequentially. Recent reviews have described that the performance of Doppler to measure PSAP has been increased with an appropriate training of the evaluators, the development of the new technology of the equipments and protocols for the measurement of pulmonary artery pressures.

Postmortem Studies

There is a lack of studies of prevalence of PAH based in findings of autopsies. When the pathologist is oriented to evaluate changes suggestive in the pulmonary arteries, the prevalence of these changes seems to be increased. Our group has found a high frequency of histological changes compatible with moderate or severe pulmonary hypertension in a group of autopsies of patients with SLE from a tertiary-care center. Interesting in only a minimum number of patients was suspected cardiovascular disease although, autopsies showed a high proportion of cardiovascular abnormalities.

An important determinant of the lower frequency of the "antemortem" diagnosis of PAH is the relative absence of symptoms in earlier stages. Most of the patients included in our cohort with pulmonary artery pressure between 30 to 40 mm Hg described only mild symptoms or they were asymptomatic [95]. Symptoms described by the patients with moderate or severe pulmonary hypertension include dyspnea, dyspnea during the performance of activities or exercise, fatigue, syncope, or an unspecified chest pain. Clinical but not early findings suggestive of PAH are data of heart failure (oedema in legs, hepatomegaly, raised jugular venous pressure, etc.). A loud pulmonic heart sound was observed in around the half of the patients with PAH in a study based in a retrospective chart review [91].

Pathogenesis

The specific mechanisms that cause pulmonary hypertension in SLE remain unknown. Although pathological findings are very similar to the primary form of pulmonary hypertension and the response to some therapies suggest similar mechanisms of development between both entities. In both, PH associated with SLE and primary PAH, the characteristic of a severe disease observed in the pulmonary vessels is the plexiform lesion that is constituted by an abnormal proliferation of endothelial cells, smooth muscle thickening and a remodeling of the adventitia (see figure 6). In SLE genetic polymorphisms, environmental factors and inflammatory mechanisms seems to participate in the pathogenesis of PAH. Some similitudes are observed between PAH associated to SLE and the primary form of PAH. In cases of the familial PAH, a variety of the primary form of PAH, there is found mutations in the bone morphogenetic protein receptor 2 (BMPR2), that is a member of the transforming growth factor- beta (TGF-β) superfamily that play a central role in the programmed cell death. Abnormalities in the regulation of this apoptosis could promote the angiogenesis developing the classical proliferation of the vascular endothelium [96, 97]. Primary PAH present abnormalities in the production and degradation of nitric oxide (NO). Increase in the expression of vascular endothelial growth factor (VEGF), angiopoietin-1, 5-lipoxygenase, 5-lipoxygenase activating factor, and endothelin-1, have been found in lungs from patients with severe pulmonary hypertension [98].

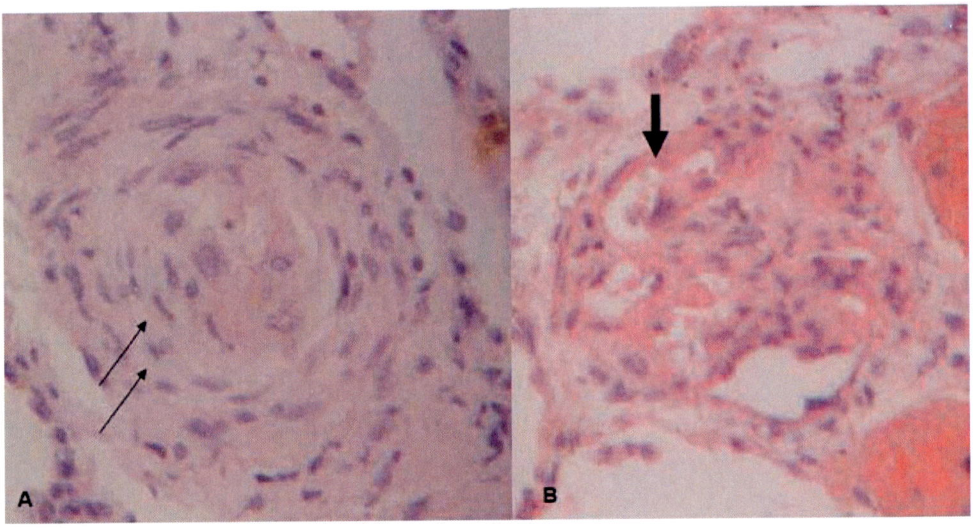

Figure 6. A. Obliteration of the pulmonary vascular lumen (thin arrows) in a case of pulmonary hypertension secondary to SLE. B. Plexiform lesions (wide arrow) in another case of pulmonary hypertension in SLE. Hematoxylin-Eosin staining 40 x (Photo Courtesy of Dr. Jose Ornelas-Aguirre, and Dr. Gonzalo Vazquez-Camacho. Department of Pathology, Centro Medico de Occidente IMSS, Guadalajara, Mexico).

In systemic lupus erythematosus, high levels of molecules that participate in the pathogenesis of primary PAH have been also found. High levels of endothelin-1 have been observed in patients with SLE and PAH [92] suggesting a common participation of endothelin in the genesis of both primary form and pulmonary hypertension associated with SLE. High levels of VGEF and its receptors have been found in active SLE [99]. Although, these levels have not been investigated in PAH in SLE and further studies should be performed to evaluate if VGEF is associated with this entity.

In both primary and secondary forms of PAH including those associated with SLE the pathological changes observed in the pulmonary arteries include medial hypertrophy, concentric intimal fibrosis, *in situ* thrombosis, pulmonary arteritis and typical plexiform lesions [100]. Inflammatory infiltrates with macrophage and lymphocytes in the lesions are observed in SLE suggesting that inflammatory cells and their products may cause these lesions. Therefore, this is the theoretical basis for the utilization of immunosuppressive therapies in PAH associated to SLE. Some cytokines such as tumor necrosis factor alpha (TNF-α), interleukin-6, interferon gamma and interleukin-2 have been associated with other forms of PAH but their role in the PAH in SLE, still have not been sufficiently evaluated. Around a decade ago was observed that patients with SLE and PAH had higher levels of IL-6 compared with controls but their effect on the pathogenesis of the disease remain unsolved [101].

Some autoantibodies have been associated with PAH associated to SLE among these the presence antiphospholipid antibodies have been with certain frequency reported by almost 2 decades in patients with SLE and PAH [102, 103]. However, a recent study did not find association of PAH with these autoantibodies [104].

Antiendothelial cell antibodies were reported increased in patients with SLE with PAH by most of a decade ago [105]. However, these have been reported in a reduced number of patients with SLE and there is a lack of studies by other authors that support these findings. Most recently the possible role for these autoantibodies has been investigated in patients with idiopathic PAH and the form associated with scleroderma [106]. In SLE patients these autoantibodies could participate in the release of endothelin-1 as response to the vascular injury [107], being an interesting hypothesis to be explored in SLE with PAH.

Diagnostic of PAH

Most of the diagnostic methods show only suggestive findings that are not pathognomonic of PAH. Therefore, the gold standard for the diagnosis continues being the invasive assessment of pulmonary pressure. There are some findings in obtained with the non-invasive methods that require further evaluation for PAH in SLE.

Chest radiograph: may show cardiomegaly with prominent pulmonary artery segments and oligaemic lung fields (see figure 7).

Electrocardiography: may show changes of right ventricular hypertrophy that are nonspecific or enlargement of the atrium.

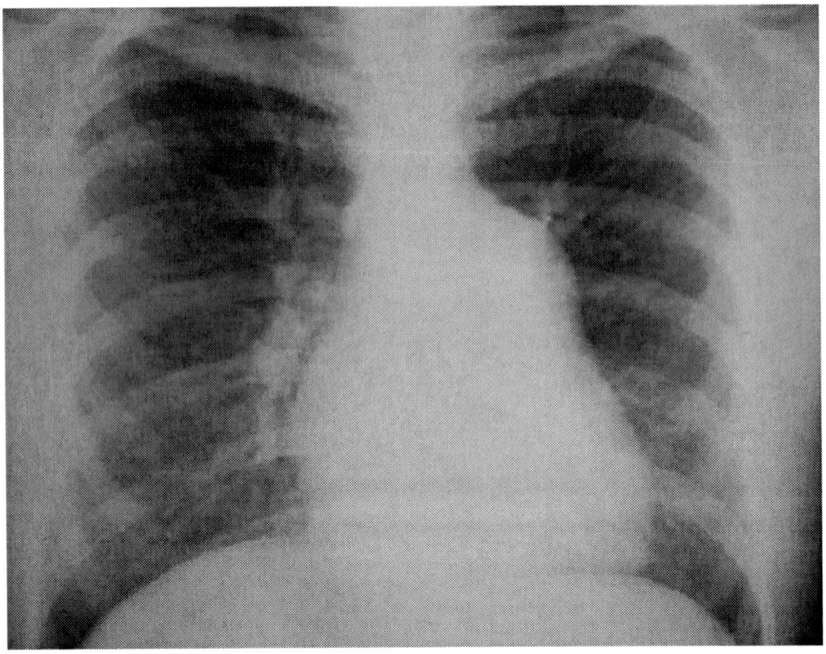

Figure 7. Plain radiograph of a woman with pulmonary artery hypertension and SLE. Note the prominence of the pulmonary arteries. The cardiac catheterization identified a pulmonary pressure of 108 mmHg.

Bidimensional-echo. The findings on the 2D-echo are unspecific and only can be used for suspicion of PAH but not confirm the presence of this entity. Most patients with symptomatic PAH present enlarged right-side chambers. In moderate - severe cases as response to pressure overload they may have a reduced right ventricular systolic function accompanied or not by a systolic flattening of the interventricular septum and thickness of the septum wall. The ratio: interventricular septum / posterior left ventricular wall is increased (>1). Usually the systolic global function is preserved excepting in cases with myocardial failure that predicts a poor prognosis.

Color-Doppler Echocardiography

Doppler echocardiography is the best non-invasive method in order to estimate the systolic pulmonary artery pressure (SPAP). Most of the patients with PAH have tricuspid regurgitation. This findings is useful to compute the sPAP using the Bernoulli formula which consist in: multiply 4 (maximum velocity tricuspid regurgitation)^2 + right atrial pressure. Different formulas have been used to calculate the right atrial pressure that ranges usually from 4 to 10 mmHg. As other measures of echocardiography the accuracy of the measurement of pulmonary artery pressure depends importantly of the experience of the personnel who perform the echocardiography. The correlation between Doppler and cardiac catheterization findings of the SPAP is considered as good [108]. There are 3 main advantages of Doppler for PAH: a) Doppler echocardiography the most reliable non-invasive method to measure PAP in patients under suspicion of PAH, b) can be useful for prevalence studies in patients with mild or absent symptomatology, c) seriated measures can be performed in order to measure response to therapy or progression of the disease. A series of studies have been now performed in order to detect PAH in SLE using Doppler echocardiography [92, 94, 95, 104, 109-112]. Interestingly, only few reports have been published about the clinical value of the measurement of PAP by Doppler-echocardiography in order to predict the evolution. Winslow et al, more a decade ago shows that the frequency of patients who develop PAH in SLE increase during the following [94]. Our group reported that patients with SLE with higher values of pulmonary systolic pressure evaluated by Doppler echocardiography develop a high incidence of cardiac failure in the following 3 years of the diagnosis [113]. Recent advances to improve the accuracy of the techniques have been developed these include the development of new ultrasound imaging equipment, use of pulsed-wave tissue Doppler imaging, contrast, tridimensional and intracardiac echocardiography. Particularly, contrast echocardiography is a useful means of enhancing the faint Doppler tricuspid flow signal that is essential for determining PAP.

Right Heart Catheterization

This method provides information about 3 important elements: a) Confirms the presence of elevated pressure with absence of pulmonary venous hypertension, b) can predict survival depending of the severity of PAH, the affectation of the right atrial pressure, and cardiac index, c) finally right heart catheterization can be useful to evaluate the response to treatment. Unfortunately this invasive method may have complications, and mortality has been observed in some patients, also requires be performed in-hospital by trained personnel and is costly. However, continue being the gold standard for the measurement of PAP and should be performed in those patients with an echocardiogram suggestive of moderate – severe PAH.

Advances in the Treatment of Pulmonary Hypertension

Several therapeutic strategies have been evaluated in SLE these strategies include calcium channel blockers, prostanoids, endothelin receptor antagonists, phosphodiesterase type 5 inhibitors, immunosuppressive drugs and combination therapy.

Table 2 synthesizes the strategies employed for the treatment of patients with PAH in SLE.

Table 2. Drug Therapy in Pulmonary Hypertension: Current and potential therapies for pulmonary hypertension in SLE

Group of drugs		
1. Vasodilators		2. Immunosuppressive drugs
Calcium channel antagonists		a) Cyclophosphamide
a) Nifedipine		
Prostacyclin therapy		3. Anticoagulants
a) Intravenous Epoprostenol		a) Warfarin
b) Beraprost		
c) Treprostinil		4. Conventional management
		a) Oxigen therapy
Endothelin Antagonists		b) Inotropic agents
a) Bosentan		c) Diuretics
b) Sitaxsentan		
c) Ambrisentan		
Nitric Oxide		
Phosphodiesterase Inhibitors		
a) Sildenafil		

Calcium Channel Blockers

Vascular tone is regulated by the entry and exit of calcium from the smooth muscle. Calcium channel blockade with calcium antagonists produces vasodilatation by decreasing calcium entry into vascular smooth muscle. Interesting there is no studies evaluating the effects of the new calcium channel blockers in PAH associated with SLE. Nifedipine has been considered as a therapeutic option although this information proceeds from case-series and still further studies are required to evaluate their benefits as concomitant therapy.

Prostanoids

Intravenous epoprostenol was one of the first drugs with substantial efficacy showed in primary PAH, thereafter, other prostanoids were subsequently developed. Other prostanoids include iloprost, and treprostinil. Prostanoids activate the cell surface prostacyclin receptors producing vasodilation. Some of the effects of prostanoids may be mediated by activation of the peroxisome proliferator-activated receptor 3, producing antiremodeling effects [114]. In SLE with PAH) only some case-series and case-reports have been described In one of these series 6 patients with moderate-severe PAH associated with SLE, the utilization of epoprestenol was associated with a decrement of both mean pulmonary artery pressure and pulmonary vascular resistance in 4 patients with an associated improvement in the New York Heart Association functional class, suggesting that this therapy can be effective in PAH secondary to SLE, although the lack of comparative studies is an important limitation in the understanding of the efficacy of the drug for these patients. Iloprost has been also only evaluated in case-reports of patients with SLE and PAH. Controlled studies with these drugs are required to demonstrate its efficacy for these patients and a careful examination of their side-effects and long- term results should be performed before to establish a conclusion of the benefits of these therapies.

Endothelin Receptor Antagonists

Bosentan is an endothelin A/B receptor antagonist. Several studies have showed clinical efficacy of bosentan in patients with primary PAH or associated with connective tissue disease [115, 116]. Recently, it has been developed ambrisentan an oral endothelin A receptor-selective antagonist. This drug has been evaluated in a randomized, placebo-controlled trial made in patients with primary PAH. Showing an improvement in exercise capacity, WHO functional class, 6-min walk distance, and hemodynamic parameters [117]. Sitaxsentan, is another selective endothelin A receptor antagonist showing benefits in patients with PAH [118]. There is no information currently available about whether a selective endothelin A receptor antagonists offer or not advantages over a nonselective endothelin A/B antagonists in patients with PAH, and data from comparative studies with both drugs are still lacking.

Phosphodiesterase Type 5 (PDE5) Inhibitors

There is currently a relevant interest about the efficacy of Sildenafil in the treatment of PAH [119]. Sildenafil has effects as vasodilator but also has antiproliferative actions on pulmonary vascular smooth muscle cells by reducing cell proliferation and inducing apoptosis [120]. In a randomized trial different doses of sildenafil (20, 40, or 80 mg three times daily) were compared with placebo showing significant improvement in 6-min walk distance, functional class and hemodynamic parameters [119]. The final results of the study showed non-significant differences in efficacy between doses, therefore, currently the recommended doses for treatment of PAH is 20 mg three times daily. In an outstanding paper Wilkins published the first double-blind study comparing bosentan versus sildenafil in patients with PAH including both the idiopathic form and the associated with connective tissue disease [121]. Although, their results showed no significant differences between both groups, there was a trend in higher improvement for the 6-min walk distances, plasma brain natriuretic peptide levels, and right ventricular muscle mass determined by magnetic resonance imaging in favor of sildenafil. Further controlled trials comparing both drugs are required to support the reliability of these findings.

Immunosuppressive Drugs

There is a lack of information from controlled studies using immunosuppressive drugs for the treatment of pulmonary hypertension in SLE. Most of the information proceed from case-series or not controlled trials. Our group reported the results of monthly administered intravenous cyclophosphamide versus oral enalapril and standard care measures in patients with pulmonary hypertension [95]. A significant improvement in functional class and a decrement in the pulmonary pressure (measured by Doppler echocardiography) were observed for patients in the arm of cyclophosphamide compared with enalapril. According to our results when the pulmonary systolic pressure is $\geq$ 35 mm Hg only 2 patients are required to be treated for obtaining an additional improvement over enalapril. Additional studies with immunosuppressive drugs are required including a comparison head to head with phosphodiesterase type 5 inhibitors or endothelin antagonists to determine the role of immunosuppressive drugs in PAH associated with SLE. Also is currently ignored if these immunosuppressive drugs are useful to increase the response when combined with bosentan or sildenafil. To date, the utilization of immunosuppressive drugs constitutes a strategy that should be considered in patients with moderate or severe pulmonary hypertension in SLE. Table 2 shows a summary of the drugs used for PAH.

Combination Therapy

There is considered that combination therapy of PAH with prostanoids, endothelin receptor antagonists, and PDE5 inhibitors will be an effective strategy for PAH when solid evidence will become available. Unfortunately, most of the current evidence of the effectiveness of combination therapy comes from uncontrolled studies and case-series. A recent study was unable to show significant differences with the combination of inhaled iloprost plus bosentan versus monotherapy [122]. The combination of bosentan and sildenafil seems to be a reasonable option in those patients without a satisfactory response with monotherapy and randomized controlled trials are required to evaluate their efficacy as first therapeutic option in patients with severe PAH.

OTHER FORMS OF CARDIAC INVOLVEMENT

Left Ventricular Diastolic Dysfunction

The cardiac cycle encompasses systole and diastole. The systolic function reflects the ability of the ventricle to contract and eject the blood to the pulmonary or systemic circulation. Instead, diastolic function reflects the ability of the ventricle to relax and fill. Diastolic dysfunction constitutes a disturbance in ventricular relaxation, distensibility or filling [123].

Diastolic dysfunction can be asymptomatic or be accompanied of symptoms or heart failure. Also patients with diastolic dysfunction can have associated or not impairment in the ejection fraction. When the patients have a preserved ejection fraction but symptoms such as dyspnea associate with efforts, venous congestion, oedema and the finding of diastolic dysfunction these patients are classified as having a diastolic heart failure. Diastolic function also depends of numerous interrelated contributing factors: including heart rate, loading conditions and contractility.

Doppler echocardiography is a noninvasive technique that provides the means to assess specific abnormalities of diastolic function. A series of indices have been provided to assess diastolic function by Doppler echocardiography. The most usually used are the mitral inflow velocities. The E wave corresponds to early flow during left ventricle relaxation whereas the A wave corresponds to the wave originated by the late ventricle filling following the atrial contraction. Under normal conditions E wave exceeds A wave velocity. In case of impaired relaxation, A wave velocity can exceeds the E wave velocity given an abnormal relation E:A, and a prolonged deceleration of the E wave. However, when the left ventricular diastolic pressure is highly increased, the contribution of the atrial contraction to the ventricular filling decrease being E wave predominant but with a rapid deceleration. These abnormalities in the contraction lead to a restrictive pattern with high E wave velocity, and an abnormal increment in the E:A relation.

Diastolic Dysfunction in SLE

Diastolic dysfunction is highly prevalent in patient with SLE. Our group has found a prevalence of diastolic dysfunction of 63% of 97 patients studied. This diastolic dysfunction was not associated with age, disease duration, disease activity or anticardiolipin antibodies [124].

In a recent report, patients with SLE and primary antiphospholipid syndrome were evaluated using Doppler echocardiography [125]. Patients with antiphospholipid syndrome primary or associated with SLE have impairment in the diastolic function compared with SLE without antiphospholipid syndrome.

Currently, there are no studies to assess the incidence and consequences of diastolic heart failure in SLE. Criteria for the diagnostic of diastolic heart failure have been proposed by the European Society of Cardiology. These are the presence of signs and symptoms of congestive heart failure, normal or mild abnormality of left ventricular systolic function and evidence of abnormal left ventricular relaxation, filling, diastolic distensibility or diastolic stiffness [126].To date there is no controlled trials to evaluate the treatment the diastolic heart failure in SLE. The objectives of the treatment for diastolic heart failure for any patient include the improvement of hemodynamic conditions, improving preload and afterload therefore, therapeutic strategies should be directed to these targets [127]. Angiotensin converting enzyme (ACE) inhibitors and angiotensin inhibitors have a beneficial because they reduce both preload and afterload, induce regression of left ventricular hypertrophy and decrease of myocardial interstitial fibrosis. Alderosterone antagonists including spironolactone and canrenone also decrease the myocardial fibrosis. B-blockers and calcium antagonists such as verapamile are useful to reduce tachycardia improving the diastolic filling.

Current recommendations for the treatment of patients with diastolic heart failure of any etiology are presented in the table 3.

Table 3. Current recommendations for the treatment of diastolic heart failure of any etiology

Drugs
Diuretics: furosemide, clortalidone, spironolactone
Long acting nitrates
ß adrenergic blockers (atenolol, carvedilol, nebivolol)
Calcium channel blockers: verapamile,
ECA-inhibitors (perindopril, rampiril)
Angiotensin II receptor blockers (irbesartan, candersartan)
Aldosterone antagonists (spironolactone)

THROMBOSIS AND AUTOANTIBODIES

Occurrence of thrombotic phenomenon in SLE patients has been recognized, as well as its close relationship with autoantibodies, mainly those so called antiphospholipid (aPL), that mainly encompass but not restricted to, anticardiolipin antibodies (aCL), anti-β2GPI antibodies, and the lupus anticoagulant. However, aCL remains an ancillary stone for the routine evaluation of SLE patients regarding serum antiphospholipid reactivity, and of interest is that several cardiovascular manifestations associates with aCL positive status even in absence of thrombotic phenomenon.

In a concise report [128] an evaluation was performed for the association of mannose-binding lectin gene polymorphisms and cardiac manifestations in SLE patients, founding that although the prevalence of cardiovascular disease in SLE patients carrying MBL-deficient genotypes was 3.3 times higher than in patients with non-deficient genotypes, the association was in fact with the coexistent antiphospholipid syndrome that these patients displayed.

Anti-Lamin B1 Autoantibodies as Major Determinant of Thromboprotection in SLE Patients Displaying Antiphospholipid Antibodies

Autoantibodies to lamins, the major polypeptide components of the nuclear lamina, have been reported in selected sera from patients with autoimmune diseases, including anti-lamin B in systemic lupus erythematosus (SLE) and anti-lamins AC in autoimmune chronic active hepatitis (CAH). In a carefully performed study, Senecal JL et al [129] studied the frequency, specificity, and isotype of autoantibodies to major and minor lamins by immunoblotting on purified rat liver lamins in 190 sera from normal controls (n = 62), rheumatic disease controls (n = 42), and autoimmune disease patients (n = 86). The frequency of anti-lamin in normal controls was 85.5%, and ranged from 77 to 100% in the other groups. In particular, anti-lamin B was not more common in SLE than in normal sera. Anti-lamin isotype were IgG and/or IgM. The highest end point titers (greater than or equal to 1:3200) were observed with chronic autoimmune hepatitis (CAH), SLE, and rheumatoid arthritis (RA) sera with IgG anti-lamins AC, B, or ABC, or with IgM anti-lamins ABC. None of these SLE and RA patients had evidence of liver disease. Reactivity with minor lamins was more frequent in CAH. They conclude from those initial works that anti-lamin autoantibodies were present in sera from most individuals and that the highest titers are found in sera from patients with autoimmune diseases and probably those patients displaying a highest titer anti-lamin antibodies could represent a special subgroup. However, the non-specificity of these western-blot detected anti-lamin antibodies was evident, and this notion was enforced by the findings of other groups [130] that identified this non-specific IgG isotype anti-lamin reactivity using immunofluorescence and western-blot techniques in sera of 60 patients with chronic fatigue syndrome. These authors speculate that occurrence of autoantibodies to a conserved intracellular protein like lamin B1 provides new laboratory evidence for an autoimmune component in chronic fatigue syndrome, however, the anti-lamin reactivity in these patients was at low titers, and it was already known that clinically healthy subjects could display this reactivity.

Research on aLB1 reached an important advance once an specific solid-phase enzyme-linked immunoassay using recombinant human LB1 was developed [131], solving the discrimination step between unspecific low-titer reactivity and the High Titers aLB1, as evidenced in the work by Senécal et al [131] determining the frequency and clinical significance of high titers of IgG autoantibodies to nuclear lamin B1 in a large number of unselected and well-characterized systemic lupus erythematosus (SLE) patients, disease controls, and normal healthy controls.

Antibodies anti lamin B 1(aLB1) and Frequency of Thrombotic Events

In this cross-sectional study [131], detection of anti-lamin B1 autoantibodies with the new immunoassay was performed on serum samples obtained at first evaluation of 238 consecutive French Canadian adults: 61 healthy control subjects, 20 patients with osteoarthritis, 22 with ankylosing spondylitis, 11 with autoimmune hepatitis, 30 with rheumatoid arthritis, and 94 with SLE. SLE patients were studied for 57 disease manifestations. A case-control study was performed to analyze the relationship between anti-lamin B1 status and thrombotic manifestations between SLE onset and last follow-up. High titers of anti-lamin B1 were strikingly restricted to a subset of 8 SLE patients (8.5%). The mean anti-lamin B1 titer was higher in this subset than in the other SLE patients or any control group ($P<0.001$). By univariate analysis and stepwise multiple logistic regression, the most striking association of anti-lamin B1 was with lupus anticoagulant (LAC) antibodies ($P = 0.00001$). Although LAC were significantly associated with thrombosis in SLE patients, anti-lamin B1 was not. The frequency of thrombosis in SLE patients expressing both LAC and anti-lamin B1 was similar to that in patients without LAC ($P = 1.0$). However, patients expressing LAC without anti-lamin B1 had a greater frequency of thrombosis ($p = 0.018$). High titers of IgG anti-lamin B1 autoantibodies are highly specific for a subset of SLE patients whose clinical characteristics include the presence of LAC and other laboratory manifestations of the antiphospholipid syndrome. The presence of LAC without anti-lamin B1 may define a subset of SLE patients at greater risk for thrombosis.

aLB1 and Thromboprotection

The fore mentioned findings introduced the concept that the expression of clinical features associated to antiphospholipid antibodies may be co-modulated, at least from the statistical approach. This hypothesis was of clinical relevance, because if confirmed, a new clinical subset of patients displaying antiphospholipid antibodies may arise, and with the presence of High-Titer aLB1 been the major determinant for thromboprotection.

The same group of researchers performed a cross-sectional study using serum samples obtained at first evaluation of 259 English Canadian and French Canadian patients from SLE registries at 3 hospitals [132] in order to demonstrate the association between autoantibodies to nuclear lamin B1 (aLB1) and protection against thrombosis ("thromboprotection") in patients with SLE, and to elucidate the mechanism by which aLB1 cause thromboprotection in vivo. Since a number of autoantigens in SLE have been localized specifically to the external surface of apoptotic blebs, it was hypothesized that circulating aLB1 may block the procoagulant effect of apoptotic blebs by binding to LB1 displayed at the external bleb surface. In a subanalysis restricted to lupus patients the relationship between aLB1 and lupus anticoagulant (LAC) status with thrombotic manifestations between onset of disease and last follow-up were evaluated. Reactivity of aLB1 with Jurkat or endothelial cells, which had been induced to undergo apoptosis, was determined by indirect immunofluorescence. Localization of LB1 in apoptotic cells and blebs was analyzed by con focal microscopy and surface labeling of cell membrane proteins. High-titer aLB1 was restricted to a subset of SLE patients (46 patients), with an overall frequency of 17.8% (range 11.6-24.3% in the 3 centers). LB1 antibodies were significantly associated with LAC but not with antibodies to cardiolipin (aCL) or beta(2)-glycoprotein I (anti-beta(2)GPI). The frequency of thrombosis differed markedly depending on aLB1 and LAC status, as follows: presence of LAC and absence of aLB1 50%, presence of both LAC and aLB1 22.7%, absence of both LAC and aLB1 25.5%, absence of LAC and presence of aLB1, 20.8%. Further subclassification of patients based on aCL and anti-beta(2)GPI status revealed that, in the presence of LAC but in the absence of aCL, anti-beta(2)GPI, and aLB1, the frequency of thrombosis was 40%, whereas in the presence of aLB1, it decreased strikingly, to 9.1%. LB1 was found to be translocated into surface membrane blebs during apoptosis and to be entirely enclosed within the apoptotic bleb plasma membrane of Jurkat and endothelial cells. The presence of aLB1 in SLE patients with LAC essentially nullifies the strong prothrombotic risk associated with LAC. Hence, aLB1 is associated with thromboprotection. Reactivity of aLB1 with apoptotic blebs does not seem to play a direct role in mediating this protection, since LB1 is buried within apoptotic blebs and inaccessible to circulating aLB1. The mechanism by which aLB1 confers thromboprotection in SLE remains to be elucidated.

Relationship between thrombophilia and cardiac manifestations in SLE are mainly restricted to those involving intracardiac thrombus formation whether as free thrombus or those aggregated over a cardiac structural abnormality.

Autoantibodies and Cardiac Involvement

Patients with SLE may display cardiac manifestations, and, in fact, several autoantibodies can mediate cardiac damage: this is the case with antiphospholipid antibodies (aPL), anti-Ro/SS-A antibodies, anti-endothelial cells antibodies, and so on [133].

Autoantibodies can directly affect heart tissue or, alternatively, can trigger mechanisms able to cause heart damage. For instance, aPL can contribute to cardiac damage enhancing atherosclerosis phenomena, causing thrombosis of coronary arteries or starting an immune complexes mediated reaction and deposition at the valves level.

The consequence of autoantibodies damage have been reported in several heart structures, such as valves, myocardium, pericardium, conduction tissue and cardiac arteries, in patients suffering from systemic lupus erythematosus (SLE), antiphospholipid syndrome (APS), Sjögrens syndrome and other connective tissue diseases.

VALVULAR ABNORMALITIES

Anatomical and functional valvular abnormalities have been described in SLE. Libman.Sacks endocarditis, also termed "atypical verrucous endocarditis", is the most characteristic lesion [134]. In a recent study [135] a frequency of 1.5% for aortic valve calcification in 199 SLE studied patients was described. Anatomical lesions were observed in 15 – 75% in necroscopy studies (136), in 40 – 50% of cases with the transthoracic echocardiography (TTE) and in 50 – 60% with transesophageal echocardiography (TEE) [137]. Therefore, TEE is more sensitive than TTE in revealing valve abnormalities.

Anatomical abnormalities are generally found in the mitral and aortic valves [137]. Histological studies have shown two types of verrucae: 1) active lesions which consists of fibrin clumps, focal necrosis and mononuclear cells infiltrates, more frequently observed in young patients with recent disease onset which rarely lead to a hemodynamically significant valvular lesion; and 2) healed lesions characterized by vascularised fibrous tissue sometimes associated with calcifications [17] found in patients with long-standing disease and with long-term corticosteroids use and frequently associated with functional valve abnormalities, especially valvular insufficiency. An association between valvular abnormalities and antiphospholipid antibodies (aPL) has also been reported, [138] but this association remains a matter of controversy. In a recent study [104], 200 SLE patients were studied to evaluate the association of aPL with cardiovascular manifestations of SLE. Antiphospholipid antibodies were present (defined as IgG or IgM anticardiolipin >40 IU/ml or the presence of lupus anticoagulant) in 42 patients (21%), mitral valve nodules and moderate-to-severe mitral regurgitation were more common in aPL-positive patients (both 14.3% versus 4.4%; P <0.02). Thirty-one percent of patients with high titers of IgG aPL (>80 IU/ml) had mitral valve nodules, compared with 20% of patients with mildly to moderately elevated levels of IgG aPL (16–80 IU/ml) and 4% of patients without IgG aPL (overall P < 0.001). Levels of soluble tumor necrosis factor receptors were higher in the presence of both aPL and mitral valve nodules. LV dimensions, systolic function, and carotid artery stiffness as well as prevalences of Raynaud's phenomenon, pulmonary hypertension, and atherosclerosis were similar in aPL-positive and aPL-negative patients. It is clear from this large cohort, that SLE patients with aPL (particularly IgG aCL) are more likely to have mitral valve lesions and consequent significant mitral regurgitation. The association of both aPL and soluble TNF receptors with mitral nodules suggests a possible pathogenic link between those antibodies, endothelial cell activation, and inflammation in the development of these lesions. In this population, aPL are not associated with abnormalities in myocardial or large artery structure and function, preclinical or clinical atherosclerosis, or other vascular manifestations such as Raynaud's phenomenon, pulmonary hypertension, or systemic hipertensión.

Several aspects of pathogenetic hypotheses involving potential association between valvular abnormalities and antiphospholipid antibodies are reviewed in a recent works by different groups [2, 133], contributing to understand the development of valvular abnormalities in SLE patients: 1) aPL and anti-endothelial antibodies bind to and activate endothelial cells, leading to platelet aggregation with thrombus formation; and 2) deposition of immunocomplexes between the endothelium and the basal membrane, leading to an infiltration of inflammatory cells.

In a work by other group verrucous endocarditis is generally asymptomatic and only occasionally leads to a cardiac murmur. In fact, the verrucae are near the edge of the valves and therefore tend not to deform the closing line, even when they are very large and protrude into the cardiac chambers. Complications due to verrucous endocarditis are rare, although embolic events can occur. Lesions are hemodynamically significant in only 3–4% of SLE patients, requiring surgical treatment in half of them. Infectious endocarditis was observed in 7% of patients with valvular disease, and stroke or peripheral embolism in 13%. Rupture of chordae tendinae was rarely observed. The risk of endocarditis is increased by dental surgical treatments. Appropriate antibiotic prophylaxis should be considered in all SLE patients with valvular abnormalities, especially if they are taking immunosuppressive drugs. Jensen-Urstad et al [139] recently reported a close association between valvular abnormalities and cardiovascular disease (CVD) as well as raised levels of homocysteine and triglycerides in SLE patients. Therefore, patients with valvular disease should be screened for clinical and subclinical atherosclerotic features.

Since Libman–Sacks endocarditis is clinically silent in the majority of cases, generally it is not treated. When it is found in an early active stage, corticosteroids (prednisone 1 mg/kg/day) are recommended, especially if antiphospholipid antibodies and lupus anticoagulant are negative. It has been reported that valvular abnormalities frequently resolved over time. When endocarditis is detected at a later stage during the course of the disease, careful clinical surveillance is necessary and, if the lesion becomes hemodynamically significant, valve surgery is needed.It is necessary to carefully evaluate the type of surgical treatment: valve repair, replacement with mechanical valve or bioprosthetic porcine graft. Anatomic valve repair does not need anticoagulation but often leads to repeated surgery and later valve replacement. Bioprosthetic porcine valves have also been hindered by complications such as valvulitis relapse. Therefore, mechanical valve replacement seems to be the best choice in lupus patients.

Rhythm and Conduction Tissue Abnormalities

Several reviews included these issues in their scope [2, 133]. Sinus tachycardia is the most frequent rhythm abnormality and is quite common in SLE patients. Atrioventricular block and bundle branch block are also observed. However, they are rare in adults and occur in only 2% of children born from mothers with anti-Ro/SSA antibodies. Rhythm and conduction abnormalities are mostly asymptomatic or may lead to some mild complaints such as palpitation or fatigue. In some cases syncope may occur. Sinus tachycardia can be due to fever, anaemia or cardiac abnormalities including pericarditis and myocarditis. Conduction defects can also be the result of antimalarial use. In SLE patients with rhythm and conduction abnormalities, electrolyte balance and thyroid hormonal status should be investigated. The treatment is based on the use of common antiarrhythmic drugs and in the most severe cases the implant of a pacemaker is necessary.

Heart Conduction Tissue and Anti-Ro/SSA Antibodies

The mothers of children born with complete heart block (CHB) are generally positive for autoantibodies, namely anti-SSA/Ro and anti-SSB/La.32. This observation is consistent with the assumption that maternal autoantibodies could affect the heart conduction tissue of the newborn.

The transplacental transfer of maternal IgG autoantibodies seems to play a major role in the pathogenic mechanism of CHB, although some questions are still debated. The facts in favour of the direct pathogenic role of anti-SSA/Ro and anti-SSB/La autoantibodies in CHB are: 1) the presence of maternal autoantibodies in fetal/neonatal circulation; 2) the elution of anti-SSA/ Ro antibodies from cardiac tissues of affected fetuses; 3) the complete AV block in pups of mice passively injected with anti-SSA/Ro 52 antibodies; and 4) the fact that anti-SSA/Ro IgG inhibits, in vitro, L-type CA2þ channel in rat and rabbit heart. On the other hand, against the role of Ro and LA antibodies in CHB is that: 1) CHB is exceptionally rare in adults with these antibodies; 2) there is a discordance of CHB in twins; and 3) there are few babies of Ro/La mothers affected by CHB.

Electrocardiographic abnormalities other than those found in CHB, have been reported in association with anti-SSA/Ro antibodies, such as bradycardia, atrioventricular (A-V) blocks of various degrees and prolongation of the QT interval. The abnormalities much closer to a direct involvement of the cardiac conduction tissue are the incomplete A-V blocks and QT prolongation. The QT interval prolongation was found to be transient, in fact it normalizes within the first year of life when maternal anti Ro/SSA antibodies disappear from neonatal circulation. In contrast with these findings, a recent case control study, comparing the electrocardiographic features of children born to anti-Ro/SSA positive and negative mothers all affected by connective tissue diseases, does not find any significant difference, showing that some interpretation problem is not yet solved. In a recent work [140], an evaluation of the QT dispersion in SLE patients without overt cardiac involvement was performed, founding that QT dispersion is significantly increased in this patients but without no correlation between QT dispersion and duration of SLE, SLEDAI-K score, corticosteroid usage, and presence of anti-SS-A antibody. More work is needed to identify if this prolonged QT dispersion can be a useful noninvasive method for early detection of cardiac involvement in SLE patients.

CONCLUSION

In summary cardiovascular disease in systemic lupus represents a very exciting area for future research being necessary to increase the number of long-term prospective cohorts and well-designed controlled trials in order to improve the clinical care of the patients with this involvement. Controlled studies evaluating the effect of modification of risk factors for atherosclerosis and other cardiovascular complications on the morbidity and mortality of the patients with SLE are still required. An adequate assessment of patients with SLE should be taken into account these risk factors in order to modify the prognosis of the patients. Also an early detection with the non-invasive methods of cardiac complications can lead to develop new strategies for the treatment. Application of new drugs and newer indications for the use of old drugs should be evaluated in controlled trials and prospective cohorts with the objective of decrease the morbidity and mortality of the patients with these complications.

Acknowledgment

The authors of this chapter thank to Dr. María Rosa Flores-Márquez, Dr. Gonzalo Vazquez-Camacho, and Dr. Jose Manuel Ornelas-Aguirre from the department of pathology in the Centro Medico Nacional de Occidente IMSS Guadalajara Mexico by the histological images for this chapter. Authors also thank Dr. Julia Dolores Sanchez-Hernandez and Dr. Alberto Muñoz-Rocha by their valuable suggestions for the pathogenesis of atherosclerosis.

References

[1] Ornelas-Aguirre JM, Vázquez-Camacho G, Velázquez-García C, González-Lopez L, García-González A, Gamez-Nava JI [Cardiac disease in Systemic Lupus Erythematosus: A retrospective study in autopsies] *Rev. Mex. Reumat.* 2001; 16: 315-321.

[2] Doria A, Iaccarino L, Sarzi-Puttini P, Atzeni F, Turriel M, Petri M. Cardiac involvement in systemic lupus erythematosus. *Lupus*. 2005;14:683-6.

[3] Man BL, Mok CC. Serositis related to systemic lupus erythematosus: prevalence and outcome. *Lupus*. 2005;14:822-6.

[4] Little WC, Freeman GL. Pericardial disease. *Circulation*. 2006;113:1622-32.

[5] Law WG, Thong BY, Lian TY, Kong KO, Chng HH. Acute lupus myocarditis: clinical features and outcome of an oriental case series. *Lupus*. 2005;14:827-31.

[6] Magnani JW, Dec GW. Myocarditis: current trends in diagnosis and treatment. *Circulation*. 2006;113:876-90.

[7] Pinamonti B, Alberti E, Cigalotto A, Dreas L, Salvi A, Silvestri F, Camerini F. Echocardiographic findings in myocarditis. *J. Cardiol.* 1988;62:285-91.

[8] Narula J, Khaw BA, Dec GW, Palacios IF, Newell JB, Southern JF, Fallon JT, Strauss HW, Haber E, Yasuda T. Diagnostic accuracy of antimyosin scintigraphy in suspected myocarditis. *J. Nucl. Cardiol.* 1996;3:371-81.

[9] Laissy JP, Messin B, Varenne O, Iung B, Karila-Cohen D, Schouman-Claeys E, Steg PG. MRI of acute myocarditis: a comprehensive approach based on various imaging sequences. *Chest*. 2002;122:1638-48.

[10] Laissy JP, Hyafil F, Feldman LJ, Juliard JM, Schouman-Claeys E, Steg PG, Faraggi M. Differentiating acute myocardial infarction from myocarditis: diagnostic value of early- and delayed-perfusion cardiac MR imaging. *Radiology*. 2005;237:75-82.

[11] Singh JA, Woodard PK, Davila-Roman VG, Waggoner AD, Gutierrez FR, Zheng J, Eisen SA. Cardiac magnetic resonance imaging abnormalities in systemic lupus erythematosus: a preliminary report. *Lupus*. 2005;14:137-44.

[12] Wu LA, Lapeyre AC 3rd, Cooper LT. Current role of endomyocardial biopsy in the management of dilated cardiomyopathy and myocarditis. *Mayo Clin. Proc.* 2001;76:1030-8.

[13] Sakaguchi Y, Nakamura Y, Sutani T, Tsuchihashi M, Yamano S, Hashimoto T, Dohi K, Hiasa Y, Kawai S, Okada R. Immunohistochemical study of the endomyocardial biopsy of systemic lupus erythematosus. *J. Cardiol.* 1995;25:181-8.

[14] Feldman AM, McNamara D. Myocarditis. *N. Engl. J. Med.* 2000;343:1388-98.

[15] Thiagarajan P. Atherosclerosis, autoimmunity, and systemic lupus erythematosus. *Circulation*. 2001;104:1876-7.

[16] Kao AH, Sabatine JM, Manzi S. Update on vascular disease in systemic lupus erythematosus. *Curr. Opin. Rheumatol.* 2003;15:519-27.

[17] Bulkley BH, Roberts WC. The heart in systemic lupus erythematosus and the changes induced in it by corticosteroid therapy. A study of 36 necropsy patients. *Am. J. Med.* 1975;58:243-64.

[18] Urowitz MB, Bookman AA, Koehler BE, Gordon DA, Smythe HA, Ogryzlo MA. The bimodal mortality pattern of systemic lupus erythematosus. *Am. J. Med.* 1976;60:221-5.

[19] Bruce IN, Gladman DD, Urowitz MB. Premature atherosclerosis in systemic lupus erythematosus. *Rheum. Dis. Clin. North Am.* 2000;26:257-78.

[20] Al-Herz A, Ensworth S, Shojania K, Esdaile JM. Cardiovascular risk factor screening in systemic lupus erythematosus. *J. Rheumatol.* 2003;30:493-6.

[21] Wajed J, Ahmad Y, Durrington PN, Bruce IN. Prevention of cardiovascular disease in systemic lupus erythematosus—proposed guidelines for risk factor management. *Rheumatology* (Oxford). 2004;43:7-12.

[22] Frostegard J. Atherosclerosis in patients with autoimmune disorders. *Arterioscler Thromb. Vasc. Biol.* 2005;25:1776-85.

[23] Svenungsson E, Gunnarsson I, Fei GZ, Lundberg IE, Klareskog L, Frostegard J. Elevated triglycerides and low levels of high-density lipoprotein as markers of disease activity in association with up-regulation of the tumor necrosis factor alpha/tumor necrosis factor receptor system in systemic lupus erythematosus. *Arthritis Rheum.* 2003;48:2533-40.

[24] Reichlin M, Fesmire J, Quintero-Del-Rio AI, Wolfson-Reichlin M. Autoantibodies to lipoprotein lipase and dyslipidemia in systemic lupus erythematosus. *Arthritis Rheum.* 2002;46:2957-63.

[25] Cervera R, Khamashta MA, Font J, Sebastiani GD, Gil A, Lavilla P, Mejia JC, Aydintug AO, Chwalinska-Sadowska H, de Ramon E, Fernandez-Nebro A, Galeazzi M, Valen M, Mathieu A, Houssiau F, Caro N, Alba P, Ramos-Casals M, Ingelmo M, Hughes GR; European Working Party on Systemic Lupus Erythematosus. Morbidity and mortality in systemic lupus erythematosus during a 10-year period: a comparison of early and late manifestations in a cohort of 1,000 patients. *Medicine* (Baltimore). 2003;82:299-308.

[26] Bessant R, Duncan R, Ambler G, Swanton J, Isenberg DA, Gordon C, Rahman A. Prevalence of conventional and lupus-specific risk factors for cardiovascular disease

in patients with systemic lupus erythematosus: A case-control study. *Arthritis Rheum.* 2006;55:892-9.

[27] Steffel J, Luscher TF, Tanner FC. Tissue factor in cardiovascular diseases: molecular mechanisms and clinical implications. *Circulation.* 2006;113:722-31).

[28] Perlstein TS, Lee RT. Smoking, metalloproteinases, and vascular disease. *Arterioscler Thromb. Vasc. Biol.* 2006;26:250-6.

[29] Urowitz MB, Ibanez D, Gladman DD. Atherosclerotic vascular events in a single large lupus cohort: prevalence and risk factors. *J. Rheumatol.* 2007;34:70-5.

[30] Toloza SM, Uribe AG, McGwin G Jr, Alarcon GS, Fessler BJ, Bastian HM, Vila LM, Wu R, Shoenfeld Y, Roseman JM, Reveille JD; LUMINA Study Group. Systemic lupus erythematosus in a multiethnic US cohort (LUMINA). XXIII. Baseline predictors of vascular events. *Arthritis Rheum.* 2004;50:3947-57.

[31] Petri M, Roubenoff R, Dallal GE, Nadeau MR, Selhub J, Rosenberg IH. Plasma homocysteine as a risk factor for atherothrombotic events in systemic lupus erythematosus. *Lancet.* 1996;348:1120-4.

[32] Refai TM, Al-Salem IH, Nkansa-Dwamena D, Al-Salem MH. Hyperhomocysteinaemia and risk of thrombosis in systemic lupus erythematosus patients. *Clin. Rheumatol.* 2002;21:457-61.

[33] Bruce IN, Urowitz MB, Gladman DD, Ibanez D, Steiner G. Risk factors for coronary heart disease in women with systemic lupus erythematosus: the Toronto Risk Factor Study. *Arthritis Rheum.* 2003;48:3159-67.

[34] Martinez-Berriotxoa A, Ruiz-Irastorza G, Egurbide MV, Rueda M, Aguirre C. Homocysteine, antiphospholipid antibodies and risk of thrombosis in patients with systemic lupus erythematosus. *Lupus.* 2004;13:927-33.

[35] MacGregor AJ, Dhillon VB, Binder A et al. Fasting lipids and anticardiolipin antibodies as risk factors for vascular disease in systemic lupus erythematosus. *Ann. Rheum. Dis.* 1992;51:152–5.

[36] Bruce IN, Urowitz MB, Gladman DD, Hallett DC. Natural history of hypercholesterolemia in systemic lupus erythematosus. *J. Rheumatol.* 1999;26:2137–43.

[37] Roman MJ, Shanker BA, Davis A et al. Prevalence and correlates of accelerated atherosclerosis in systemic lupus erythematosus. *N. Engl. J. Med.* 2003;349:2399–406.

[38] Liuzzo G, Goronzy JJ, Yang H et al. Monoclonal T-cell proliferation and plaque instability in acute coronary syndromes. *Circulation.* 2000;101:2883–8.

[39] Hansson GK, Libby P, Schonbeck U, Yan ZQ. Innate and adaptive immunity in the pathogenesis of atherosclerosis. *Circ. Res.* 2002; 91281–91.

[40] Maksimowicz-McKinnon K, Bhatt DL, Calabrese LH. Recent advances in vascular inflammation: C-reactive protein and other inflammatory biomarkers. *Curr. Opin. Rheumatol.* 2004;16:18-24.

[41] Hansson GK. Immune mechanisms in atherosclerosis. *Arterioscler. Thromb. Vasc. Biol.* 2001;21:1876-90.

[42] Svenungsson E, Fei GZ, Jensen-Urstad K, de Faire U, Hamsten A, Frostegard J. TNF-alpha: a link between hypertriglyceridaemia and inflammation in SLE patients with cardiovascular disease. *Lupus.* 2003;12:454-61.

[43] van Leuven SI, Kastelein JJ, D'Cruz DP, Hughes GR, Stroes ES. Atherogenesis in rheumatology. *Lupus*. 2006;15:117-21.

[44] Chisolm GM, Steinberg D. The oxidative modification hypothesis of atherogenesis: an overview. *Free Radic. Biol. Med.* 2000;28:1815-26.

[45] Chisolm GM 3rd, Chai Y. Regulation of cell growth by oxidized LDL. *Free Radic. Biol. Med.* 2000;28:1697-707.

[46] Matsuura E, Kobayashi K, Hurley BL, Lopez LR. Atherogenic oxidized low-density lipoprotein/beta2-glycoprotein I (oxLDL/beta2GPI) complexes in patients with systemic lupus erythematosus and antiphospholipid syndrome. *Lupus*. 2006;15:478-83.

[47] Matsuura E, Kobayashi K, Tabuchi M, Lopez LR. Oxidative modification of low-density lipoprotein and immune regulation of atherosclerosis. *Prog. Lipid. Res.* 2006;45:466-86.

[48] Vaarala O, Manttari M, Manninen V, Tenkanen L, Puurunen M, Aho K, Palosuo T. Anti-cardiolipin antibodies and risk of myocardial infarction in a prospective cohort of middle-aged men. *Circulation.* 1995;91:23-7.

[49] Erkkila AT, Narvanen O, Lehto S, Uusitupa MI, Yla-Herttuala S. Antibodies against oxidized LDL and cardiolipin and mortality in patients with coronary heart disease. *Atherosclerosis*. 2005;183:157-62.

[50] Akimoto T, Kobayashi S, Tamura N, Ohsawa T, Kawano T, Tanaka M, Hashimoto H. Risk factors for recurrent thrombosis: prospective study of a cohort of Japanese systemic lupus erythematosus. *Angiology*. 2005;56:601-9.

[51] Petri M. The lupus anticoagulant is a risk factor for myocardial infarction (but not atherosclerosis): Hopkins Lupus Cohort. *Thromb. Res*. 2004;114:593-5.

[52] Petri M. Detection of coronary artery disease and the role of traditional risk factors in the Hopkins Lupus Cohort. *Lupus.* 2000;9:170-5.

[53] Toubi E, Shoenfeld Y. Predictive and protective autoimmunity in cardiovascular diseases: is vaccination therapy a reality? *Lupus.* 2005;14:665-9.

[54] Hirono S, Dibrov E, Hurtado C, Kostenuk A, Ducas R, Pierce GN. Chlamydia pneumoniae stimulates proliferation of vascular smooth muscle cells through induction of endogenous heat shock protein 60. *Circ. Res*. 2003;93:710-6.

[55] Mayr M, Metzler B, Kiechl S, Willeit J, Schett G, Xu Q, Wick G. Endothelial cytotoxicity mediated by serum antibodies to heat shock proteins of Escherichia coli and Chlamydia pneumoniae: immune reactions to heat shock proteins as a possible link between infection and atherosclerosis. *Circulation*. 1999;99:1560-6.

[56] Xu Q, Kiechl S, Mayr M, Metzler B, Egger G, Oberhollenzer F, Willeit J, Wick G. Association of serum antibodies to heat-shock protein 65 with carotid atherosclerosis : clinical significance determined in a follow-up study. *Circulation*. 1999;100:1169-74.

[57] Zhu J, Katz RJ, Quyyumi AA, Canos DA, Rott D, Csako G, Zalles-Ganley A, Ogunmakinwa J, Wasserman AG, Epstein SE. Association of serum antibodies to

heat-shock protein 65 with coronary calcification levels: suggestion of pathogen-triggered autoimmunity in early atherosclerosis. *Circulation*. 2004;109:36-41.

[58] Kitumnuaypong T, Scalzi LV, Nalbant S, Von Feldt JM, Schumacher HR Jr. Is there a role for Chlamydia pneumoniae infection in systemic lupus erythematosus and in the associated atherosclerotic cardiovascular disease? *Clin. Exp. Rheumatol.* 2004;22:339-42.

[59] Sarkissian T, Beyene J, Feldman B, McCrindle B, Silverman ED. Longitudinal examination of lipid profiles in pediatric systemic lupus erythematosus. *Arthritis Rheum.* 2007;56:631-8.

[60] Karrar A, Sequeira W, Block JA. Coronary artery disease in systemic lupus erythematosus: A review of the literature. *Semin. Arthritis Rheum*. 2001;30:436-43.

[61] Casscells W, Naghavi M, Willerson JT. Vulnerable atherosclerotic plaque: a multifocal disease. *Circulation*. 2003;107:2072-5.

[62] MacNeill BD, Lowe HC, Takano M, Fuster V, Jang IK. Intravascular modalities for detection of vulnerable plaque: current status. *Arterioscler. Thromb. Vasc. Biol.* 2003;23:1333-42.

[63] Guerci AD, Arad Y. Potential use of Ca++ scanning to determine the need for and intensity of lipid-lowering therapy in asymptomatic adults. *Curr. Cardiol. Rep.* 2001;3:408-15.

[64] Chung CP, Oeser A, Avalos I, Raggi P, Stein CM. Cardiovascular risk scores and the presence of subclinical coronary artery atherosclerosis in women with systemic lupus erythematosus. *Lupus*. 2006;15:562-9.

[65] Von Feldt JM, Scalzi LV, Cucchiara AJ, Morthala S, Kealey C, Flagg SD, Genin A, Van Dyke AL, Nackos E, Chander A, Gehrie E, Cron RQ, Whitehead AS. Homocysteine levels and disease duration independently correlate with coronary artery calcification in patients with systemic lupus erythematosus. *Arthritis Rheum*. 2006;54:2220-7.

[66] Baller D, Notohamiprodjo G, Gleichmann U, Holzinger J, Weise R, Lehmann J. Improvement in coronary flow reserve determined by positron emission tomography after 6 months of cholesterol-lowering therapy in patients with early stages of coronary atherosclerosis. *Circulation*. 1999;99:2871-5.

[67] Greenland P, Abrams J, Aurigemma GP, Bond MG, Clark LT, Criqui MH, Crouse JR 3rd, Friedman L, Fuster V, Herrington DM, Kuller LH, Ridker PM, Roberts WC, Stanford W, Stone N, Swan HJ, Taubert KA, Wexler L. Prevention Conference V: Beyond secondary prevention: identifying the high-risk patient for primary prevention: noninvasive tests of atherosclerotic burden: Writing Group III. *Circulation*. 2000;101:E16-22.

[68] Ahmad Y, Shelmerdine J, Bodill H, Lunt M, Pattrick MG, Teh LS, Bernstein RM, Walker MG, Bruce IN. Subclinical atherosclerosis in systemic lupus erythematosus (SLE): the relative contribution of classic risk factors and the lupus phenotype. *Rheumatology* (Oxford). 2007 Mar 23; [Epub ahead of print] PMID: 17384179.

[69] Sella EM, Sato EI, Leite WA, Oliveira Filho JA, Barbieri A. Myocardial perfusion scintigraphy and coronary disease risk factors in systemic lupus erythematosus. *Ann. Rheum. Dis*. 2003;62:1066-70.

[70] Dimitrow PP. Transthoracic Doppler echocardiography - noninvasive diagnostic window for coronary flow reserve assessment. *Cardiovasc. Ultrasound.* 2003;1:4. PMID: 12740038.

[71] Bruce IN, Gladman DD, Urowitz MB. Detection and modification of risk factors for coronary artery disease in patients with systemic lupus erythematosus: a quality improvement study. *Clin. Exp. Rheumatol.* 1998;16:435-40.

[72] Urowitz MB, Gladman DD, Ibanez D, Berliner Y. Modification of hypertension and hypercholesterolaemia in patients with systemic lupus erythematosus: a quality improvement study. *Ann. Rheum. Dis.* 2006;65:115-7.

[73] Tam LS, Gladman DD, Hallett DC, Rahman P, Urowitz MB. Effect of antimalarial agents on the fasting lipid profile in systemic lupus erythematosus. *J. Rheumatol.* 2000;27:2142-5.

[74] Rahman P, Gladman DD, Urowitz MB, Yuen K, Hallett D, Bruce IN. The cholesterol lowering effect of antimalarial drugs is enhanced in patients with lupus taking corticosteroid drugs. *J. Rheumatol.* 1999;26:325-30.

[75] Petri M. Hydroxychloroquine use in the Baltimore Lupus Cohort: effects on lipids, glucose and thrombosis. *Lupus.* 1996;5 Suppl 1:S16-22.

[76] Sachet JC, Borba EF, Bonfa E, Vinagre CG, Silva VM, Maranhao RC. Chloroquine increases low-density lipoprotein removal from plasma in systemic lupus patients. *Lupus.* 2007;16:273-8.

[77] Borba EF, Bonfa E. Longterm beneficial effect of chloroquine diphosphate on lipoprotein profile in lupus patients with and without steroid therapy. *J. Rheumatol.* 2001;28:780-5.

[78] Albert MA, Danielson E, Rifai N, Ridker PM; PRINCE Investigators. Effect of statin therapy on C-reactive protein levels: the pravastatin inflammation/CRP evaluation (PRINCE): a randomized trial and cohort study. *JAMA.* 2001;286:64-70.

[79] Riboldi P, Gerosa M, Meroni PL. Statins and autoimmune diseases. *Lupus.* 2005;14:765-8.

[80] Jury EC, Ehrenstein MR. Statins: immunomodulators for autoimmune rheumatic disease? *Lupus.* 2005;14:192-6.

[81] Costenbader KH, Karlson EW, Gall V, de Pablo P, Finckh A, Lynch M, Bermas B, Schur PH, Liang MH. Barriers to a trial of atherosclerosis prevention in systemic lupus erythematosus. *Arthritis Rheum.* 2005;53:718-23.

[82] Costenbader KH, Liang MH, Chibnik LB, Aizer J, Kwon H, Gall V, Karlson EW. A pravastatin dose-escalation study in systemic lupus erythematosus. *Rheumatol Int.* 2007 Apr 3; [Epub ahead of print] PMID: 17404733 [PubMed - as supplied by publisher].

[83] Costenbader KH, Brome D, Blanch D, Gall V, Karlson E, Liang MH. Factors determining participation in prevention trials among systemic lupus erythematosus patients: a qualitative study. *Arthritis Rheum.* 2007;57:49-55.

[84] Ridker PM, Cook NR, Lee IM, Gordon D, Gaziano JM, Manson JE, Hennekens CH, Buring JE. A randomized trial of low-dose aspirin in the primary prevention of cardiovascular disease in women. *N. Engl. J. Med.* 2005;352:1293-304.

[85] Kurth T, Glynn RJ, Walker AM, Chan KA, Buring JE, Hennekens CH, Gaziano JM. Inhibition of clinical benefits of aspirin on first myocardial infarction by nonsteroidal antiinflammatory drugs. *Circulation*. 2003;108:1191-5.

[86] Bosch J, Lonn E, Pogue J, Arnold JM, Dagenais GR, Yusuf S; HOPE/HOPE-TOO Study Investigators. Long-term effects of ramipril on cardiovascular events and on diabetes: results of the HOPE study extension. *Circulation*. 2005;112:1339-46.

[87] Yusuf S, Sleight P, Pogue J, Bosch J, Davies R, Dagenais G. Effects of an angiotensin-converting-enzyme inhibitor, ramipril, on cardiovascular events in high-risk patients. The Heart Outcomes Prevention Evaluation Study Investigators. *N. Engl. J. Med.* 2000;342:145-53.

[88] Ward MM. Outcomes of hospitalizations for myocardial infarctions and cerebrovascular accidents in patients with systemic lupus erythematosus. *Arthritis Rheum.* 2004;50:3170-6.

[89] Bruce IN. 'Not only...but also': factors that contribute to accelerated atherosclerosis and premature coronary heart disease in systemic lupus erythematosus. *Rheumatology* (Oxford). 2005;44:1492-502.

[90] Chemla D, Castelain V, Herve P, Lecarpentier Y, Brimioulle S. Haemodynamic evaluation of pulmonary hypertension. *Eur. Respir. J.* 2002;20:1314-31.

[91] Pan TL, Thumboo J, Boey ML. Primary and secondary pulmonary hypertension in systemic lupus erythematosus. *Lupus*. 2000;9:338-42.

[92] Shen JY, Chen SL, Wu YX, Tao RQ, Gu YY, Bao CD, Wang Q. Pulmonary hypertension in systemic lupus erythematosus. *Rheumatol Int.* 1999;18:147-51.

[93] Simonson JS, Schiller NB, Petri M, Hellmann DB. Pulmonary hypertension in systemic lupus erythematosus. *J. Rheumatol.* 1989;16:918-25.

[94] Winslow TM, Ossipov MA, Fazio GP, Simonson JS, Redberg RF, Schiller NB. Five-year follow-up study of the prevalence and progression of pulmonary hypertension in systemic lupus erythematosus. *Am. Heart J.* 1995;129:510-5.

[95] Gonzalez-Lopez L, Cardona-Munoz EG, Celis A, Garcia-de la Torre I, Orozco-Barocio G, Salazar-Paramo M, Garcia-Gonzalez C, Garcia-Gonzalez A, Sanchez-Ortiz A, Trujillo-Hernandez B, Gamez-Nava JI. Therapy with intermittent pulse cyclophosphamide for pulmonary hypertension associated with systemic lupus erythematosus. *Lupus*. 2004;13:105-12.

[96] Rubin LJ. Pulmonary arterial hypertension. *Proc. Am. Thorac. Soc.* 2006;3:111-5.

[97] Hoeper MM, Rubin LJ. Update in pulmonary hypertension 2005. *Am. J. Respir. Crit. Care Med.* 2006;173:499-505.

[98] Cool CD, Groshong SD, Oakey J, Voelkel NF. Pulmonary hypertension: cellular and molecular mechanisms. *Chest.* 2005;128(6 Suppl):565S-571S.

[99] Robak E, Sysa-Jedrzejewska A, Robak T. Vascular endothelial growth factor and its soluble receptors VEGFR-1 and VEGFR-2 in the serum of patients with systemic lupus erythematosus. *Mediators Inflamm*. 2003;12:293-8.

[100] Dorfmuller P, Perros F, Balabanian K, Humbert M. Inflammation in pulmonary arterial hypertension. *Eur. Respir. J.* 2003;22:358-63.

[101] Yoshio T, Masuyama JI, Kohda N, Hirata D, Sato H, Iwamoto M, Mimori A, Takeda A, Minota S, Kano S. Association of interleukin 6 release from endothelial cells and pulmonary hypertension in SLE. *J. Rheumatol.* 1997;24:489-95.

[102] Asherson RA, Cervera R. Review: antiphospholipid antibodies and the lung. *J. Rheumatol.* 1995;22:62-6.

[103] Asherson RA, Higenbottam TW, Dinh Xuan AT, Khamashta MA, Hughes GR. Pulmonary hypertension in a lupus clinic: experience with twenty-four patients. *J. Rheumatol.* 1990;17:1292-8.

[104] Farzaneh-Far A, Roman MJ, Lockshin MD, Devereux RB, Paget SA, Crow MK, Davis A, Sammaritano L, Levine DM, Salmon JE. Relationship of antiphospholipid antibodies to cardiovascular manifestations of systemic lupus erythematosus. *Arthritis Rheum.* 2006;54:3918-25.

[105] Yoshio T, Masuyama J, Sumiya M, Minota S, Kano S. Antiendothelial cell antibodies and their relation to pulmonary hypertension in systemic lupus erythematosus. *J. Rheumatol.* 1994;21:2058-63.

[106] Tamby MC, Chanseaud Y, Humbert M, Fermanian J, Guilpain P, Garcia-de-la-Pena-Lefebvre P, Brunet S, Servettaz A, Weill B, Simonneau G, Guillevin L, Boissier MC, Mouthon L. Anti-endothelial cell antibodies in idiopathic and systemic sclerosis associated pulmonary arterial hypertension. *Thorax.* 2005;60:765-72.

[107] Yoshio T, Masuyama J, Mimori A, Takeda A, Minota S, Kano S. Endothelin-1 release from cultured endothelial cells induced by sera from patients with systemic lupus erythematosus. *Ann. Rheum. Dis.* 1995;54:361-5.

[108] Raeside D, Peacock A. Making measurements in the pulmonary circulation: when and how? *Thorax.* 1997;52:9-11.

[109] Gin PL, Wang WC, Yang SH, Hsiao SH, Tseng JC. Right heart function in systemic lupus erythematosus: insights from myocardial Doppler tissue imaging. *J. Am. Soc. Echocardiogr.* 2006;19:441-9.

[110] Chung SM, Lee CK, Lee EY, Yoo B, Lee SD, Moon HB. Clinical aspects of pulmonary hypertension in patients with systemic lupus erythematosus and in patients with idiopathic pulmonary arterial hypertension. *Clin. Rheumatol.* 2006;25:866-72.

[111] Morelli S, Giordano M, De Marzio P, Priori R, Sgreccia A, Valesini G. Pulmonary arterial hypertension responsive to immunosuppressive therapy in systemic lupus erythematosus. *Lupus.* 1993;2:367-9.

[112] Crozier IG, Li E, Milne MJ, Nicholls MG. Cardiac involvement in systemic lupus erythematosus detected by echocardiography. *Am. J. Cardiol.* 1990;65:1145-8.

[113] Gonzalez-Lopez L, Gamez-Nava JI, Cardona-Muñoz EG, Blanco-Turbay R, Suarez-Almazor ME, Ramos-Remus C. Impact of pulmonary hypertension (PH) on patients with systemic lupus erythematosus (SLE), compared with controls. Results of a 3.5 year prospective cohort. *Arthritis Rheum.* 1997; 40: S106 (abstract).

[114] Ali FY, Egan K, Fitzgerald GA, Desvergne B, Wahli W, Bishop-Bailey D, Warner TD, Mitchell JA. Role of prostacyclin versus peroxisome proliferator-activated receptor βreceptors in prostacyclin sensing by fibroblasts. *Am. J. Respir. Cell Mol. Biol.* 2006;34:242–246.

[115] Rubin LJ, Badesch DB, Barst RJ, Galie N, Black CM, Keogh A, Pulido T, Frost A, Roux S, Leconte I, *et al.* Bosentan therapy for pulmonary arterial hypertension. *N. Engl. J. Med.* 2002;346:896–903.

[116] Channick RN, Simonneau G, Sitbon O, Robbins IM, Frost A, Tapson VF, Badesch DB, Roux S, Rainisio M, Bodin F, *et al.* Effects of the dual endothelin-receptor antagonist bosentan in patients with pulmonary hypertension: a randomised placebo-controlled study. *Lancet* 2001;358:1119–1123.

[117] Galiè N, Badesch D, Oudiz R, Simonneau G, McGoon MD, Keogh AM, Frost AE, Zwicke D, Naeije R, Shapiro S, *et al.* Ambrisentan therapy for pulmonary arterial hypertension. *J. Am. Coll Cardiol.* 2005;46:529–535.

[118] Barst RJ, Langleben D, Frost A, Horn EM, Oudiz R, Shapiro S, McLaughlin V, Hill N, Tapson VF, Robbins IM, *et al.* Sitaxsentan therapy for pulmonary arterial hypertension. *Am. J. Respir. Crit Care Med.* 2004;169:441–447.

[119] Galiè N, Ghofrani HA, Torbicki A, Barst RJ, Rubin LJ, Badesch D, Fleming T, Parpia T, Burgess G, Branzi A, *et al.* Sildenafil citrate therapy for pulmonary arterial hypertension. *N. Engl. J. Med.* 2005;353:2148–2157.

[120] Wharton J, Strange JW, Moller GM, Growcott EJ, Ren X, Franklyn AP, Phillips SC, Wilkins MR. Antiproliferative effects of phosphodiesterase type 5 inhibition in human pulmonary artery cells. *Am. J. Respir. Crit. Care Med.* 2005;172:105–113.

[121] Wilkins MR, Paul GA, Strange JW, Tunariu N, Gin-Sing W, Banya WA, Westwood MA, Stefanidis A, Ng LL, Pennell DJ, *et al.* Sildenafil versus Endothelin Receptor Antagonist for Pulmonary Hypertension (SERAPH) study. *Am. J. Respir. Crit. Care Med.* 2005;171:1292–1297.

[122] Hoeper MM, Leuchte H, Halank M, Wilkens H, Meyer FJ, Seyfarth HJ, Wensel R, Ripken F, Bremer H, Kluge S, Hoeffken G, Behr J. Combining inhaled iloprost with bosentan in patients with idiopathic pulmonary arterial hypertension. *Eur. Respir. J.* 2006;28:691-4.

[123] Leite-Moreira AF. Current perspectives in diastolic dysfunction and diastolic heart failure. *Heart.* 2006;92:712-8.

[124] Gonzalez-Lopez L, Gamez- Nava JI, Ramos –Remus C, Cardona-Muñoz E, Herrera-Esparza R, Alvarado-Flores E, Suarez-Almazor M, et all. Ventricular diastolic dysfunction in patients with systemic lupus erythematosus population (SLE). *Arthritis Rheum.* 1994;37: Suppl no.9 :S322 (abstract).

[125] Paran D, Caspi D, Levartovsky D, Elkayam O, Kaufman I, Litinsky I, Keren G, Koifman B. Cardiac dysfunction in patients with systemic lupus erythematosus and antiphospholipid syndrome. *Ann. Rheum. Dis.* 2007;66:506-10.

[126] Paulus WJ, Tschope C, Sanderson JE, Rusconi C, Flachskampf FA, Rademakers FE, Marino P, Smiseth OA, De Keulenaer G, Leite-Moreira AF, Borbely A, Edes I, Handoko ML, Heymans S, Pezzali N, Pieske B, Dickstein K, Fraser AG, Brutsaert DL. How to diagnose diastolic heart failure: a consensus statement on the diagnosis of heart failure with normal left ventricular ejection fraction by the Heart Failure and Echocardiography Associations of the European Society of Cardiology. *Eur. Heart J.* 2007; [Epub ahead of print] PMID: 17428822.

[127] Galderisi M. Diastolic dysfunction and diastolic heart failure: diagnostic, prognostic and therapeutic aspects. *Cardiovasc. Ultrasound.* 2005;3:9.

[128] Font J, Ramos-Casals M, Brito-Zeron P, Nardi N, Ibanez A, Suarez B, Jimenez S, Tassies D, Garcia-Criado A, Ros E, Sentis J, Reverter JC, Lozano F. Association of mannose-binding lectin gene polymorphisms with antiphospholipid syndrome, cardiovascular disease and chronic damage in patients with systemic lupus erythematosus. *Rheumatology* (Oxford). 2007;46:76-80.

[129] Senecal JL, Raymond Y. Autoantibodies to major and minor nuclear lamins are not restricted to autoimmune diseases. *Clin. Immunol. Immunopathol.* 1992;63:115-25.

[130] Konstantinov K, von Mikecz A, Buchwald D, Jones J, Gerace L, Tan EM. Autoantibodies to nuclear envelope antigens in chronic fatigue syndrome. *J. Clin. Invest.* 1996;98:1888-96.

[131] Senecal JL, Rauch J, Grodzicky T, Raynauld JP, Uthman I, Nava A, Guimond M, Raymond Y. Strong association of autoantibodies to human nuclear lamin B1 with lupus anticoagulant antibodies in systemic lupus erythematosus. *Arthritis Rheum.* 1999;42:1347-53.

[132] Dieude M, Senecal JL, Rauch J, Hanly JG, Fortin P, Brassard N, Raymond Y. Association of autoantibodies to nuclear lamin B1 with thromboprotection in systemic lupus erythematosus: lack of evidence for a direct role of lamin B1 in apoptotic blebs. *Arthritis Rheum.* 2002;46:2695-707.

[133] Tincani A, Biasini-Rebaioli C, Cattaneo R, Riboldi P. Nonorgan specific autoantibodies and heart damage. *Lupus.* 2005;14:656-9.

[134] Libman E, Sacks B. A hitherto undescribed form of valvular and mural endocarditis. *Arch. Intern. Med.* 1924; 33: 701–737.

[135] Kiani AN, Fishman EK, Petri M. Aortic valve calcification in systemic lupus erythematosus. *Lupus* 2006;15:873-6.

[136] Doria A, Petri M. Cardiac involvement in systemic lupus erythematosus. In Doria A, Pauletto P, eds. *The heart in systemic autoimmune disease.* Amsterdam: Elsevier, Amsterdam, 2004: 146–162.

[137] Omdal R, Lunde P, Rasmussen K et al. Transesophageal and transthoracic echocardiography and Doppler-examination in systemic lupus erythematosus. *Scand. J. Rheumatol.* 2001; 30: 275–281.

[138] Leszczynski P, Straburzynska-Migaj E, Korczowska I, Lacki JK, Mackiewicz S. Cardiac valvular disease in patients with systemic lupus erythematosus. Relationship with anticardiolipin antibodies. *Clin. Rheumatol.* 2003; 22: 405–408.

[139] Jensen-Urstad K, Svenungsson E, de Faire U et al. Cardiac valvular abnormalities are frequent in systemic lupus erythematosus with manifest arterial disease. *Lupus* 2002; 11: 744–752.

[140] Yavuz B, Atalar E, Karadag O, Tulumen E, Ozer N, Akdogan A, Ertenli I, Kiraz S, Calguneri M, Ozmen F. QT dispersion increases in patients with systemic lupus erythematosus. *Clin. Rheumatol.* 2007;26:376-9.

In: Progress in Systemic Lupus Erythematosus Research
Editor: Tomas I. Seward, pp. 77-103
ISBN 978-1-60021-861-3

Chapter 2

COMORBIDITY IN SYSTEMIC LUPUS ERYTHEMATOSUS: ASPECTS OF CARDIOVASCULAR DISEASE, OSTEOPOROSIS AND INFECTIONS

Irene E. M. Bultink**, *Ben A. C. Dijkmans* and *Alexandre E. Voskuyl
Department of Rheumatology, VU University Medical Center,
Room 4A49, PO box 7057, 1007 MB Amsterdam, The Netherlands

ABSTRACT

Over the last decades, the survival of patients with systemic lupus erythematosus (SLE) has improved dramatically. Having improved treatment for active lupus disease, the challenge is now to understand and prevent the long-term complications of the disease, which may be due to the disease itself or the therapies used. To date, long-term complications of SLE are now considered to be important, including cardiovascular disease, osteoporosis and infections.

Cardiovascular disease in patients with SLE, including coronary artery disease, ischemic cerebrovascular disease, and peripheral vascular disease, is the result of premature atherosclerosis. Besides the traditional risk factors (like hypertension, hypercholesterolaemia and smoking), renal insufficiency, raised homocysteine levels, and the presence of anti-phospholipid, antibodies have been recognized as additional risk factors for cardiovascular disease in SLE. Recent studies have demonstrated that the nitric oxide pathway and its endogenous inhibitor asymmetric dimethylarginine may also be involved in the pathogenesis of cardiovascular organ damage in SLE. The metabolic syndrome and insulin resistance in SLE patients are current topics of research in this field.

* Tel: +31-20-4443432; Fax: +31-20-4442138.

Several studies have demonstrated a high prevalence of low bone mineral density in patients with SLE, especially in females. In the last few years, more attention is paid to osteoporotic fractures, one of the items of the organ damage index for SLE, and likely the most preventable form of musculoskeletal organ damage in SLE patients. Recent studies have demonstrated an increased frequency of symptomatic vertebral and nonvertebral fractures in patients with SLE. Moreover, a high prevalence of mostly asymptomatic vertebral fractures in patients with SLE was detected. These vertebral fractures were associated with previous use of intravenous methylprednisolone. The importance of identifying vertebral fractures in SLE patients is illustrated by the observed association between prevalent vertebral fractures and reduced quality of life as well as an increased risk of future vertebral and nonvertebral fractures in the general population.

Infection imposes a serious burden on patients with SLE. In case series, infectious complications were found in 25% to 45% of SLE patients, and infection as primary cause of death has been demonstrated in up to 50% of SLE patients. Defects of immune defence and treatment with corticosteroids and other immunosuppressive agents are supposed to play a role in the pathogenesis of infections in SLE. Recently, research has focused on the role of the lectin pathway of complement activation in the occurrence of infections in SLE.

In this review the results of recent studies on cardiovascular disease, osteoporosis and infectious complications in SLE will be discussed.

INTRODUCTION

Systemic lupus erythematosus (SLE) is a chronic autoimmune disorder that usually affects multiple organ systems and may be associated with considerable morbidity and mortality.

Over the last 3 decades, the survival of patients with SLE has improved dramatically. A 60% decrease in the standardized all-cause mortality rate (SMR) from 1970-1979 (SMR 4.9) to 1990-2001 (SMR 2.0) has been demonstrated in a large international multicenter study [1]. The improved health outcome in patients with SLE has been attributed to earlier and better diagnostic methods as well as better immunosuppressive treatment strategies. Despite the improved survival, mortality rates in patients with SLE are still significantly higher than those in the general population, across countries, and throughout the course of the disease, up to 20 years disease duration [1]. The most important causes of death in patients with SLE are disease activity (complicated by organ system involvement), treatment related complications such as infections, and long-term disease complications (particularly cardiovascular disease). From 1970 to 2001, a change in death causes in SLE patients has been observed [1-3]. In this period of time, a decrease in the rate of death primarily due to disease activity has occurred [1, 4], while death due to cardiovascular disease remained unchanged [4] or slightly increased, [1] and cardiovascular death is currently probably the commonest cause of death in lupus patients in the Western world [1, 4]. Despite improvements in immunosuppressive treatment strategies for active disease, infections are still an important cause of death in SLE patients, both early and late in the disease course [1-3, 5-7].

Apart from mortality, prognosis in SLE has also aspects with regard to morbidity. The prolonged survival of patients with SLE is also associated with considerable morbidity due to long-term complications of the disease. These long-term complications in SLE patients may be due to the disease itself, the therapies used, or comorbid diseases, and are associated with functional limitations and a reduced quality of life.

In this review, recent research in the field of three important long-term complications in patients with SLE will be discussed. First atherosclerotic cardiovascular disease, which is the major cause of cardiovascular, neuropsychiatric, and peripheral vascular organ damage in SLE patients, as assessed with the Systemic Lupus International Collaborating Clinics/American College of Rheumatology (SLICC/ACR) damage index score [8]. Secondly, osteoporosis and fractures, which contribute to damage in the most frequently involved system in SLE patients: the musculoskeletal system. In the third item, results of recent research on infectious complications in SLE will be highlighted.

Cardiovascular Disease in SLE

Over the last decades, accelerated atherosclerosis and premature cardiovascular disease (CVD), including coronary heart disease [9], ischaemic cerebrovascular disease [10], and peripheral vascular disease [11] has been identified as a major contributor to the morbidity and mortality of patients with SLE. In female SLE patients, the risk of myocardial infarction is 10-fold increased [12], the risk of stroke 8 to 10-fold [12, 13] and the risk of heart failure may be increased as much as 13-fold [13] as compared to age- and sex-matched healthy controls. Atherosclerotic events also tend to occur at younger ages in patients with SLE. In patients with SLE, the first myocardial infarction occurs at a mean age of 49 years as compared to 65 to 74 years in the general population, which illustrates the premature occurrence of CVD in SLE [9].

In addition, several studies have demonstrated a high prevalence of subclinical atherosclerosis in 17% to 40% of SLE patients, as measured by myocardial perfusion scans, presence of atherosclerotic plaques in the carotid artery and assessment of coronary artery calcifications by computer tomography [14-16]. Endothelial dysfunction, as defined by impaireded flow-mediated dilatation of the brachial artery, was present in 55% of SLE patients as compared to 26% of healthy persons in a recent study [17]. Data from an autopsy study performed in patients with SLE demonstrated that 52% of patients had moderate to severe atherosclerosis at the time of death, regardless of the cause of death [2].

Risk factors for CVD in SLE

The mechanisms underlying the accelerated atherosclerosis in SLE are not fully understood, but endothelial dysfunction and/or atherosclerosis in combination with prothrombotic factors are supposed to be important contributors to this process [18] . In recent years, both traditional and non-traditional risk factors have been identified, which play a role in the pathogenesis of CVD in SLE.

1. Traditional Risk Factors

Patients with SLE have an increased prevalence of several traditional risk factors for atherosclerosis, such as hypertension [12, 19, 20], diabetes mellitus [19], obesity [19, 20], inactivity [19-21], hypercholesterolaemia [20] and hypertriglyceridaemia [19] and these risk factors are, also in SLE patients, associated with an increased risk for CVD. However, even after adjustment for the presence of the traditional Framingham risk factors, the risk for cardiovascular events in patients with SLE is still 7 to 17-fold increased [12, 22]. Therefore, additional metabolic, inflammatory, medication related and lifestyle factors are suggested to contribute to the development of atherosclerosis and vascular disease in SLE.

2. Antiphospholipid Antibodies

The occurrence of a secondary antiphospholipid antibody syndrome in SLE patients is common and is characterized by both arterial and venous thrombosis [23].

The presence of lupus anticoagulant has been recognized as an independent risk factor for myocardial infarction [24] and cerebral arterial occlusion [25] in SLE patients. These findings support the idea that thrombosis plays a role in the increased risk of CVD in SLE. Studies of the relationship between the presence of lupus anticoagulant and atherosclerosis in SLE demonstrate conflicting results. In a Swedish study, the presence of lupus anticoagulant was associated with an increased intima-media thickness of the carotid artery [26], but in a recent study in the USA the presence of lupus anticoagulant or anticardiolipin (aCL) antibodies was not associated with coronary or carotid atherosclerosis [27].

The role of aCL and anti-ß2-glycoprotein 1 (ß2GP1) antibodies in the development of CVD in SLE is not completely clear. In the general population, the presence of aCL antibodies has been associated with an increased risk for future myocardial infarction [28, 29], but this finding has not been confirmed in SLE yet. In the study of Svenungsson and colleagues, both aCL antibodies and anti-ß2GP1 antibodies tended to be associated with arterial disease in lupus patients, but these associations were not statistically significant [26].

However, several other studies have suggested that aCL and anti-ß2GP1 antibodies might play a role in the atherosclerotic process in SLE [30-33]. The low-density lipoprotein (LDL) particle is susceptible to oxidative modification, which accounts for its atherogenic properties. Oxidized LDL (ox-LDL) contributes to the formation of foam cells in atherosclerotic lesions [30]. Ox-LDL can bind anti-ß2GP1, which results in ß2GP1-ox-LDL complexes [31]. Antibodies against these complexes are supposed to increase LDL uptake by macrophages, which contributes to foam cell formation, a process considered important in atherosclerotic plaque formation [33]. Moreover, it was demonstrated that binding of these antibodies to ß2GP1 on endothelial cells induces expression of adhesion molecules, which further enhances leukocyte adhesion to the endothelium [32]. The role of antibodies to ox-LDL in the pathogenesis of atherosclerosis in SLE is still under debate. The occurrence and high titres of these antibodies have been associated with the extent of atherosclerosis and CVD in reports, but other studies suggested that antibodies to ox-LDL play a protective role in the atherosclerotic process [33, 34]. Future research might provide more insight in the subtle interplay between thrombogenesis and atherogenesis and in the role of antiphospholipid antibodies in the pathogenesis of CVD in lupus.

3. SLE Related Risk Factors

Several diseases related factors have been recognized as independent risk factors for CVD in SLE.

In SLE patients, longer disease duration [9, 20, 21] and premature menopause [19] have been associated with an increased risk of CVD.

In addition, renal disease is an important contributor to CVD in lupus. Nephritis is a highly frequent complication in SLE and may cause proteinuria and renal failure. Nephrotic syndrome and proteinuria are associated with un unfavourable lipid profile [35] and atherosclerosis in SLE [36, 37]. Moreover, an elevated serum creatinine or history of renal disease are associated with atherosclerosis [38, 39].

Dyslipidaemia in SLE is characterized by a reduced high-density lipoprotein (HDL) cholesterol as well as an increased LDL cholesterol, VLDL cholesterol, triglycerides [40] and increased lipoprotein a (Lp(a)) [26, 41]. Dyslipidaemia occurs especially in active disease [40] and is associated with atherosclerosis and cardiovascular events [19, 26, 36]. The mechanisms underlying the dyslipidaemia in SLE are not well known, but tumor necrosis factor-α (TNF-α) induced de novo hepatic lipogenesis and inhibition of LDL are two possible mechanisms [18]. This hypothesis is supported by the strong associations found between elevated circulating levels of TNF-α, high triglycerides and low HDL levels in SLE patients [42]. Recently, the presence of anti-lipoprotein lipase antibodies (anti-LPL) in association with dyslipidaemia and increased inflammatory parameters have been demonstrated in patients with SLE [43]. Further research is necessary to unravel the role of these antibodies in the pathogenesis of atherosclerosis in lupus.

The role of antibodies against endothelial cells (aEC) in the development of CVD in SLE is not clear. These antibodies have been associated with vasculitis and disease activity [44] and direct stimulation of endothelial cells in SLE [45], but no correlation between aEC antibodies and CVD was found in one study [46].

Atherosclerosis can be considered to have an important inflammatory component and several inflammatory factors are supposed to promote atherosclerosis in SLE. In the general population, raised serum concentrations of C-reactive protein (CRP) are a strong predictor of future coronary events [47]. In line with this finding, raised serum levels of CRP were associated with subclinical atherosclerosis [39] and cardiovascular arterial events in SLE patients [48]. Moreover, serum levels of complement increase in response to inflammation and studies in the general population have demonstrated associations between high complement C3 levels and traditional cardiovascular risk factors and coronary heart disease [49, 50]. In lupus patients, increased complement C3 levels were correlated with increased vascular stiffness of the aorta [39] and with coronary calcifications in SLE [36]. Furthermore, we found an association between high C3 levels and metabolic syndrome score in female lupus patients [51]. This finding is in line with the results of a study by Chung et al, demonstrating an association between higher levels of inflammation and prevalence of the metabolic syndrome in patients with SLE [52]. In lupus, the systemic inflammatory response is accompanied by systemic complement activation and immune complex deposition in specific tissues. Complement activation induces endothelial cell activation, the release of monocyte chemoattractant protein-1 (MCP-1), and the release of IL-6 from vascular smooth muscle cells, which promote recruitment of leukocytes and atherosclerosis [53, 54]. Recently,

Asanuma and colleagues found increased concentrations of IL-6 and MCP-1 in lupus patients and these cytokines were associated with inflammation, disease activity, body mass index and low HDL levels [14]. Moreover, IL-6 concentrations were correlated with coronary calcification [14]. Inflammation in SLE might also contribute to the dyslipidaemia associated with lupus by IL-6 mediated inhibition of lipoprotein lipase (LPL), the key enzyme in the metabolism of LDL and VLDL [15]. Reduced LPL activity has been demonstrated in lupus patients and was strongly associated with high triglyceride levels [55].

Recently, decreased binding of annexin V to endothelial cells has been proposed as a possible mechanism contributing to atherosclerosis in SLE [56]. Annexin V has anti-thrombotic properties and decreased binding of this plasma protein to endothelial cells, caused by antiphospholipid antibodies, might promote atherosclerosis. Associations between annexin V binding and carotid intima media thickness in lupus patients with a history of CVD have been demonstrated [56]. Further research is necessary to elucidate the role of annexin V and other inflammatory factors in the atherosclerotic process in lupus.

4. Oxidative Stress

Several studies have demonstrated increased oxidative stress in patients with SLE [57, 58]. In lupus patients with a history of cardiovascular events, raised plasma levels of ox-LDL have been demonstrated [26]. The contribution of ox-LDL to foam cell formation in atherosclerotic plaques has been debated. However, ox-LDL levels have also been associated with renal manifestations in SLE, and it is well known that nephritis and renal failure are risk factors for CVD. Therefore, the exact role of ox-LDL in the atherosclerotic process in SLE is still under debate and will be subject of more research.

The hypothesis that oxidative stress contributes to the atherosclerotic process in SLE is supported by a study demonstrating reduced activity of the antioxidant enzyme paraoxanase in SLE [59].

Recently, the role of the nitric oxide pathway and its endogenous inhibitor asymmetric dimethylarginine (ADMA) has been investigated in SLE. In the general population, high plasma ADMA levels are associated with endothelial dysfunction [60]. Moreover, high ADMA levels are a predictor of acute coronary events [61] and a risk factor for cardiovascular events and mortality in patients with end stage renal disease [62]. In patients with SLE, AMDA levels were significantly higher in patients with a history of cardiovascular events than in patients without a CVD history [63]. Moreover, high ADMA levels in SLE were associated with disease activity, high titers of anti-dsDNA antibodies [63, 64] and with coronary calcification [64]. The observed association between high ADMA levels and high titers of anti-dsDNA antibodies is in line with results from in vitro studies. Anti-dsDNA antibodies were shown to be reactive with the arginine-glycine-rich domains in recombinant heterogeneous nuclear ribonucleoprotein A2 (hnRNP A2) [65]. These domains are also preferred sites for the methylation of arginine to ADMA by type 1 protein arginine methyltransferase (PRMT1) [66]. In the presence of anti-dsDNA, methylation of hnRNP A2 by PRMT1 was increased to 3.5 times that of the control level. Therefore, anti-dsDNA antibodies might be a trigger for increased ADMA production by up regulating methylation of arginine residues by PRMT1. Furthermore, anti-dsDNA monoclonal antibodies were demonstrated to augment the inflammatory reaction by the release of proinflammatory cytokines from mononuclear cells [67]. These studies suggest that anti-dsDNA antibodies might play a role in the development of CVD in SLE by enhancing ADMA production and by enhancing the inflammatory reaction. However, a prospective study is required to answer definitively the question of whether high ADMA levels are an independent risk factor for future cardiovascular events in SLE.

5. Metabolic Risk Factors

In a prospective study in 337 patients with SLE from the Hopkins lupus cohort, raised plasma homocysteine levels were found in 15% of the patients and high homocysteine levels were an independent risk factor for stroke and arterial thrombosis [68]. This finding was confirmed by a Dutch study, reporting an increased risk for arterial thrombosis in SLE patients with high homocysteine levels [69].

The metabolic syndrome is a condition characterized by the clustering of cardiovascular risk factors, including hypertension, obesity, insulin resistance and dyslipidaemia, and is associated with an increased risk of diabetes mellitus and cardiovascular mortality in the general population, especially in women [70, 71]. Recently, research has focused on insulin resistance and the associated metabolic syndrome in SLE. In patients with SLE, an increased prevalence of insulin resistance was demonstrated [72, 73]. A study in the United Kingdom reported that 18% of female SLE patients, as compared with 2.5% of healthy female controls, fulfilled the criteria of the National Cholesterol Education Program (NCEP) metabolic syndrome [72]. A study by Chung et al in the United States reported that the metabolic syndrome was present in 29.4% of male and female SLE patients and 19.8% of healthy controls, using the NCEP definition [52]. In a recent study in 141 Dutch female SLE patients, the prevalence of the metabolic syndrome was 16% and a high metabolic syndrome score was associated with previous treatment with intravenous methylprednisolone, renal insufficiency, older age, higher erythrocyte sedimentation rate and higher C3 levels [51]. Moreover, the mean metabolic syndrome score was significantly higher in SLE patients with a history of cardiovascular events than in those without a previous cardiovascular event [51]. In both the Dutch and the USA study, associations were found between the metabolic syndrome and high levels of inflammation. Therefore, the metabolic syndrome might provide a link between inflammation and the increased vascular risk in SLE. A prospective study is necessary to investigate whether the metabolic syndrome is a predictor of cardiovascular events and mortality in patients with SLE.

6. The Role of Anti-Rheumatic Drugs

The role of corticosteroid treatment in the development of CVD in SLE has been investigated in many studies. Corticosteroids have a negative effect on blood pressure, glucose metabolism and body fat distribution. On the other hand, corticosteroids have an anti-inflammatory effect, which might be beneficial with respect to the atherosclerotic process. The evaluation of the effect of corticosteroids on CVD in SLE is complicated, since corticosteroids are usually prescribed in patients with more active disease. Therefore, a history of corticosteroid treatment might reflect a higher inflammatory disease state, which is supposed to be an important risk factor for CVD per se [47]. Associations between increased exposure to corticosteroids and atherosclerosis and cardiovascular events have been reported in patients with SLE [9, 20, 38], but other studies failed to find such an association [16, 74]. The benefit or harm of corticosteroids might be dose-dependent. In SLE patients, a daily dose of < 10 mg corticosteroids did not have an adverse effect on lipid levels [75], but a dose of > 10 mg daily was associated with increased cholesterol and triglyceride levels [75, 76]. The conflicting results of the studies on this subject illustrate the dual role of corticosteroid therapy with respect to the development of CVD in SLE.

Antimalarial drugs reduce the atherosclerotic risk in SLE by several mechanisms. First, antimalarials have an anti-inflammatory effect in mild to moderate disease activity. Secondly, a beneficial effect of antimalarials on the dyslipidaemia in SLE, especially in case of concomitant treatment with corticosteroids, has been reported in several studies [77-80]. In the third place, antimalarials may have a beneficial effect on insulin sensitivity, because these drugs prolong the half-life of the active insulin-receptor complex through the inhibition of insulin dissociation from its receptor [81]. However, the effect of antimalarials on insulin resistance has not been investigated in SLE patients yet.

Despite the great number of studies performed in the context of CVD and its risk factors in SLE, little is known about the role of other antirheumatic drugs. However, a negative association between previous cyclophosphamide use and the prevalence of carotid plaque was demonstrated in one study [16], suggesting that tight control of disease activity might be beneficial in the prevention of atherosclerosis in SLE.

Prevention and Treatment of CVD in SLE

Traditional risk factors, disease-related factors and the associated metabolic changes, immunologic factors, anti-phospholipid antibodies, lifestyle factors and use of antirheumatic drugs all contribute to the accelerated atherosclerosis and premature CVD in subgroups of patients with SLE. Prospective studies in large patient groups are necessary to evaluate the relative influence of each of these factors. In the meantime, physicians should use a proactive approach to suppress disease activity and other modifiable risk factors for atherosclerosis in these high-risk patients. Screening for risk factors in SLE patients is very important for several reasons. First, in patients with SLE, a high prevalence of multiple risk factors has been demonstrated [19, 20]. Secondly, a recent quality improvement study in Canada has demonstrated that hypertension and especially hypercholesterolaemia are not managed adequately in the majority of SLE patients [82]. In the third place, many of the risk factors mentioned may be relatively easily recognized and managed in clinical practice by lifestyle advices (stop smoking, physical activity, weight reduction) or medication (anti-hypertensive treatment, lipid lowering agents, anti-diabetic medication, anticoagulants, supplementation with folic acid and vitamin B12 in case of increased homocysteine levels). It was suggested by Bruce, that the diagnosis of SLE can be regarded as a risk factor for CVD itself, like diabetes, which has implications for the ideal targets for blood pressure, lipid levels and glucose levels in SLE patients [15].

The identification of biological markers of disease activity associated with atherosclerosis might be a tool to improve therapy and prevent cardiovascular complications in SLE.

In addition, physicians eagerly await the definitive results of current large-scale prospective studies evaluating the effect of different intervention strategies to reduce the risk for CVD in SLE. The preliminary results of a Canadian intervention study are promising [83].

Osteoporosis and Fractures in SLE

In recent years, osteoporosis and fractures have been recognized as important disease complications in patients with SLE. The growing interest in these unfortunate disease complications is justified for several reasons. First, in studies from 1990 to 2007, a high prevalence of low bone mineral density (BMD) in patients with SLE has been demonstrated, especially in female patients [84-101]. Secondly, osteoporotic fractures are an item of the SLICC/ACR organ damage index for SLE. In the third place, it was demonstrated in studies in the general population, that osteoporotic fractures are associated with a reduced quality of life [102], an increased risk of future fractures [103, 104], and an increased mortality rate [103].

Osteoporosis in SLE

A reduced BMD, as measured by Dual Energy X-ray absorptiometry (DEXA), is highly frequent in patients with SLE. Osteopenia is reported in 25-74% of SLE patients [93, 95, 101] and osteoporosis, defined as a T score less than -2.5 SD, is reported in 1-23% [84, 96, 98, 100]. The great majority of studies of BMD performed in patients with SLE had a cross-sectional study design [84, 86, 88-95, 97-100, 105-112]. Only a few longitudinal studies have been published [85, 113-116]. The prevalence of osteopenia and osteoporosis reported in studies in lupus patients differs widely as a consequence of differences between study populations with respect to size, mean age, ethnic background, menstrual status, disease severity and treatments used. The aetiology of bone loss in SLE is supposed to be multifactorial, involving both non-disease related and disease related factors.

Non-Disease Related Risk Factors for Osteoporosis in SLE

Higher age [84, 90, 93, 96, 101], low body-mass index [84, 86, 93], postmenopausal status [84, 86, 93, 94, 101], and non-Afro-Caribbean race [101] have been recognized as significant non-disease related risk factors for reduced BMD in patients with SLE. Two small studies in men demonstrated no increased prevalence of osteoporosis in male SLE patients [106, 109]. Several studies have evaluated the effects of smoking and alcohol use, but no significant associations with low BMD in patients with SLE have been reported [86, 90, 93, 101, 112, 113]. Data on other possible risk factors for low BMD (e.g. family history of osteoporosis and reduced mobility) are generally not available.

Disease Related Risk Factors for Osteoporosis in SLE

Disease duration, inflammation, renal failure, deficiency of 25(OH) vitamin D, reduced physical activity, hormonal factors and medication related factors have been suggested to play a role in the development of osteoporosis in SLE.

In contrast to two studies [98, 105] reporting an association between disease duration and BMD in SLE patients, most studies did not find such an association [84, 86, 88, 90, 94, 108, 112].

Disease activity is supposed to play a role in the development of osteoporosis in SLE [117]. Serum levels of pro-inflammatory cytokines, such as TNF-α, IL-1 and IL-6, are increased in patients with SLE [118] and production of bone-resorbing lymphokines by B-cells in SLE patients has been described [119]. These findings suggest that disease activity might be a risk factor for osteoporosis in SLE. Indeed, Petri and colleagues reported that disease activity, as measured by low serum C4 levels, was an independent predictor of low BMD in the lumbar spine [120]. However, no association between disease activity and BMD was found in all recent studies, including studies using cumulative measures for disease activity over time [86, 90, 94-96, 98, 100, 105, 106, 109, 115].

The relationship between BMD and organ damage in patients with SLE has been investigated in several studies, with conflicting results. In four studies [94, 98, 105, 111], higher organ damage score was significantly associated with low BMD in patients with SLE, but in four other studies [86, 90, 91, 93] no association between BMD and organ damage score in SLE patients was found. The reasons for this discrepancy are unclear.

Renal failure might contribute to the development of low BMD in patients with SLE through several mechanisms. Renal damage due to SLE may result in an impairment of vitamin D 1-hydroxylation by the kidneys, secondary hyperparathyroidism and increased osteoclastic bone resorption. However, no significant association between renal function and BMD was reported in recent studies [86, 90, 94], which might be explained by the relatively small number of patients with renal failure included in most recent studies and exclusion of patients with renal failure in several other studies [88, 92, 95, 98, 100, 106, 109, 110, 112].

Deficiency of 25(OH) vitamin D might be regarded as a non-disease related as well as a disease related risk factor for osteoporosis in SLE. However, the increased prevalence of 25(OH) vitamin D deficiency reported in patients with SLE, as compared to healthy controls [121] is usually ascribed to the disease related conscious avoidance of exposure to sunlight and/or the use of sunscreens [99, 105, 106, 121]. In a study in 107 Dutch SLE patients, deficiency of 25(OH) vitamin D was significantly associated with low BMD in the lumbar spine, but not at the hip [86].

Reduced physical activity is considered an important risk factor for the development of osteoporosis in several rheumatic disorders [117]. Bhattoa et al [84] reported a significant negative association between Steinbrocker functional classification and lumbar spine and hip BMD in SLE patients, but other studies failed to demonstrate an association between physical activity and BMD in SLE patients [86, 90, 91, 115].

Several hormonal factors may be involved in the pathogenesis of low BMD in lupus. SLE is characterized by enhanced hydroxylation of estradiol, increased oxidation of testosterone and relatively low plasma levels of androgens, such as dehydroepiandrosterone sulphate (DHEAS). In addition, hyperprolactinaemia has been reported in patients with SLE, which may further decrease serum levels of estradiol and androgens [122]. In a study in 37 premenopausal SLE patients, a significant positive relationship between serum DHEAS levels and BMD was demonstrated [89]. In a small study in 20 male SLE patients, no association between hyperprolactinemia and low BMD was found [109]. Premature ovarian dysfunction as a result of active disease or caused by medication, is common in female SLE patients and contributes to bone loss by a reduction of overall estrogen exposure. In a study by Gordon et al [91], significantly decreased BMD values in SLE patients with a disordered menstrual history were found. These findings support the viewpoint that hormonal factors contribute to the development of low BMD in SLE.

The role of corticosteroids in the development of osteoporosis in SLE is still under debate. Various studies reported a relationship between corticosteroid use and low BMD [84, 85, 90, 91, 93, 94, 98, 100, 110], but several other studies did not find a significant relationship between corticosteroid treatment and BMD in SLE patients [86-89, 92, 96, 105, 106, 108, 109, 111-113]. The reasons for this discrepancy are unclear, but may be related to differences in patient populations in size, mean age and menstrual status, as well as differences between centers in treatment strategies for osteoporosis and use of corticosteroids. Moreover, corticosteroids might play a dual role with respect to the development of osteoporosis in SLE. On the one hand corticosteroid therapy may induce bone loss, but on the other hand corticosteroids might have a beneficial effect on bone mass by suppressing inflammation. Bone loss in patients with SLE might also be induced by other drugs which are commonly used in these patients. Cyclophosphamide may induce osteoporosis by induction of premature ovarian failure. In addition, long-term exposure to oral anticoagulation, and to a lesser extent, low-molecular-weight heparin, has been associated with increased bone loss in the general population [123], but this has not been investigated in patients with SLE.

Fractures in SLE

In contrast to the large number of studies on BMD, only a few studies on osteoporotic fractures in SLE have been published. In 4 studies, symptomatic vertebral and peripheral fractures occurring since disease onset were reported in 9-16.5% of SLE patients [84, 91, 93, 124]. The incidence of symptomatic vertebral and peripheral fractures was demonstrated to be 5 times higher in female SLE patients as compared to age-matched healthy women, and higher age and prolonged use of corticosteroids were identified as the most important risk factors for fractures [124]. In this large study, 10% of the symptomatic fractures were reported to be vertebral fractures.

Only two studies on prevalent vertebral fractures in SLE patients, using a standardized method to assess vertebral fractures, have been performed and in these studies at least 1 vertebral fracture was detected in 20-21% of the patients [86, 107]. In both studies, vertebral fractures were defined as a reduction of ≥ 20% of the vertebral body height. The frequency of vertebral fractures (20%) in 90 Dutch SLE patients with mean age 41 years, was high in comparison to the 12% prevalence of vertebral fractures in the general population of Europe with an age between 65 and 69 years [125]. Interestingly, in both studies on prevalent vertebral fractures in SLE, no association between oral corticosteroid use and vertebral fractures was found, but in the Dutch study, previous use of intravenous methylprenisolone was associated with prevalent vertebral fractures [86]. In both studies, BMD was not different between SLE patients with and without prevalent vertebral fractures [86, 107]. This finding is in line with results of a previous study in the general population, which reported that the proportion of fractures attributable to osteoporosis is modest, ranging from 10% to 44% [126]. These data suggest that bone quality contributes more to bone strength than bone quantity and point to the limited value of BMD measurement by DEXA in the assessment of future fracture risk. The high frequency of both peripheral and vertebral fractures demonstrated in SLE patients highlights the need to develop better strategies for the prevention and treatment of osteoporosis and fractures as important disease complications in lupus patients. The need for better prevention and treatment strategies is also illustrated by the relative high frequency of undertreatment of SLE patients with manifest osteoporosis or at high risk of the development of osteoporosis, as demonstrated in the Dutch study [86].

Prevention and Treatment of Osteoporosis in SLE

Prevention strategies directed toward SLE patients at risk for osteoporosis and fractures include advice for maintaining a normal body weight and daily performance of weight-baring physical activity. In addition, physicians should encourage a healthy diet and strongly advice against smoking. Moreover, adequate calcium and vitamin D supplementation should be prescribed. We advocate to perform BMD measurement by DEXA in SLE patients treated with corticosteroids and/or in postmenopausal patients with SLE. Moreover, as a consequence of the high prevalence of vertebral fractures demonstrated in SLE patients, physicians should consider to perform spine X-rays (analyzed using a standardized method for assessing vertebral deformities) next to BMD measurement of the spine and hip in the assessment of osteoporosis and future fracture risk. Postmenopausal women with osteoporosis and/or fractures and women on corticosteroids should be treated with appropriate antiosteoporosis medication, eg bisphosphonates. Results of a recent study in postmenopausal women in the general population have demonstrated a significant beneficial effect on BMD and a significantly reduced risk for symptomatic vertebral fractures (but not for other fractures) in patients continuing bisphosphonate therapy for 10 years as compared to patients who discontinued bisphosphonates after 5 years [127]. Moreover, the safety of long-term treatment with bisphosphonates up to 10 years was demonstrated in this study [127]. Bisphosphonates are contraindicated in patients with renal failure and in premenopausal lupus women planning pregnancy. Bisphosphonates are maintained in bone for a long period of time even after discontinuation of therapy, and fetal abnormalities due to bisphosphonates were demonstrated in animal studies [128]. Hormonal replacement therapy may be useful in postmenopausal women without an increased risk of thrombosis.

Infections in SLE

Importance of Infections in SLE

Infections are an important cause of morbidity and mortality in patients with SLE. Infections occur in 25% to 50% of SLE patients in case series [129-132] and a third of the infections in SLE patients were demonstrated to be major infections for which hospital admission is required [129, 130, 133]. Infection as primary cause of death has been reported in up to 50% of patients with SLE [5, 7].

Spectrum of Infections in SLE

SLE patients suffer from a broad spectrum of infections caused predominantly by community-acquired bacteria [129-131, 133], but also opportunistic infections are reported [5]. Among Indian SLE patients, tuberculosis was demonstrated to be the commonest infection [134]. Moreover, a high incidence (up to 21%) of Herpes zoster infection was found in several studies in SLE patients [129, 130, 135-139].

Risk Factors for Infections in SLE

Treatment with corticosteroids and immunosuppressive agents and defects in immune function (which may result from the disease itself and its therapy) are supposed to play a role in the pathogenesis [5], but also disease activity [7, 133, 140-142], disease duration [129, 143], active nephritis [135, 144] and decreased renal function [142] have been linked to an increased risk of infection in lupus patients.

The role of corticosteroid use as an independent risk factor for infections in SLE was demonstrated in several studies [130-132, 135, 145], but other studies failed to find such an association [129, 133, 140-142]. The impact of immunosuppressive drugs, such as cyclophosphamide, azathioprine and methotrexate, on the immune system is well established. Use of immunosuppressive drugs was identified as an independent risk factor for infections in some studies in SLE [131, 132, 142, 145], but not in other studies in patients with SLE [7, 86, 133, 140]. Some studies failed to demonstrate an additive effect of cytotoxic drugs in increasing the overall infection rate, but showed an increased incidence of Herpes zoster infections in patients using cyclophosphamide [136, 146] or azathioprine [135]. Since corticosteroids and immunosuppressive drugs are used mostly in patients with more severe disease, it is likely that both disease activity and drug therapy contribute to the increased infection risk in SLE. In a recent study, a strong negative association between hydroxychloroquine use and the occurrence of major infections was demonstrated [129]. This finding might be explained by the frequent use of hydroxychloroquine in the treatment of patients with mild lupus disease activity. Another explanation might be protection against infections due to the antimicrobial properties of hydroxychloroquine. However, antimalarials act against pathogenic organisms that are very uncommon in Western European countries [129].

Defects in the Complement System and Infections in SLE

Several defects in both humoral and cellular immunity have been described in lupus patients, which might contribute to an inadequate immune defence [5]. The potential role of macrophage defects, polymorphonuclear cell defects, defects in number and function of natural killer cells, T cells and B cells, immunoglobulin defects and dysfunction of the reticuloendothelial system in the pathogenesis of infections in SLE has been extensively described by Iliopoulos and Tsokos [5]. This chapter is restricted to the results of recent research on the contribution of the complement system to the increased infection risk in SLE.

The complement system plays an important role in host defence against microorganisms and the increased infection rate in SLE patients has been attributed in part to defects in the complement system [5]. A strong association between genetic deficiencies of early components of the classical pathway of complement activation and the development of SLE has been demonstrated [147]. In particular, deficiency of C1q is a major risk factor for the development of SLE. Moreover, deficiency of C1q might play a role in the susceptibility to infections in SLE, since C1q plays a role in the recognition and clearance of apoptotic material [148] and binds predominantly to antibodies and protein structures on bacteria and viruses, resulting in complement activation. The consumption of complement proteins by circulating and tissue-fixed immune complexes might also limit the amount of complement that is available for host defence against invading pathogens.

Deficiency of Mannose-Binding Lectin and Infections in SLE

Recently, the lectin pathway of complement activation has also been suggested to play a role in the pathogenesis of SLE [149] and in the occurrence of infections in SLE patients [150-152]. Mannose-binding lectin (MBL) is a serum protein that shares many features with C1q [153]. In contrast to C1q, which is a recognition molecule in the classical pathway of complement activation, MBL serves as one of the recognition molecules in the lectin pathway of complement activation [154]. MBL may activate complement through the lectin pathway by interacting with MBL-associated serine proteases (MASP). In addition, MBL can directly opsonise pathogenic microorganisms and enhance the activity of phagocytes [154].

In a meta-analysis of all available case-control studies, homozygosity for variant MBL alleles was demonstrated to be a minor risk factor for the presence of SLE [155]. A significant association between MBL codon 54 variant B and SLE was reported in that study.

In two Danish studies [150, 151] and a Japanese study [152], SLE patients homozygous for MBL variant alleles were at an increased risk for serious infections in comparison with patients who were heterozygous or homozygous for the normal allele. In contrast, in a study in Dutch SLE patients, no association between the biological activity of MBL and the occurrence of infections was found [129]. In this study, functional MBL activity was determined using three different assays: 1) an assay measuring functional MBL serum levels which is dependent only on the amount of functional protein, 2) an assay measuring activity of the MBL/MASP complex by assessing MBL-induced C4 deposition and 3) an assay measuring the complete MBL pathway activity in serum, which is sensitive to defects in all components of the MBL pathway. None of these assays demonstrated an association between deficient MBL activity and the occurrence of infections or major infections in patients with SLE [129]. There are two possible explanations for the discrepancy between the results of the genetic and the phenotypic studies. First, functional activity of MBL in serum not only is determined by mutations in the gene encoding MBL, but is also dependent on promoter polymorphisms, MASP activity, serum levels of other complement factors, and environmental factors [156, 157]. Therefore, measurement of functional MBL activity is supposed to be a better estimation of the in vivo situation than assessment of MBL genotypes when evaluating the association between the MBL pathway of complement activation and the occurrence of infections in SLE. Secondly, the discrepancy between the genotypic and phenotypic data could be explained by unidentified linkages between mutations or polymorphisms in the MBL gene with mutations or polymorphisms in other genes, which might influence the genetic approach. The results of this study suggest that deficiency of functional MBL activity does not play a role in the susceptibility to infections or major infections in SLE. However, this does not exclude an influence of defects in the complement system on the occurrence of infections in SLE. Therefore, future research will be focused on the role of defects of other complement factors and complement inhibitors in the pathogenesis of infections in SLE.

Diagnostic and Therapeutic Considerations

It is often difficult to distinguish infection from disease flare in febrile patients with SLE. As a consequence of an inadequate inflammatory response, signs and symptoms of infection may be subtle or absent, especially in patients treated with immunosuppressive drugs. On the other hand, clinical symptoms of lupus activity may simulate infection. Physicians should be aware that false-positive serological tests for several infections (e.g. Lyme disease, toxoplasmosis, syphilis), which are caused by polyclonal hypergammaglobulinaemia, are often found in SLE patients [5]. In addition, skin tests may be false-negative in case of corticosteroid use [5]. Chills and leukocytosis are markers favouring infection. Moreover, in a study in SLE patients, high C-reactive protein levels were associated with infection, in the absence of serositis [158]. Another study demonstrated increased serum procalcitonine levels in lupus patients with bacterial or fungal infections as compared to patients with viral infections or with lupus flare [159]. The presence of low complement levels and high serum anti-DNA antibody titers suggests lupus flare.

Strategies to reduce the morbidity and mortality related to infections in SLE include hygienic measures, prophylactic use of antimicrobial agents and immunisations.

Prophylaxis against *Pneumocystis carinii,* using a regimen of low-dose trimethoprim/sulfamethoxazole or inhaled pentamidine should be considered in selected SLE patients being treated with immunosuppressive agents [160]. Moreover, prophylaxis with isoniazide is recommended in SLE patients with positive tuberculin skin test requiring high dose corticosteroids [161].

Although initial reports suggested that pneumococcal vaccinations in patients with SLE might induce disease exacerbations [162], recent studies demonstrated that vaccinations against influenza en pneumococcus are safe in this patient group [163, 164], although influenza vaccination was less effective in SLE patients than in controls [163].

Early diagnosis and treatment of infections in patients with SLE remains a difficult challenge for physicians. More research is necessary to develop laboratory tests that will improve differentiating between infections and disease exacerbations in patients with SLE.

Conclusion

The importance of CVD, osteoporosis, and infections as long-term complications in patients with SLE, can not be over emphasized. The aetiology of these complications in SLE is supposed to be multifactorial, including risk factors that also apply to the general population, disease-related and treatment-related risk factors. The relative contributions of these risk factors are not fully understood. Ongoing research should attempt to further unravel the pathogenic mechanisms, applying especially to SLE patients. Physicians treating patients with SLE should be aware of the long-term complications that might develop in their patients. In addition, SLE patients themselves need to understand how to modify lifestyle factors that increase the risk of premature atherosclcrosis, osteoporosis, fractures and infectious complications. Treatment regimens will benefit from the results of large scale prospective studies evaluating the effect of different intervention strategies to reduce the risk of CVD, osteoporosis and infections in patients with SLE.

References

[1] Bernatsky S, Boivin JF, Joseph L, Manzi S, Ginzler E, Gladman DD et al. Mortality in systemic lupus erythematosus. *Arthritis Rheum.* 2006;54(8):2550-7.

[2] Abu-Shakra M, Urowitz MB, Gladman DD, Gough J. Mortality studies in systemic lupus erythematosus. Results from a single center. I. Causes of death. *J. Rheumatol.* 1995;22(7):1259-64.

[3] Urowitz MB, Gladman DD. How to improve morbidity and mortality in systemic lupus erythematosus. *Rheumatology (Oxford)* 2000;39(3):238-44.

[4] Bjornadal L, Yin L, Granath F, Klareskog L, Ekbom A. Cardiovascular disease a hazard despite improved prognosis in patients with systemic lupus erythematosus: results from a Swedish population based study 1964-95. *J. Rheumatol.* 2004;31(4):713-9.

[5] Iliopoulos AG, Tsokos GC. Immunopathogenesis and spectrum of infections in systemic lupus erythematosus. *Semin Arthritis Rheum.* 1996;25(5):318-36.

[6] Moss KE, Ioannou Y, Sultan SM, Haq I, Isenberg DA. Outcome of a cohort of 300 patients with systemic lupus erythematosus attending a dedicated clinic for over two decades. *Ann. Rheum Dis.* 2002;61(5):409-13.

[7] Nossent JC. Course and prognostic value of Systemic Lupus Erythematosus Disease Activity Index in black Caribbean patients. *Semin. Arthritis Rheum.* 1993;23(1):16-21.

[8] Gladman D, Ginzler E, Goldsmith C, Fortin P, Liang M, Urowitz M et al. The development and initial validation of the Systemic Lupus International Collaborating Clinics/American College of Rheumatology damage index for systemic lupus erythematosus. *Arthritis Rheum.* 1996;39(3):363-9.

[9] Manzi S, Meilahn EN, Rairie JE, Conte CG, Medsger TA, Jr., Jansen-McWilliams L et al. Age-specific incidence rates of myocardial infarction and angina in women with systemic lupus erythematosus: comparison with the Framingham Study. *Am. J. Epidemiol.* 1997;145(5):408-15.

[10] Kitagawa Y, Gotoh F, Koto A, Okayasu H. Stroke in systemic lupus erythematosus. *Stroke* 1990;21(11):1533-9.

[11] McDonald J, Stewart J, Urowitz MB, Gladman DD. Peripheral vascular disease in patients with systemic lupus erythematosus. *Ann. Rheum Dis.* 1992;51(1):56-60.

[12] Esdaile JM, Abrahamowicz M, Grodzicky T, Li Y, Panaritis C, du Berger R et al. Traditional Framingham risk factors fail to fully account for accelerated atherosclerosis in systemic lupus erythematosus. *Arthritis Rheum.* 2001;44(10):2331-7.

[13] Ward MM. Premature morbidity from cardiovascular and cerebrovascular diseases in women with systemic lupus erythematosus. *Arthritis Rheum.* 1999;42(2):338-46.

[14] Asanuma Y, Chung CP, Oeser A, Shintani A, Stanley E, Raggi P et al. Increased concentration of proatherogenic inflammatory cytokines in systemic lupus erythematosus: relationship to cardiovascular risk factors. *J. Rheumatol.* 2006;33(3):539-45.

[15] Bruce IN. 'Not only...but also': factors that contribute to accelerated atherosclerosis and premature coronary heart disease in systemic lupus erythematosus. *Rheumatology (Oxford)* 2005;44(12):1492-502.

[16] Roman MJ, Shanker BA, Davis A, Lockshin MD, Sammaritano L, Simantov R et al. Prevalence and correlates of accelerated atherosclerosis in systemic lupus erythematosus. *N. Engl. J. Med.* 2003;349(25):2399-406.

[17] El-Magadmi M, Bodill H, Ahmad Y, Durrington PN, Mackness M, Walker M et al. Systemic lupus erythematosus: an independent risk factor for endothelial dysfunction in women. *Circulation* 2004;110(4):399-404.

[18] Frostegard J. SLE, atherosclerosis and cardiovascular disease. *J. Intern. Med.* 2005;257(6):485-95.

[19] Bruce IN, Urowitz MB, Gladman DD, Ibanez D, Steiner G. Risk factors for coronary heart disease in women with systemic lupus erythematosus: the Toronto Risk Factor Study. *Arthritis Rheum.* 2003;48(11):3159-67.

[20] Petri M, Perez-Gutthann S, Spence D, Hochberg MC. Risk factors for coronary artery disease in patients with systemic lupus erythematosus. *Am. J. Med.* 1992;93(5):513-9.

[21] Manzi S, Selzer F, Sutton-Tyrrell K, Fitzgerald SG, Rairie JE, Tracy RP et al. Prevalence and risk factors of carotid plaque in women with systemic lupus erythematosus. *Arthritis Rheum.* 1999;42(1):51-60.

[22] Bessant R, Hingorani A, Patel L, MacGregor A, Isenberg DA, Rahman A. Risk of coronary heart disease and stroke in a large British cohort of patients with systemic lupus erythematosus. *Rheumatology (Oxford)* 2004;43(7):924-9.

[23] Harris EN, Gharavi AE, Boey ML, Patel BM, Mackworth-Young CG, Loizou S et al. Anticardiolipin antibodies: detection by radioimmunoassay and association with thrombosis in systemic lupus erythematosus. *Lancet* 1983;2(8361):1211-4.

[24] Petri M. The lupus anticoagulant is a risk factor for myocardial infarction (but not atherosclerosis): Hopkins Lupus Cohort. *Thromb. Res.* 2004;114(5-6):593-5.

[25] Jouhikainen T, Stephansson E, Leirisalo-Repo M. Lupus anticoagulant as a prognostic marker in systemic lupus erythematosus. *Br. J. Rheumatol.* 1993;32(7):568-73.

[26] Svenungsson E, Jensen-Urstad K, Heimburger M, Silveira A, Hamsten A, de Faire U et al. Risk factors for cardiovascular disease in systemic lupus erythematosus. *Circulation* 2001;104(16):1887-93.

[27] Farzaneh-Far A, Roman MJ, Lockshin MD, Devereux RB, Paget SA, Crow MK et al. Relationship of antiphospholipid antibodies to cardiovascular manifestations of systemic lupus erythematosus. *Arthritis Rheum.* 2006;54(12):3918-25.

[28] Vaarala O, Manttari M, Manninen V, Tenkanen L, Puurunen M, Aho K et al. Anti-cardiolipin antibodies and risk of myocardial infarction in a prospective cohort of middle-aged men. *Circulation* 1995;91(1):23-7.

[29] Wu R, Nityanand S, Berglund L, Lithell H, Holm G, Lefvert AK. Antibodies against cardiolipin and oxidatively modified LDL in 50-year-old men predict myocardial infarction. *Arterioscler. Thromb. Vasc. Biol.* 1997;17(11):3159-63.

[30] Haberland ME, Olch CL, Folgelman AM. Role of lysines in mediating interaction of modified low density lipoproteins with the scavenger receptor of human monocyte macrophages. *J. Biol. Chem.* 1984;259(18):11305-11.

[31] Kobayashi K, Kishi M, Atsumi T, Bertolaccini ML, Makino H, Sakairi N et al. Circulating oxidized LDL forms complexes with beta2-glycoprotein I: implication as an atherogenic autoantigen. *J. Lipid Res.* 2003;44(4):716-26.

[32] Matsuura E, Koike T. Accelerated atheroma and anti-beta2-glycoprotein I antibodies. *Lupus* 2000;9(3):210-6.

[33] van Leuven SI, Kastelein JJ, D'Cruz DP, Hughes GR, Stroes ES. Atherogenesis in rheumatology. *Lupus* 2006;15(3):117-21.

[34] Shoenfeld Y, Wu R, Dearing LD, Matsuura E. Are anti-oxidized low-density lipoprotein antibodies pathogenic or protective? *Circulation* 2004;110(17):2552-8.

[35] Leong KH, Koh ET, Feng PH, Boey ML. Lipid profiles in patients with systemic lupus erythematosus. *J. Rheumatol.* 1994;21(7):1264-7.

[36] Manger K, Kusus M, Forster C, Ropers D, Daniel WG, Kalden JR et al. Factors associated with coronary artery calcification in young female patients with SLE. *Ann. Rheum. Dis.* 2003;62(9):846-50.

[37] Theodoridou A, Bento L, D'Cruz DP, Khamashta MA, Hughes GR. Prevalence and associations of an abnormal ankle-brachial index in systemic lupus erythematosus: a pilot study. *Ann. Rheum. Dis.* 2003;62(12):1199-203.

[38] Doria A, Shoenfeld Y, Wu R, Gambari PF, Puato M, Ghirardello A et al. Risk factors for subclinical atherosclerosis in a prospective cohort of patients with systemic lupus erythematosus. *Ann. Rheum. Dis.* 2003;62(11):1071-7.

[39] Selzer F, Sutton-Tyrrell K, Fitzgerald SG, Pratt JE, Tracy RP, Kuller LH et al. Comparison of risk factors for vascular disease in the carotid artery and aorta in women with systemic lupus erythematosus. *Arthritis Rheum.* 2004;50(1):151-9.

[40] Borba EF, Bonfa E. Dyslipoproteinemias in systemic lupus erythematosus: influence of disease, activity, and anticardiolipin antibodies. *Lupus* 1997;6(6):533-9.

[41] Borba EF, Santos RD, Bonfa E, Vinagre CG, Pileggi FJ, Cossermelli W et al. Lipoprotein(a) levels in systemic lupus erythematosus. *J. Rheumatol.* 1994;21(2):220-3.

[42] Svenungsson E, Gunnarsson I, Fei GZ, Lundberg IE, Klareskog L, Frostegard J. Elevated triglycerides and low levels of high-density lipoprotein as markers of disease activity in association with up-regulation of the tumor necrosis factor alpha/tumor necrosis factor receptor system in systemic lupus erythematosus. *Arthritis Rheum.* 2003;48(9):2533-40.

[43] de Carvalho JF, Borba EF, Viana VS, Bueno C, Leon EP, Bonfa E. Anti-lipoprotein lipase antibodies: a new player in the complex atherosclerotic process in systemic lupus erythematosus? *Arthritis Rheum.* 2004;50(11):3610-5.

[44] D'Cruz DP, Houssiau FA, Ramirez G, Baguley E, McCutcheon J, Vianna J et al. Antibodies to endothelial cells in systemic lupus erythematosus: a potential marker for nephritis and vasculitis. *Clin. Exp. Immunol.* 1991;85(2):254-61.

[45] Carvalho D, Savage CO, Isenberg D, Pearson JD. IgG anti-endothelial cell autoantibodies from patients with systemic lupus erythematosus or systemic vasculitis stimulate the release of two endothelial cell-derived mediators, which enhance adhesion molecule expression and leukocyte adhesion in an autocrine manner. *Arthritis Rheum.* 1999;42(4):631-40.

[46] Cederholm A, Svenungsson E, Stengel D, Fei GZ, Pockley AG, Ninio E et al. Platelet-activating factor-acetylhydrolase and other novel risk and protective factors for cardiovascular disease in systemic lupus erythematosus. *Arthritis Rheum.* 2004;50(9):2869-76.

[47] Ridker PM, Hennekens CH, Buring JE, Rifai N. C-reactive protein and other markers of inflammation in the prediction of cardiovascular disease in women. *N. Engl. J. Med.* 2000;342(12):836-43.

[48] Toloza SM, Uribe AG, McGwin G, Jr., Alarcon GS, Fessler BJ, Bastian HM et al. Systemic lupus erythematosus in a multiethnic US cohort (LUMINA). XXIII. Baseline predictors of vascular events. *Arthritis Rheum.* 2004;50(12):3947-57.

[49] Muscari A, Bastagli L, Poggiopollini G, Tomassetti V, Massarelli G, Cappelletti O et al. Different associations of C-reactive protein, fibrinogen and C3 with traditional risk factors in middle-aged men. *Int. J. Cardiol.* 2002;83(1):63-71.

[50] Onat A, Uzunlar B, Hergenc G, Yazici M, Sari I, Uyarel H et al. Cross-sectional study of complement C3 as a coronary risk factor among men and women. *Clin. Sci. (Lond)* 2005;108(2):129-35.

[51] Bultink IEM, Turkstra F, Diamant M, Dijkmans BAC, Voskuyl AE. Metabolic syndrome in women with systemic lupus erythematosus: Prevalence and association of metabolic syndrome score with disease characteristics and cardiovascular events. *Arthritis Rheum.* 2006;54(9):S270.

[52] Chung CP, Avalos I, Oeser A, Gebretsadik T, Shintani A, Raggi P et al. High prevalence of the metabolic syndrome in patients with systemic lupus erythematosus: association with disease characteristics and cardiovascular risk factors. *Ann. Rheum. Dis.* 2007;66(2):208-14.

[53] de Lemos JA, Morrow DA, Sabatine MS, Murphy SA, Gibson CM, Antman EM et al. Association between plasma levels of monocyte chemoattractant protein-1 and long-term clinical outcomes in patients with acute coronary syndromes. *Circulation* 2003;107(5):690-5.

[54] Schieffer B, Selle T, Hilfiker A, Hilfiker-Kleiner D, Grote K, Tietge UJ et al. Impact of interleukin-6 on plaque development and morphology in experimental atherosclerosis. *Circulation* 2004;110(22):3493-500.

[55] Reichlin M, Fesmire J, Quintero-Del-Rio AI, Wolfson-Reichlin M. Autoantibodies to lipoprotein lipase and dyslipidemia in systemic lupus erythematosus. *Arthritis Rheum.* 2002;46(11):2957-63.

[56] Cederholm A, Svenungsson E, Jensen-Urstad K, Trollmo C, Ulfgren AK, Swedenborg J et al. Decreased binding of annexin v to endothelial cells: a potential mechanism in atherothrombosis of patients with systemic lupus erythematosus. *Arterioscler. Thromb. Vasc. Biol.* 2005;25(1):198-203.

[57] Ames PR, Alves J, Murat I, Isenberg DA, Nourooz-Zadeh J. Oxidative stress in systemic lupus erythematosus and allied conditions with vascular involvement. *Rheumatology (Oxford)* 1999;38(6):529-34.

[58] Nuttall SL, Heaton S, Piper MK, Martin U, Gordon C. Cardiovascular risk in systemic lupus erythematosus--evidence of increased oxidative stress and dyslipidaemia. *Rheumatology (Oxford)* 2003;42(6):758-62.

[59] Delgado AJ, Ames PR, Donohue S, Stanyer L, Nourooz-Zadeh J, Ravirajan C et al. Antibodies to high-density lipoprotein and beta2-glycoprotein I are inversely correlated with paraoxonase activity in systemic lupus erythematosus and primary antiphospholipid syndrome. *Arthritis Rheum.* 2002;46(10):2686-94.

[60] Boger RH, Bode-Boger SM, Szuba A, Tsao PS, Chan JR, Tangphao O et al. Asymmetric dimethylarginine (ADMA): a novel risk factor for endothelial dysfunction: its role in hypercholesterolemia. *Circulation* 1998;98(18):1842-7.

[61] Valkonen VP, Paiva H, Salonen JT, Lakka TA, Lehtimaki T, Laakso J et al. Risk of acute coronary events and serum concentration of asymmetrical dimethylarginine. *Lancet* 2001;358(9299):2127-8.

[62] Zoccali C, Bode-Boger S, Mallamaci F, Benedetto F, Tripepi G, Malatino L et al. Plasma concentration of asymmetrical dimethylarginine and mortality in patients with end-stage renal disease: a prospective study. *Lancet* 2001;358(9299):2113-7.

[63] Bultink IE, Teerlink T, Heijst JA, Dijkmans BA, Voskuyl AE. Raised plasma levels of asymmetric dimethylarginine are associated with cardiovascular events, disease activity, and organ damage in patients with systemic lupus erythematosus. *Ann. Rheum. Dis.* 2005;64(9):1362-5.

[64] Kiani AN, Post W, Mahoney JA, Petri M. ADMA in SLE is associated with serologic activity, cardiovascular risk factors, and coronary calcium. *Arthritis Rheum.* 2005;52(9):S603.

[65] Sun KH, Tang SJ, Wang YS, Lin WJ, You RI. Autoantibodies to dsDNA cross-react with the arginine-glycine-rich domain of heterogeneous nuclear ribonucleoprotein A2 (hnRNP A2) and promote methylation of hnRNP A2. *Rheumatology (Oxford)* 2003;42(1):154-61.

[66] Gary JD, Clarke S. RNA and protein interactions modulated by protein arginine methylation. *Prog. Nucleic. Acid. Res. Mol. Biol*.1998;61:65-131.

[67] Sun KH, Yu CL, Tang SJ, Sun GH. Monoclonal anti-double-stranded DNA autoantibody stimulates the expression and release of IL-1beta, IL-6, IL-8, IL-10 and TNF-alpha from normal human mononuclear cells involving in the lupus pathogenesis. *Immunology* 2000;99(3):352-60.

[68] Petri M, Roubenoff R, Dallal GE, Nadeau MR, Selhub J, Rosenberg IH. Plasma homocysteine as a risk factor for atherothrombotic events in systemic lupus erythematosus. *Lancet* 1996;348(9035):1120-4.

[69] Fijnheer R, Roest M, Haas FJ, De Groot PG, Derksen RH. Homocysteine, methylenetetrahydrofolate reductase polymorphism, antiphospholipid antibodies, and thromboembolic events in systemic lupus erythematosus: a retrospective cohort study. *J. Rheumatol.* 1998;25(9):1737-42.

[70] Hanson RL, Imperatore G, Bennett PH, Knowler WC. Components of the "metabolic syndrome" and incidence of type 2 diabetes. *Diabetes* 2002;51(10):3120-7.

[71] Wilson PW, Kannel WB, Silbershatz H, D'Agostino RB. Clustering of metabolic factors and coronary heart disease. *Arch. Intern. Med*.1999;159(10):1104-9.

[72] El Magadmi M, Ahmad Y, Turkie W, Yates AP, Sheikh N, Bernstein RM et al. Hyperinsulinemia, insulin resistance, and circulating oxidized low density lipoprotein in women with systemic lupus erythematosus. *J. Rheumatol.* 2006;33(1):50-6.

[73] Sada KE, Yamasaki Y, Maruyama M, Sugiyama H, Yamamura M, Maeshima Y et al. Altered levels of adipocytokines in association with insulin resistance in patients with systemic lupus erythematosus. *J. Rheumatol.* 2006;33(8):1545-52.

[74] Asanuma Y, Oeser A, Shintani AK, Turner E, Olsen N, Fazio S et al. Premature coronary-artery atherosclerosis in systemic lupus erythematosus. *N. Engl. J. Med.* 2003; 349(25):2407-15.

[75] MacGregor AJ, Dhillon VB, Binder A, Forte CA, Knight BC, Betteridge DJ et al. Fasting lipids and anticardiolipin antibodies as risk factors for vascular disease in systemic lupus erythematosus. *Ann. Rheum. Dis.* 1992;51(2):152-5.

[76] Petri M, Spence D, Bone LR, Hochberg MC. Coronary artery disease risk factors in the Johns Hopkins Lupus Cohort: prevalence, recognition by patients, and preventive practices. *Medicine (Baltimore)* 1992;71(5):291-302.

[77] Borba EF, Bonfa E. Longterm beneficial effect of chloroquine diphosphate on lipoprotein profile in lupus patients with and without steroid therapy. *J. Rheumatol.* 2001;28(4):780-5.

[78] Petri M, Lakatta C, Magder L, Goldman D. Effect of prednisone and hydroxychloroquine on coronary artery disease risk factors in systemic lupus erythematosus: a longitudinal data analysis. *Am. J. Med.* 1994;96(3):254-9.

[79] Rahman P, Gladman DD, Urowitz MB, Yuen K, Hallett D, Bruce IN. The cholesterol lowering effect of antimalarial drugs is enhanced in patients with lupus taking corticosteroid drugs. *J. Rheumatol.* 1999;26(2):325-30.

[80] Wallace DJ, Metzger AL, Stecher VJ, Turnbull BA, Kern PA. Cholesterol-lowering effect of hydroxychloroquine in patients with rheumatic disease: reversal of deleterious effects of steroids on lipids. *Am. J. Med.* 1990;89(3):322-6.

[81] Bevan AP, Krook A, Tikerpae J, Seabright PJ, Siddle K, Smith GD. Chloroquine extends the lifetime of the activated insulin receptor complex in endosomes. *J. Biol. Chem.* 1997;272(43):26833-40.

[82] Urowitz MB, Gladman DD, Ibanez D, Berliner Y. Modification of hypertension and hypercholesterolaemia in patients with systemic lupus erythematosus: a quality improvement study. *Ann. Rheum. Dis.* 2006;65(1):115-7.

[83] Fortin PR, Abahamowicz M, Cymet A, Neville C, Harvey P, Su J et al. The health improvement and prevention program (HIPP) in systemic lupus erythematosus (SLE) shows preliminary benefits in reducing the estimated 8-year risk of cardiovascular disease. *Arthritis Rheum.* 2006;54(9):S791.

[84] Bhattoa HP, Bettembuk P, Balogh A, Szegedi G, Kiss E. Bone mineral density in women with systemic lupus erythematosus. *Clin. Rheumatol.* 2002;21(2):135-41.

[85] Boyanov M, Robeva R, Popivanov P. Bone mineral density changes in women with systemic lupus erythematosus. *Clin. Rheumatol.* 2003;22(4-5):318-23.

[86] Bultink IE, Lems WF, Kostense PJ, Dijkmans BA, Voskuyl AE. Prevalence of and risk factors for low bone mineral density and vertebral fractures in patients with systemic lupus erythematosus. *Arthritis Rheum.* 2005;52(7):2044-50.

[87] Chong HC, Chee SS, Goh EM, Chow SK, Yeap SS. Dietary calcium and bone mineral density in premenopausal women with systemic lupus erythematosus. *Clin. Rheumatol.* 2007;26(2):182-5.

[88] Formiga F, Moga I, Nolla JM, Pac M, Mitjavila F, Roig-Escofet D. Loss of bone mineral density in premenopausal women with systemic lupus erythematosus. *Ann. Rheum. Dis.* 1995;54(4):274-6.

[89] Formiga F, Moga I, Nolla JM, Navarro MA, Bonnin R, Roig-Escofet D. The association of dehydroepiandrosterone sulphate levels with bone mineral density in systemic lupus erythematosus. *Clin. Exp. Rheumatol.* 1997;15(4):387-92.

[90] Gilboe IM, Kvien TK, Haugeberg G, Husby G. Bone mineral density in systemic lupus erythematosus: comparison with rheumatoid arthritis and healthy controls. *Ann. Rheum. Dis.* 2000;59(2):110-5.

[91] Gordon C. Long-term complications of systemic lupus erythematosus. *Rheumatology (Oxford)* 2002;41(10):1095-100.

[92] Kalla AA, Fataar AB, Jessop SJ, Bewerunge L. Loss of trabecular bone mineral density in systemic lupus erythematosus. *Arthritis Rheum.* 1993;36(12):1726-34.

[93] Kipen Y, Buchbinder R, Forbes A, Strauss B, Littlejohn G, Morand E. Prevalence of reduced bone mineral density in systemic lupus erythematosus and the role of steroids. *J. Rheumatol.* 1997;24(10):1922-9.

[94] Lakshminarayanan S, Walsh S, Mohanraj M, Rothfield N. Factors associated with low bone mineral density in female patients with systemic lupus erythematosus. *J. Rheumatol.* 2001;28(1):102-8.

[95] Mok CC, Mak A, Ma KM. Bone mineral density in postmenopausal Chinese patients with systemic lupus erythematosus. *Lupus* 2005;14(2):106-12.

[96] Pineau CA, Urowitz MB, Fortin PJ, Ibanez D, Gladman DD. Osteoporosis in systemic lupus erythematosus: factors associated with referral for bone mineral density studies, prevalence of osteoporosis and factors associated with reduced bone density. *Lupus* 2004;13(6):436-41.

[97] Redlich K, Ziegler S, Kiener HP, Spitzauer S, Stohlawetz P, Bernecker P et al. Bone mineral density and biochemical parameters of bone metabolism in female patients with systemic lupus erythematosus. *Ann. Rheum. Dis.* 2000;59(4):308-10.

[98] Sinigaglia L, Varenna M, Binelli L, Zucchi F, Ghiringhella D, Gallazzi M et al. Determinants of bone mass in systemic lupus erythematosus: a cross sectional study on premenopausal women. *J. Rheumatol.* 1999;26(6):1280-4.

[99] Teichmann J, Lange U, Stracke H, Federlin K, Bretzel RG. Bone metabolism and bone mineral density of systemic lupus erythematosus at the time of diagnosis. *Rheumatol. Int.* 1999;18(4):137-40.

[100] Uaratanawong S, Deesomchoke U, Lertmaharit S, Uaratanawong S. Bone mineral density in premenopausal women with systemic lupus erythematosus. *J Rheumatol* 2003;30(11):2365-8.

[101] Yee CS, Crabtree N, Skan J, Amft N, Bowman S, Situnayake D et al. Prevalence and predictors of fragility fractures in systemic lupus erythematosus. *Ann. Rheum. Dis.* 2005;64(1):111-3.

[102] Oleksik A, Lips P, Dawson A, Minshall ME, Shen W, Cooper C et al. Health-related quality of life in postmenopausal women with low BMD with or without prevalent vertebral fractures. *J. Bone Miner Res.* 2000;15(7):1384-92.

[103] Hasserius R, Karlsson MK, Nilsson BE, Redlund-Johnell I, Johnell O. Prevalent vertebral deformities predict increased mortality and increased fracture rate in both men and women: a 10-year population-based study of 598 individuals from the Swedish cohort in the European Vertebral Osteoporosis Study. *Osteoporos Int.* 2003;14(1):61-8.

[104] Klotzbuecher CM, Ross PD, Landsman PB, Abbott TA, III, Berger M. Patients with prior fractures have an increased risk of future fractures: a summary of the literature and statistical synthesis. *J. Bone Miner Res.* 2000;15(4):721-39.

[105] Becker A, Fischer R, Scherbaum WA, Schneider M. Osteoporosis screening in systemic lupus erythematosus: impact of disease duration and organ damage. *Lupus* 2001;10(11):809-14.

[106] Bhattoa HP, Kiss E, Bettembuk P, Balogh A. Bone mineral density, biochemical markers of bone turnover, and hormonal status in men with systemic lupus erythematosus. *Rheumatol Int.* 2001;21(3):97-102.

[107] Borba VZ, Matos PG, da Silva Viana PR, Fernandes A, Sato EI, Lazaretti-Castro M. High prevalence of vertebral deformity in premenopausal systemic lupus erythematosus patients. *Lupus* 2005;14(7):529-33.

[108] Dhillon VB, Davies MC, Hall ML, Round JM, Ell PJ, Jacobs HS et al. Assessment of the effect of oral corticosteroids on bone mineral density in systemic lupus erythematosus: a preliminary study with dual energy x ray absorptiometry. *Ann. Rheum. Dis* 1990;49(8):624-6.

[109] Formiga F, Nolla JM, Mitjavila F, Bonnin R, Navarro MA, Moga I. Bone mineral density and hormonal status in men with systemic lupus erythematosus. *Lupus* 1996;5(6):623-6.

[110] Houssiau FA, Lefebvre C, Depresseux G, Lambert M, Devogelaer JP, Nagant de DC. Trabecular and cortical bone loss in systemic lupus erythematosus. *Br. J. Rheumatol.* 1996;35(3):244-7.

[111] Lee C, Almagor O, Dunlop DD, Manzi S, Spies S, Chadha AB et al. Disease damage and low bone mineral density: an analysis of women with systemic lupus erythematosus ever and never receiving corticosteroids. *Rheumatology (Oxford)* 2006;45(1):53-60.

[112] Li EK, Tam LS, Young RP, Ko GT, Li M, Lau EM. Loss of bone mineral density in Chinese pre-menopausal women with systemic lupus erythematosus treated with corticosteroids. *Br. J. Rheumatol.* 1998;37(4):405-10.

[113] Hansen M, Halberg P, Kollerup G, Pedersen-Zbinden B, Horslev-Petersen K, Hyldstrup L et al. Bone metabolism in patients with systemic lupus erythematosus. Effect of disease activity and glucocorticoid treatment. *Scand. J. Rheumatol.* 1998;27(3):197-206.

[114] Jardinet D, Lefebvre C, Depresseux G, Lambert M, Devogelaer JP, Houssiau FA. Longitudinal analysis of bone mineral density in pre-menopausal female systemic lupus erythematosus patients: deleterious role of glucocorticoid therapy at the lumbar spine. *Rheumatology (Oxford)* 2000;39(4):389-92.

[115] Kipen Y, Briganti E, Strauss B, Will R, Littlejohn G, Morand E. Three year followup of bone mineral density change in premenopausal women with systemic lupus erythematosus. *J Rheumatol* 1999;26(2):310-7.

[116] Pons F, Peris P, Guanabens N, Font J, Huguet M, Espinosa G et al. The effect of systemic lupus erythematosus and long-term steroid therapy on bone mass in pre-menopausal women. *Br. J. Rheumatol.* 1995;34(8):742-6.

[117] Star VL, Hochberg MC. Osteoporosis in patients with rheumatic diseases. *Rheum Dis Clin. North Am.* 1994;20(3):561-76.

[118] Al-Janadi M, al-Balla S, al-Dalaan A, Raziuddin S. Cytokine profile in systemic lupus erythematosus, rheumatoid arthritis, and other rheumatic diseases. *J. Clin. Immunol.* 1993;13(1):58-67.

[119] Tanaka Y, Watanabe K, Suzuki M, Saito K, Oda S, Suzuki H et al. Spontaneous production of bone-resorbing lymphokines by B cells in patients with systemic lupus erythematosus. *J. Clin. Immunol.* 1989;9(5):415-20.

[120] Petri M. Musculoskeletal complications of systemic lupus erythematosus in the Hopkins Lupus Cohort: an update. *Arthritis Care Res.* 1995; 8(3):137-45.

[121] Muller K, Kriegbaum NJ, Baslund B, Sorensen OH, Thymann M, Bentzen K. Vitamin D3 metabolism in patients with rheumatic diseases: low serum levels of 25-hydroxyvitamin D3 in patients with systemic lupus erythematosus. *Clin. Rheumatol.* 1995;14(4):397-400.

[122] Lukert BP, Raisz LG. Glucocorticoid-induced osteoporosis. *Rheum. Dis. Clin. North Am.* 1994;20(3):629-50.

[123] Resch H, Pietschmann P, Krexner E, Willvonseder R. Decreased peripheral bone mineral content in patients under anticoagulant therapy with phenprocoumon. *Eur. Heart J.* 1991;12(3):439-41.

[124] Ramsey-Goldman R, Dunn JE, Huang CF, Dunlop D, Rairie JE, Fitzgerald S et al. Frequency of fractures in women with systemic lupus erythematosus: comparison with United States population data. *Arthritis Rheum.* 1999;42(5):882-90.

[125] Lips P. Epidemiology and predictors of fractures associated with osteoporosis. *Am. J. Med.* 1997;103(2A):3S-8S.

[126] Stone KL, Seeley DG, Lui LY, Cauley JA, Ensrud K, Browner WS et al. BMD at multiple sites and risk of fracture of multiple types: long-term results from the Study of Osteoporotic Fractures. *J. Bone Miner Res.* 2003;18(11):1947-54.

[127] Black DM, Schwartz AV, Ensrud KE, Cauley JA, Levis S, Quandt SA et al. Effects of continuing or stopping alendronate after 5 years of treatment: the Fracture Intervention Trial Long-term Extension (FLEX): a randomized trial. *JAMA* 2006;296(24):2927-38.

[128] Patlas N, Golomb G, Yaffe P, Pinto T, Breuer E, Ornoy A. Transplacental effects of bisphosphonates on fetal skeletal ossification and mineralization in rats. *Teratology* 1999;60(2):68-73.

[129] Bultink IE, Hamann D, Seelen MA, Hart MH, Dijkmans BA, Daha MR et al. Deficiency of functional mannose-binding lectin is not associated with infections in patients with systemic lupus erythematosus. *Arthritis Res. Ther.* 2006; 8(6):R183.

[130] Gladman DD, Hussain F, Ibanez D, Urowitz MB. The nature and outcome of infection in systemic lupus erythematosus. *Lupus* 2002;11(4):234-9.

[131] Noel V, Lortholary O, Casassus P, Cohen P, Genereau T, Andre MH et al. Risk factors and prognostic influence of infection in a single cohort of 87 adults with systemic lupus erythematosus. *Ann. Rheum. Dis.* 2001;60(12):1141-4.

[132] Pryor BD, Bologna SG, Kahl LE. Risk factors for serious infection during treatment with cyclophosphamide and high-dose corticosteroids for systemic lupus erythematosus. *Arthritis Rheum.* 1996;39(9):1475-82.

[133] Zonana-Nacach A, Camargo-Coronel A, Yanez P, Sanchez L, Jimenez-Balderas FJ, Fraga A. Infections in outpatients with systemic lupus erythematosus: a prospective study. *Lupus* 2001;10(7):505-10.

[134] Shyam C, Malaviya AN. Infection-related morbidity in systemic lupus erythematosus: a clinico-epidemiological study from northern India. *Rheumatol Int.* 1996;16(1):1-3.

[135] Ginzler E, Diamond H, Kaplan D, Weiner M, Schlesinger M, Seleznick M. Computer analysis of factors influencing frequency of infection in systemic lupus erythematosus. *Arthritis Rheum.* 1978;21(1):37-44.

[136] Kahl LE. Herpes zoster infections in systemic lupus erythematosus: risk factors and outcome. *J. Rheumatol.* 1994;21(1):84-6.

[137] Moutsopoulos HM, Gallagher JD, Decker JL, Steinberg AD. Herpes zoster in patients with systemic lupus erythematosus. *Arthritis Rheum.* 1978;21(7):789-802.

[138] Pope JE, Krizova A, Ouimet JM, Goodwin JL, Lankin M. Close association of herpes zoster reactivation and systemic lupus erythematosus (SLE) diagnosis: case-control study of patients with SLE or noninflammatory nusculoskeletal disorders. *J. Rheumatol.* 2004;31(2):274-9.

[139] Wong KL. Pattern of SLE in Hong Kong Chinese: a cohort study. *Scand. J. Rheumatol.* 1992;21(6):289-96.

[140] Duffy KN, Duffy CM, Gladman DD. Infection and disease activity in systemic lupus erythematosus: a review of hospitalized patients. *J. Rheumatol.* 1991;18(8):1180-4.

[141] Nived O, Sturfelt G, Wollheim F. Systemic lupus erythematosus and infection: a controlled and prospective study including an epidemiological group. *Q. J. Med.* 1985;55(218):271-87.

[142] Petri M, Genovese M. Incidence of and risk factors for hospitalizations in systemic lupus erythematosus: a prospective study of the Hopkins Lupus Cohort. *J. Rheumatol.* 1992;19(10):1559-65.

[143] Jonsson H, Nived O, Sturfelt G. Outcome in systemic lupus erythematosus: a prospective study of patients from a defined population. *Medicine (Baltimore)* 1989;68(3):141-50.

[144] Lee P, Urowitz MB, Bookman AA, Koehler BE, Smythe HA, Gordon DA et al. Systemic lupus erythematosus. A review of 110 cases with reference to nephritis, the nervous system, infections, aseptic necrosis and prognosis. *Q. J. Med.* 1977;46(181):1-32.

[145] Hellmann DB, Petri M, Whiting-O'Keefe Q. Fatal infections in systemic lupus erythematosus: the role of opportunistic organisms. *Medicine (Baltimore)* 1987;66(5):341-8.

[146] Austin HA, III, Klippel JH, Balow JE, le Riche NG, Steinberg AD, Plotz PH et al. Therapy of lupus nephritis. Controlled trial of prednisone and cytotoxic drugs. *N. Engl. J.* 1986;Med 314(10):614-9.

[147] Reveille JD. The molecular genetics of systemic lupus erythematosus and Sjogren's syndrome. *Curr. Opin. Rheumatol.* 1991;3(5):722-30.

[148] Nauta AJ, Daha MR, van Kooten C, Roos A. Recognition and clearance of apoptotic cells: a role for complement and pentraxins. *Trends Immunol.* 2003;24(3):148-54.

[149] Davies EJ, Snowden N, Hillarby MC, Carthy D, Grennan DM, Thomson W et al. Mannose-binding protein gene polymorphism in systemic lupus erythematosus. *Arthritis Rheum.* 1995;38(1):110-4.

[150] Garred P, Madsen HO, Halberg P, Petersen J, Kronborg G, Svejgaard A et al. Mannose-binding lectin polymorphisms and susceptibility to infection in systemic lupus erythematosus. *Arthritis Rheum.* 1999;42(10):2145-52.

[151] Garred P, Voss A, Madsen HO, Junker P. Association of mannose-binding lectin gene variation with disease severity and infections in a population-based cohort of systemic lupus erythematosus patients. *Genes Immun.* 2001;2(8):442-50.

[152] Takahashi R, Tsutsumi A, Ohtani K, Muraki Y, Goto D, Matsumoto I et al. Association of mannose binding lectin (MBL) gene polymorphism and serum MBL concentration with characteristics and progression of systemic lupus erythematosus. *Ann. Rheum. Dis.* 2005;64(2):311-4.

[153] Turner MW. Mannose-binding lectin: the pluripotent molecule of the innate immune system. *Immunol. Today* 1996;17(11):532-40.

[154] Turner MW, Hamvas RM. Mannose-binding lectin: structure, function, genetics and disease associations. *Rev. Immunogenet.* 2000;2(3):305-22.

[155] Lee YH, Witte T, Momot T, Schmidt RE, Kaufman KM, Harley JB et al. The mannose-binding lectin gene polymorphisms and systemic lupus erythematosus: two case-control studies and a meta-analysis. *Arthritis Rheum.* 2005;52(12):3966-74.

[156] Crosdale DJ, Ollier WE, Thomson W, Dyer PA, Jensenious J, Johnson RW et al. Mannose binding lectin (MBL) genotype distributions with relation to serum levels in UK Caucasoids. *Eur. J. Immunogenet* 2000;27(3):111-7.

[157] Hansen TK, Thiel S, Dall R, Rosenfalck AM, Trainer P, Flyvbjerg A et al. GH strongly affects serum concentrations of mannan-binding lectin: evidence for a new IGF-I independent immunomodulatory effect of GH. *J. Clin. Endocrinol. Metab.* 2001;86(11):5383-8.

[158] ter Borg EJ, Horst G, Limburg PC, van Rijswijk MH, Kallenberg CG. C-reactive protein levels during disease exacerbations and infections in systemic lupus erythematosus: a prospective longitudinal study. *J. Rheumatol.* 1990;17(12):1642-8.

[159] Shin KC, Lee YJ, Kang SW, Baek HJ, Lee EB, Kim HA et al. Serum procalcitonin measurement for detection of intercurrent infection in febrile patients with SLE. *Ann. Rheum. Dis.* 2001;60(10):988-9.

[160] Porges AJ, Beattie SL, Ritchlin C, Kimberly RP, Christian CL. Patients with systemic lupus erythematosus at risk for Pneumocystis carinii pneumonia. *J. Rheumatol.* 1992;19(8):1191-4.

[161] Gilliland WR, Tsokos GC. Prophylactic use of antibiotics and immunisations in patients with SLE. *Ann. Rheum. Dis.* 2002;61(3):191-2.

[162] Croft SM, Schiffman G, Snyder E, Herrmann K, James K, Jarrett MP. Specific antibody response after in vivo antigenic stimulation in systemic lupus erythematosus. *J. Rheumatol.* 1984;11(2):141-6.

[163] Holvast A, Huckriede A, Wilschut J, Horst G, De Vries JJ, Benne CA et al. Safety and efficacy of influenza vaccination in systemic lupus erythematosus patients with quiescent disease. *Ann. Rheum. Dis.* 2006;65(7):913-8.

[164] McDonald E, Jarrett MP, Schiffman G, Grayzel AI. Persistence of pneumococcal antibodies after immunization in patients with systemic lupus erythematosus. *J. Rheumatol.* 1984;11(3):306-8.

In: Progress in Systemic Lupus Erythematosus Research
Editor: Tomas I. Seward, pp. 105-129
ISBN 978-1-60021-861-3

Chapter 3

SEVERE TISSUE TRAUMA TRIGGERS LUPUS AUTOIMMUNE DISEASE

Khairul Anam[1], Mihret Amare[1], Shruti Naik[1], Kathleen A. Szabo[2] and Thomas A. Davis[1,*]

[1]From the Regenerative Medicine Department at the Naval Medical Research Center
[2]Department of Diagnostic Pathology at the Walter Reed Army Institute of Research, Silver Spring, 20910-7500

ABSTRACT

Systemic lupus erythematosus (SLE) is a chronic, complex autoimmune disease characterized by high levels of non-organ-specific, self-reactive antibody production leading to immune complex formation. The etiology of this autoimmune disease remains elusive. The disease results in multiple health problems including increased infection, renal and skin disorders, neurological complications, osteoporosis, rheumatoid arthritis, osteoarthritis, and fibromylagias. Tissue damage associated with severe injury can result in profound immune dysfunction that involves suppressive cell types and a cascade of inflammatory and tissue reparative mediators. Mice from MRL strains have been used as models to study SLE pathogenesis. Wild type MRL/MpJ mice exhibit SLE autoimmune disorders but symptoms are manifested much later in life (70-90 weeks) compared to MRL/MpJ-Fas^{lpr} mice (17-22 weeks) which possess a lymphoproliferative mutation. Based on our preliminary findings, we hypothesize that following traumatic tissue injury, the activation of specific cell types, cytokines and other mediators involved in wound healing and repair processes may be critical in triggering lupus-like disease. We investigated the role of a severe (15% total body surface area) full-thickness cutaneous burn on the early onset of lupus-like autoimmune disease in young adult, lupus prone wild type MRL/MpJ mice, and control BALB/c mice. MRL/MpJ mice develop autoimmune disease 4-15 weeks post injury, manifested by skin lesions, vasculitis,

* Address correspondence and reprint requests to: Thomas A. Davis, Ph.D.[1,3] Regenerative Medicine Department, Naval Medical Research Center, room 2A10, 503 Robert Grant Avenue, Silver Spring, MD USA 20910. Tel. 301-319-9528, Fax 301-319-7210, E-mail: davist@nmrc.navy.mil

epidermal ulcers, cellular infiltration, splenomegaly, lymphadenopathy, hypergammaglobulinemia, elevated autoantibodies, and renal pathologies including proteinuria, glomerulonephritis, and immune complex deposition. Post-injury survival rate of injured MRL/MpJ mice is significantly reduced due to autoimmune related complications. In contrast, neither uninjured MRL/MpJ mice nor burned BALB/c displayed signs of autoimmunity or premature death. We analyzed mRNA expression of numerous cytokines at the wound margins in the skin at days 1-7 post injury. Our results do not reveal an early or clear Th1 or Th2 cytokine expression pattern during the early wound repair process but demonstrate a correlation between the pathogenic effects of dysregulated interleukin-beta (IL-1β), interleukin-6 (IL-6), tumor necrosis factor alpha (TNF-α) and prostaglandin-E2 (PGE2) synthesis and the early onset of lupus-like disease. Interestingly, we found that normal skin isografts transplanted onto the dorsum of MRL/MpJ mice with healed wounds (30- 40 days post burn injury) are rejected within 7 days after transplantation. In contrast, skin grafts transplanted onto uninjured age-matched MRL/MpJ achieved long-term survival. Collectively, these findings suggest that traumatic injury exacerbates inflammatory skin disease and the early onset of severe multi-organ SLE pathogenesis.

Keywords: SLE, autoimmunity, lupus, trauma, and burns.

INTRODUCTION

Autoimmune disease is estimated to affect at least 2% of the population in the United States [1]. Systemic lupus erythromatosus (SLE) is a chronic, complex, multi-organ, autoimmune disease characterized by high levels of non-organ-specific, self-reactive antibodies directed to cellular DNA, RNA, and histone components [2, 3]. Although SLE primarily afflicts pre-menopausal females (ages 12-40) it can occur in males, and disproportionately affects African Americans [4, 5]. Several genes have been implicated in the development of lupus; however, not all individuals with a genetic predisposition develop SLE. Extreme physical and emotional stress, psychosocial, physiologic, hormonal, and other factors are likely involved as triggers for SLE [3, 6-8]. Such factors have been linked to the manifestation of Gulf War Illness, a lupus-like condition [9-14]. Moreover, exposure to chemicals, vaccines, medications, drugs, UV radiation, and other ubiquitous environmental factors may promote SLE in otherwise healthy individuals [15-18]. A number of studies have suggested that the immune response to infectious agents and foreign antigens (bacterial, viral, and allergen) play a key role in triggering the activation of autoreactive T and B lymphocytes and induction of anti-DNA responses [19-21]. Immune reactivity may cause tissue damage without the classical signs of an autoimmune disease.

Individuals diagnosed with SLE are at increased risk of significant health problems, including deteriorating renal dysfunction, skin pathologies, increased infections, seizures and other neurological complications, and chronic musculoskeletal pain syndromes such as osteoporosis, rheumatoid arthritis, osteoarthritis, and fibromyalgia [2, 22]. Many of these individuals require long-term clinical care and systemic immunosuppressive/immunotherapy. Warfighters, for example, experience exposure to extreme environments and as a result endure physical and emotional stress making them particularly susceptible to SLE.

Furthermore, an increase in the number of women in combat situations could lead to increased incidence of lupus in the U.S. fighting force, because SLE afflicts women on average more than men [23]. Warfighters with SLE may be unable to continue their military service, therefore, greatly impacting U.S. military force strength.

Tissue trauma is a leading cause of disease experienced by military personnel and as accidents in civilian populations. The time course of wound repair and the amount of scar tissue formed depend on several factors including the type of wound, the extent of the tissue damage, inflammation, the presence of devitalized tissue and nonviable foreign tissue, and infection. More specifically, repair of damaged tissue involves a well-orchestrated sequence of events, initiated by platelet aggregation and fibrin polymerization, followed by infiltration of leukocytes [24-26]. Among the earliest cues for initiation of the wound repair response is the release of chemokines and growth factors by infiltrating degranulating platelets, keratinocytes, resident mast cells, and damaged tissue. Neutrophils, macrophages, and other inflammatory cells are recruited to the area of damaged tissue in response to chemokines and growth factors released at the site of the wound [27]. Leukocyte infiltration is also essential for removal of necrotic cellular debris, whereas many cell types participate in the removal of apoptotic cells and in subsequent reparative and remodeling processes [27-29].

Tissue damage associated with severe tissue injury can result in profound immune dysfunction and induction of adaptive immune response [30, 31]. While inflammatory cytokines are indispensable in wound healing and the restoration of homeostasis, it is often the excessive activity of either proinflammatory or anti-inflammatory cytokines that causes injury to the host or renders the host immunocompromised. Aberrant shifts in immune reactivity can result in delayed wound healing and in serious systemic complications such as hypermetabolism and catabolism leading to peripheral protein waste, systemic inflammatory response syndrome (SIRS), multiple organ dysfunction (MOD), sepsis, shock, and even death [32-35].

The adaptive immune response has evolved to recognize and attack foreign agents while maintaining tolerance to self-antigens. Adaptive immunity is induced by activation of T lymphocytes. Loss of T helper cell function and cytokine production after severe tissue damage is evident in the switch from Th1 inflammatory responses (augmented IL-2, TNFα and IFNγ production) towards counterinflammatory Th2-reactivity (IL-4 and IL-10) mediated by macrophages, $CD4^+$ and $CD8^+$ T cells [36]. Dysregulation of proinflammatory cytokines has been shown to play a pivotal role in SLE etiology [37-39].

Wild type MRL/MpJ mice exhibit SLE autoimmune disorders but symptoms are manifested much later in life (70-90 weeks) compared to MRL/MpJ-*Fas*^{lpr} mice (17-22 weeks) which possess a lymphoproliferative mutation [40,41]. In this study, we demonstrate accelerated development of lupus-like autoimmune disease in young adult, wild type MRL/MpJ mice following tissue trauma (cutaneous burn wound). Results from our studies indicate that these mice develop severe SLE, 10-15 weeks post injury, with characteristic skin lesions, cellular infiltration, hypergammaglobulinemia, anti-DNA autoantibodies, immune complex formation, glomerulonephritis, and lymphadenopathy. Our results also demonstrate a correlation between the pathogenic effects of dysregulated cytokine production (IL-1β, IL-6, TNF-α, PGE2) and the early onset of SLE. Taken together, results from this study suggest that traumatic injury exacerbates inflammatory skin disease and the early onset of severe multi-organ SLE pathogenesis.

Material and Methods

Animals

Five to six-week-old female MRL/MpJ mice and BALB/c mice were purchased from The Jackson Laboratory (Bar Harbor, ME) and maintained at the Armed Forces Radiobiology Research Institute or the Walter Reed Army Institute of Research (WRAIR, Silver Spring, MD) animal facility, which are both accredited by the Association for the Assessment and Accreditation of Laboratory Animal Care International. All procedures were conducted using facilities and protocols approved by the Animal Care and Use Committee of AFRRI (#2004-02-001) and WRAIR (protocol #K06-005). Mice were housed five animals per cage prior to surgery or any treatment, and individually caged post burn injury in standard micro-isolator polycarbonate caging. Mice were used for experimentation at 8 to 12 weeks of age. Animal rooms were maintained at 21° ± 2°C with 50% ± 10% humidity on a 12-hr light/dark cycle. Commercial rodent ration (Harlan Teklad Rodent Diet 8604) was available freely, as was acidified (pH=2.5) water to control opportunistic infections.

Experimental Design

At 12 weeks of age, mice received either 15% TSBA full-thickness burn or were sham-treated. Two sets of experiments were conducted; the first set (twenty-one animals for each experimental and control group) was for examination of survival rate, urine proteinuria, and the development of "lupus like" cutaneous lesion formations on the ears, neck and dorsum until the mice reached 9 months of age (6 months post injury). At days 1, 3, and 7 post injury, skin biopsies from another cohort of mice (n = 3 mice per group at each time point) were excised from the wound margin and screened using a custom made RT-PCR microarrays (Applied Biosystems Foster City, CA) containing oligo sequences for 184 inflammatory cytokine and wound repair gene transcripts. Mice that developed severe skin lesions and/or those with proteinuria levels of > 500 dm/dl were euthanized by $C0_2$ inhalation followed by cervical dislocation. Immediately, post euthanasia, blood samples were collected by cardiac puncture for examination of serum IgG levels. Spleen and kidneys were removed for evaluating splenomegaly, and immunopathology, respectively. Skin lesions and adjacent normal skin were excised, fixed with 10% formalin, embedded in paraffin, and sectioned. After deparaffinization and rehydration, 5 μm sections were washed (3x) with PBS and stained with hematoxylin and eosin (HandE). In the latter set of experiments (n=5 mice per group), isogeneic skin graft experiments were conducted on mice 30-40 days post burn injury or sham-treatment. Graft survival was examined three times weekly for 1 month. Photographs of skin lesions, skin grafts, and histological sections were taken with a digital Fuji Finepix

Camera or a Nikon DXM 1200 Digital Camera mounted on a Nikon Eclipse E800 microscope. Images were imported into Adobe Photoshop CS2 for reproduction.

Burn Injury Model

Mice were anesthetized using either an intraperitoneal injection of ketamine (75 mg/kg), xylazine (15 mg/kg), acepromazine (2.5 mg/kg) or isoflurane inhalation. After shaving the dorsum, the exposed skin was washed gently with room temperature sterile water and prepped with Betadine (a 10% povidone-iodine solution for skin disinfection). The Betadine solution from the prepped area was wiped off using 3 series of sponge gauzes containing 70% isopropyl alcohol. In a few selected studies, mice were further treated with a depilatory agent (Nair) to remove remaining hair stubble. Using a surgical skin marker, a 15mm diameter circular area along the dorsal midline region was outlined. A full thickness burn (10-15% total body) was introduced with an electrocautery bovie (370-400°C for 1.5 sec: Bovie Aaron Medical, St. Petersburg, FL). This protocol causes a well demarcated, full thickness, injury in anesthetized mice that is nonlethal with < 0.5% mortality. Wounds became covered with eschar, and there was no macroscopic evidence of infection. Wounds were topically treated with Bacitracin immediately after the burn and left uncovered without a dressing. Once mice recovered from anesthesia, they were placed in separate cages and maintained under standard conditions in the animal facility. With the exception of pain medication (Buprenorphine 0.1 mg/kg SC BID; Reckitt Benckiser Pharmaceuticals, Richmond, VA) for the first two days post burn, no other treatment or topical wound care was administered. At various time points post injury mice were euthanized by CO_2 inhalation followed by cervical dislocation.

Skin Lesions, Splenomegaly and Lymphadenopathy

Following wounding and sham treatment, mice were observed weekly for skin lesions and protruding lymph nodes (cervical, brachial and inguinal). At the time of death or euthanasia, skin lesions were scored by gross pathology using the following scale: 0= none, 1= small and localized to one site (face or ears), 2 = moderate, more than one site involved, < 2 cm (face, ears, dorsum); and 3 = severe, > 2 cm (face, ears and dorsum). Spleens were weighed and enlarged lymph nodes scored on a scale of 0-3 (0= none; 1 = small, at one site; 2 = moderate, more than one site; and 3 = large, more than two sites).

Proteinuria

Urine was tested for proteinuria using commercially available kits (Multistix, Bayer , Elkhart, IN). Proteinuria scored as 0 (negative), <30mg/dl (trace 0.5+), 30 mg/dl (1+), 100 mg/dl (2+) and >500 mg/dl (3+). Animals were considered to have proteinuria if they scored 2+ for two consecutive urine samples.

Measurement of Serum IgG Antibodies

Total serum IgG, IgG1, IgG2a, IgG2b and IgG3 isotype concentrations were determined by ELISA. Polystyrene plates precoated with goat anti-mouse Fc specific IgG capture antibody and blocked were commercially purchased (RandD Systems, Minneapolis, MN). 100 μl of Ig standards (Southern Biotechnology Associates, Birmingham, AL) were added per well in a series of 2-fold dilutions (125ng/ml – 3.9ng/ml), and serum Ig concentrations were assessed at a 1:200,000 dilution (100 μl per well). After two hours of incubation at room temperature, the plates were washed three times with phosphate-buffered saline solution (PBS) containing 0.05% Tween-20 (wash buffer). Bound Ig was detected with 100 μl per well of appropriately diluted horseradish peroxidase conjugated anti-IgG (Chemicon, Temecula, CA), IgG1, IgG2a, IgG2b, and IgG3 antibodies (Southern Biotechnology Associates, Birmingham, AL). Secondary antibodies were added to the plates for one hour at room temperature, followed by 3 washes. Then, 100 μl per well of freshly prepared substrate solution containing equal volumes of 0.4g/L 3,3',5,5' tetramethylbenzidine and 0.02% hydrogen peroxide was used to develop the assay (Pierce, Rockford, IL). Reaction was stopped with 100 μl per well of 2N sulfuric acid (Sigma, St Louis, MO) and the absorbance was measured at 450 nm using a 680 Microplate reader (BioRad, Hercules, CA). Results are denoted as the Ig concentration (mg/ml) at various time points.

Measurement of Autoantibodies

Ig class specific anti-DNA antibodies were measured by ELISA. Polystyrene covalink 96-well microtitre plates (Fisher, Pittsburgh, PA) were coated with 50 μl per well of 10 μg/ml Calf Thymus DNA (Sigma, St Louis, MO) and allowed to incubate overnight at 4°C. After washing three times with wash buffer, 300 μl of blocking solution (3% bovine serum albumin, BSA, in PBS) were added per well and incubated for two hours at room temperature. The plates were washed three times with wash buffer and 100 μl of diluted sera were added to each well, (dilutions ranged from 1:50 to 1:100,000). After two hours of incubation at room temperature, plates were washed three times with wash buffer. Then, 100 μl of appropriately diluted horseradish peroxidase conjugated anti- IgG (Chemicon, Temecula, CA), IgG1, IgG2a, IgG2b, and IgG3 antibodies (Southern Biotechnology Associates, Birmingham, AL) were added per well to the plates for one hour, and followed by three washes. 100 μl per well of freshly prepared substrate solution containing equal volumes of 0.4g/L 3,3',5,5' tetramethylbenzidine and 0.02% hydrogen peroxide were used to develop the assay (Pierce, Rockford, IL). Reaction was stopped with 2N sulfuric acid (Sigma, St Louis, MO) and the absorbance was measured at 450 nm using a 680 Microplate reader (BioRad, Hercules, CA). Results are denoted as the OD_{450} at various dilutions.

Renal Pathological Assessment

Mice were euthanized by CO_2 inhalation followed by cervical dislocation, and the kidneys were removed. One kidney was fixed with buffered formalin for > 48 hr, embedded in paraffin blocks, sectioned and stained with hematoxylin and eosin (HandE) or periodic acid Schiff (PAS) by standard methods. Glomerular pathologies were evaluated morphometrically by light microscopy. The glomerular lesion (mesangial hypercellularity, increase in mesangial matrix, crescent formation, and necrosis) was graded on a semiquantitative scale from 0 to 3 (0 = normal, 1 = mild, 2 = moderate, 3 = severe) for more than 20 glomeruli per mouse. Scores assigned to each of these elements were added together to yield a mean renal score. Values were reported as the mean $\pm$ standard deviation (SD) of seven specimens. For immunofluorescence studies of deposition of Ig's, the second kidney was embedded in optimal cutting temperature (OCT) compound (Miles Inc, Elkhart, IN) and snap-frozen in a solution of 2-methylbutane and dry ice. Tissue samples were stored at -80°C.

Immunoflorescence Staining

Snap frozen kidneys were cut into 3μm thick cryosections and frozen tissue sections mounted on glass slides. A DAKO Autostainer Plus Universal Staining System (DAKO, Carpenteria, CA) was used for the immunohistochemical and immunofluorescent staining. Immunofluorescent detection of IgG was performed on sections of frozen blocks of mouse kidney using a FITC-conjugated goat-antimouse Ig antibody (Jackson Immunoresearch Laboratories Inc., West Grove, PA), incubated for 30 minutes at room temperature using a 1:250 dilution prepared with background reducing antibody diluent (DAKO),and visualized by dark field microscopy. Immunohistochemical detection of C3 was performed on sections of frozen blocks of mouse kidney using a labeled polymer (EnVision plus rabbit, DAKO, Carpenteria, CA) for visualization by light field microscopy. Rabbit polyclonal antibody for C3 (Abcam, Cambridge, MA) was used at a dilution of 1:10 with background reducing antibody diluent (DAKO) and incubated for 30 minutes at room temperature. The chromogen 3,3' Diaminobenzidine (DAKO) was used. The sections were counterstained with Hematoxylin (DAKO) and then cover-slipped. Negative tissue controls included normal mouse kidney. Negative reagent controls consisted of a serial section (the second unstained frozen slide), processed identical to the first unstained frozen slide, but normal rabbit serum was substituted for the primary antibody in every assay.

RNA Extraction

Mice were euthanized by CO_2 inhalation followed by cervical dislocation on days 1, 3 and 7 post-burn injury. Total RNA was extracted from skin excised from the wound margin and stored in RNAlater (Ambion, Austin, TX). Briefly, skin tissue was homogenized in Trizol reagent (Invitrogen, Carlsbad, CA) and total RNA was isolated using Qiagen RNeasy Lipid Tissue Mini Kit (QIAGEN Inc. Valencia, CA) according to manufacturer's instructions. RNA's were resuspended in 30 μl of 10 mM Tris buffer, pH 7.5. Sample purity, quantity, and quality was assessed by determining the $A_{260/280}$, $A_{260/230}$ ratio on an Nanodrop Spectrophotometer (NanoDrop Technologies Inc. Wilmington, DE) and by measuring 28S/18S ribosomal RNA ratio and RNA Integrity Number (RIN) using a Agilent 2100 BioAnalyzer (Agilent Technologies Inc. Santa Clara, CA). All Agilent RNA integrity values were ≥ 8.5. Reverse transcription was performed with Roche 1st Strand Synthesis kit (Roche Diagnostics Corporation, Indianapolis, IN). Briefly, 2.5 μg of RNA sample was added to a master mix containing 1x reaction buffer, 5 mM $MgCl_2$, 1 mM deoxynucleotide mix, 6.4 μg random primers, 100 units RNase inhibitor, and 40 units AMV reverse transcriptase. 10 mM Tris buffer, pH 7.5 was used to reach 40 μl final reaction volume. Then, final reaction mixture was subjected to a single reverse-transcription cycle of 25 °C for 10 min, 42 °C for 60 min, 99 °C for 5 min, and 4 °C for at least 10 min.

Real-Time quantitative PCR (RT-PCR) Gene Profiling for Proinflammatory Transcripts

Quantitative real-time polymerase chain reaction (RT-PCR) was performed using the ABI Prism 7900HT Sequence Detection System (Applied Biosystems, Foster City, CA). Custom designed 'Wound Repair' TaqMan® Low Density Array (TLDA) cards (Applied Biosystems, Foster City, CA) were used to assess gene expression. The set of TLDA cards were comprised of 184 individual target assays (including respective forward and reverse primers and a dual labeled probe (5'-6-FAM; 3'-MGB)) in quadruplicate on a 384-well card (96 genes per card). Amplification parameters were as follows: one cycle of 50 °C for 2 min and 95 °C for 10 min followed by 40 cycles of 95 °C for 30 sec and 60 °C for 1 min. Two samples were processed on each card.

RT-PCR Data Analysis

RT-PCR data was analyzed using the Sequence Detection System version 2.1 included with the ABI Prism 7900HT SDS and using Microsoft Excel. The threshold cycle (C_t) for each sample was manually set to 0.2 and the baseline was set between 3 and 15 cycles. 18S ribosomal RNA was used as an endogenous housekeeping control gene for normalization and the comparative C_t method was used to calculate the relative fold expression by $2^{-\Delta\Delta C_T}$ [42, 43]. Assays with C_t values greater than 35 cycles were excluded from analysis.

Skin Transplantation

Full-thickness skin specimens for transplantation were obtained from naïve female MRL/MpJ mice, 8-10 weeks of age, and grafted onto syngeneic naive (8-10 weeks of age) and experimental (15-17 weeks of age) recipient female MRL/MpJ mice which had fully recovered from a previous 15% full-thickness TSBA burn injury. Briefly, full thickness donor skin (3 cm x 3 cm) was harvested from the dorsal skin of euthanized and shaved MRL/MpJ donor mice, and the underside was gently scraped with a scalpel to remove fat and muscle. Skin was immersed in cold PBS prior to transplantation. The dorsal surfaces of anesthetized (i.p. injection of 150 mg/kg ketamine) recipient mice were shaved and washed with 70% ethanol. A graft bed was prepared with fine curved scissors by removing an area of epidermis and dermis down to the level of the intrinsic muscle. Grafts, 3 cm^2 in area, were fitted to the prepared bed without suturing and then covered with an adhesive plastic bandage. After 7 days, the adhesive bandage was removed. Graft survival was then followed by daily visual inspection. Rejection was defined as complete necrosis and loss of viable skin tissue.

Statistics

Mann-Whitney's *U* test was used to determine the statistical significance of differences between groups. Survival, incidence of proteinuria, and skin graft rejection-survival was analyzed by the Kaplan-Meier method and the Log-rank test was used to determine the statistical significances. P-values less than 0.05 were considered significant.

RESULTS

Severely Injured MRL/MpJ Mice Develop a "Lupus-Like" Syndrome

To assess the role of wound trauma on SLE-like disease development in MRL/MpJ mice and control BALB/c were subjected to either a full-thickness 15% TSBA burn on the dorsum or sham-treated. Mice were examined at least twice a week for 6 months the development of gross skin rashes, ear necrosis, or lymphadenopathy. Results illustrated in Figures 1A-1C show that within a 1-2 months timeframe post burn injury MRL/MpJ mice started to spontaneously develop a lupus-like phenotype characterized by severe, excoriating dermatitis-vasculitis in the dorsum and scapular regions $\pm$ ear necrosis. Histological sections of MRL/MpJ skin lesions demonstrate mixed acute and chronic inflammatory cell infiltrates extending from the epidermis to the subcutis with abnormal hair follicle proliferation (data not shown). In contrast, no such lesions were observed in either sham-treated or wounded BALB/c mice.

To assess the effect of burn injury on renal disease development, we monitored urine protein levels on a weekly basis as an index of proteinuria. Mice were considered to have proteinuria if they scored >100 mg/dl (>2+) for two consecutive urine samples within a 2 week timeframe.The cumulative incidence of proteinuria (> 100 mg/dl) for each group of mice is shown in Figure 2A. The incidence and severity of urinary protein scores (Figure 2B) increased in injured MLR/MpJ mice over time compared to sham-treated MRL/MpJ mice, wherein only 1 mouse developed severe proteinuria at day 135 post treatment. In contrast, minimal protein levels were detected in the urine collected from burn injured or sham-treated BALB/c mice throughout the study interval (data not shown).

As shown in Figure 1C, the observed occurrence of severe skin lesions and proteinuria results in death 1-2 months later. MRL/MpJ presenting with a SLE lupus-like syndrome died significantly earlier, with a median survival rate of 103 days, when compared to the 100% survival of sham-treated BALB/c mice during the 6 month evaluation time period. Six months after the severe burn injury (mice 8 months of age) only 2 of 21 of the burned MRL/MpJ mice were alive and showed no gross macroscopic evidence of cutaneous autoimmune disease.

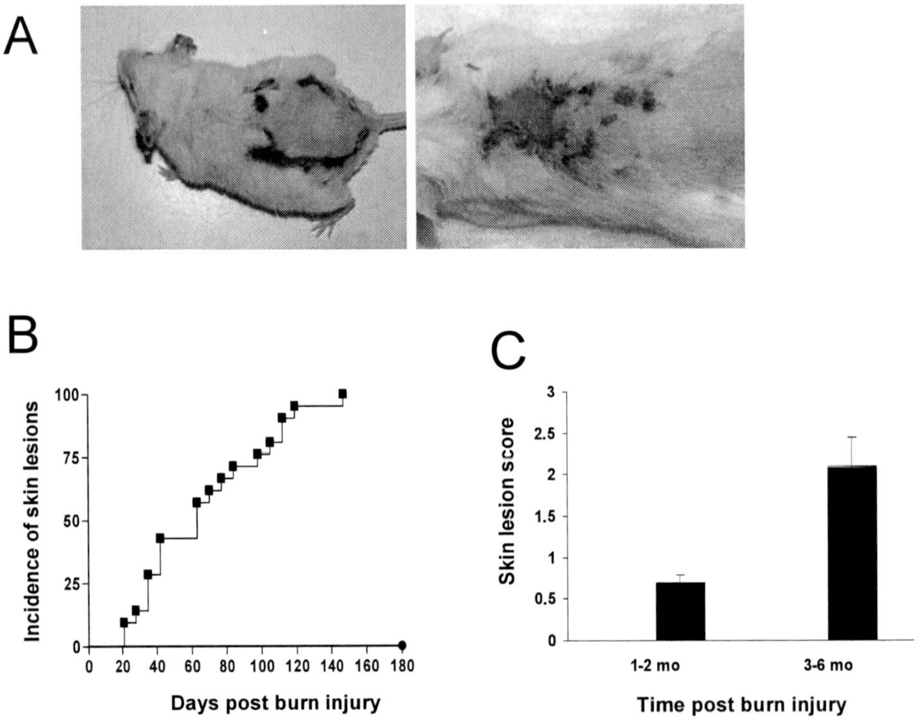

Figure 1. Burn trauma augments SLE development in lupus-prone MRL/MpJ mice. A. Photographs of typical skin and ear lesions in MRL/MpJ mice exhibiting lupus-like symptoms at 2-6 months post burn injury. In contrast, no lesions were observed in burned BALB/c mice or age-matched sham-treated MRL/MpJ mice. B. Cumulative incidence burn injured MRL/MpJ mice [■] and sham-treated MRL/MpJ mice [●] exhibiting skin lesions. C. Mean skin lesion score (*see Material and Methods*) of burninjured mice [■] and sham-treated mice [□].

As depicted in Figures 1C, a biphasic survival response ensued with a cohort of MRL/MpJ mice that displayed autoimmunity within 1-2 months post burn injury and a separate cohort of MRL/MpJ mice that developed cutaneous lupus-like lesions 4-6 months post burn injury.

For this reason, data from these two groupings were pooled and evaluated separately. In sharp contrast, 19 of 21 sham-treated age-matched control MRL/MpJ mice survived to greater than 36 weeks of age and showed no incidence of cutaneous disease and minimal proteinuria during the same observation period. One sham-treated MRL/MpJ mouse spontaneously died at 3 month of age and the other at 5 month of age with unknown causes of deaths. Sham-treated (21 of 21) and burn injured BALB/c mice (21 of 21) appeared normal and healthy throughout the study period, showed no signs of proteinuria or premature death and thus were not evaluated rigorously. Notably, at the time of euthanasia the comparison of spleen weights between wounded MRL/MpJ mice at 4-6 months post injury and sham-treated mice at 6 months post injury, revealed a mild splenomegaly (~1.7-fold increase) in mice exhibiting lupus-like disease (393 $\pm$ 90mg, n=10 versus 231 $\pm$ 60 mg, n=13, $P< 0.05$, Figure 3A). Similar increases were noted in the size of some of the cervical, brachial and inguinal lymph nodes. Approximately, 30% of the mice with skin lesions had enlarged lymph nodes at 4-6 months post burn injury, while sham-treated MRL/MpJ mice did not exhibit visible signs of enlarged lymph nodes (Figure 3B). In comparison, no significant differences in spleen weight and lymph nodes size between sham-treated and wounded BALB/c mice was observed (data not shown).

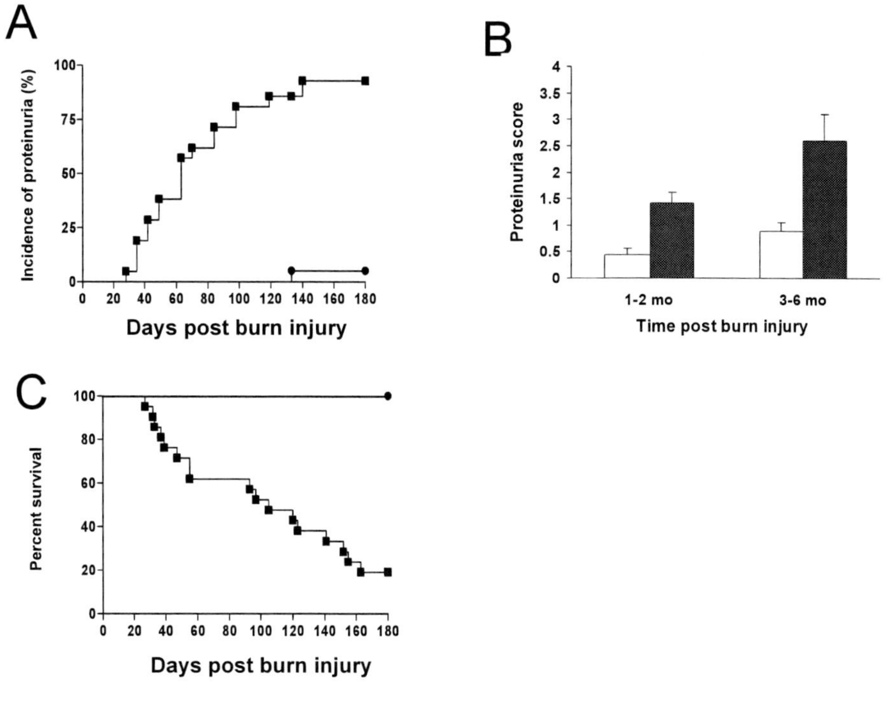

Figure 2. Wounded lupus-prone MLR/MpJ develop proteinuria and have marked decrease survival in comparison either to age-matched sham-treated MRL/MpJ mice or control BALB/c mice (data not shown). (A) Cumulative incidence of proteinuria (> 100mg/dl) (B) Mean proteinuria score (*see Material and Methods*) of burn injured mice [■] and sham-treated mice [□]. (C) Percent survival rate of burn injured MRL/MpJ mice (■) and sham-treated MRL/MpJ mice [●].

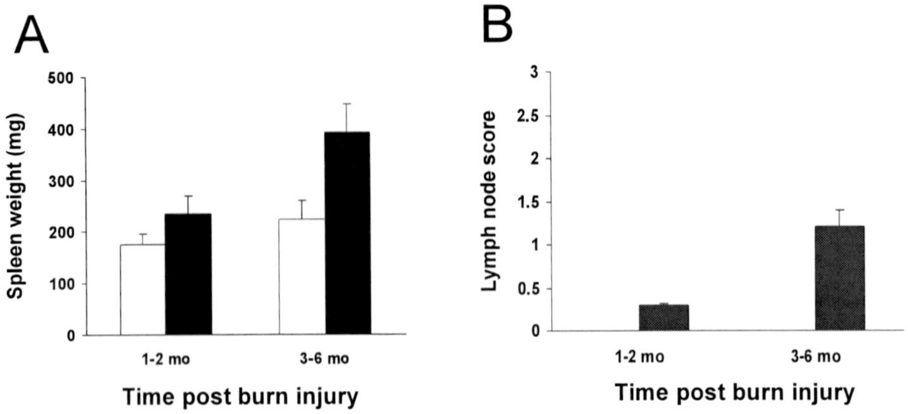

Figure 3. Spleen weights (A) and lymph node scores (B) in burn injured mice [■] and sham-treated mice [□] MRL/MpJ lupus prone mice. * $p < 0.05$.

Serum Hypergammaglobulinemia and Anti-DNA Antibodies

Hypergammaglobulinemia and elevated levels of autoantibodies, such as anti-dsDNA antibody, in the serum are characteristic of autoimmune disease in lupus-prone mice. To determine whether burn injury affected serum Ig concentrations in MRL/MpJ mice, we measured serum IgG1, IgG2a, IgG2b and IgG3 isotype specific anti-dsDNA antibodies by ELISA at 0-1, 2-3 and 4-6 months post burn injury and in sham-treated mice at 6 months (end of study). As shown in Table 1, burn injury in MRL/MpJ mice induced a significant elevation (up to threefold increase) of serum IgG1, IgG2a, IgG2b and IgG3 isotypes in comparison to Ig levels in the serum of sham-treated MRL/MpJ mice after 6 months of time. Isotypic analysis of serum anti-dsDNA antibodies revealed significant elevations in serum anti-dsDNA IgG2a, IgG2b and IgG3 levels were differentially induced between wounded MRL/MpJ mice and sham-treated MRL/MpJ mice at 4-6 months post wounding (Figure 4). The ratio of the anti-dsDNA IgG2a to anti-dsDNA IgG1, a parameter of Th1/Th2 balance, was significantly increased in the wounded MRL/MpJ mice at 4-6 months post injury. Notably, the frequency of IgG2a, IgG2b and IgG3 anti-dsDNA antibodies was significantly lower in sham-treated MRL/MpJ mice. As expected, no significant difference in serum IgG isotypes and IgG specific anti-DNA antibodies were detected in either burned or sham-treated BALB/C mice at the end of the study period (data not shown). Thus indicating wound trauma promotes production of anti-dsDNA autoantibodies in lupus-prone mice.

Table 1. Serum IgG subclasses in sham-treated controls and burned MRL/MpJ mice at the time of euthanasia[a]

		Sham-treated	Burned
IgG1	0-2 wks	ND	0.43 ± 0.259
	2-3 mo	ND	5.52 ± 0.77*
	4-6 mo	1 .46 ± 0.18*	4.41 ± 1.88*
IgG2a	0-2 wks	ND	0.14 ± 0.13
	1-2 mo	ND	1.59 ± 0.34*
	3-6 mo	0.64 ± 0.29*	2.16 ± 0.51*
IgG2b	0-2 wks	ND	< 0.014
	1-2 mo	ND	0.17 ± 0.6*
	3-6 mo	0.09 ± 0.03	0.27 ± 0.08*
IgG3	0-2 wks	ND	< 0.01
	1-2 mo	ND	0.17 ± 0.06*
	3-6 mo	0.01 ± 0.01	0.27 ± 0.07*

[a]Sera IgG isotypes were measured by ELISA at 1:200,000 dilution. Results are expressed as the Ig concentration in mg/ml ± SEM.
*$p < 0.05$ versus 0-2 week post burn measurements.

Renal Histopathology

Glomerulonephritis is a characteristic pathological feature of murine SLE. To investigate the effects of burn injury on renal disease progression, kidney sections obtained at the time of necropsy were examined by standard histopathological and immunohistochemical techniques for evidence of glomerular inflammation and immune complex deposition.

The photomicrographs in Figure 4 are representative glomeruli from a wounded MRL/MpJ mouse exhibiting lupus-like syndrome 90 days post injury and glomeruli from an age-matched sham-treated control MRL/MpJ mouse. PAS stained glomeruli from mice presenting with lupus like syndrome typically showed a marked increase in glomerular cellularity with histopathological evidence of diffuse proliferative glomerulonephritis, segmented glomeruli, proliferative changes in mesangial and endothelial cells of the glomeruli, increase in mesangial matrix, capillary basement membrane thickening, mononuclear cell infiltrates in interstitium, and often the presence of intratubular proteinaceous casts. All these findings are indicative of glomerular dysfunction. Kidneys from age-matched sham-injured MRL/MpJ mice revealed glomeruli with normal cellularity, mesangium, and glomerular basement membranes. The average renal lesion score in mice exhibiting lupus-like syndrome was significantly greater than that of uninjured age-matched control MRL/MpJ mice (Figure 4B).

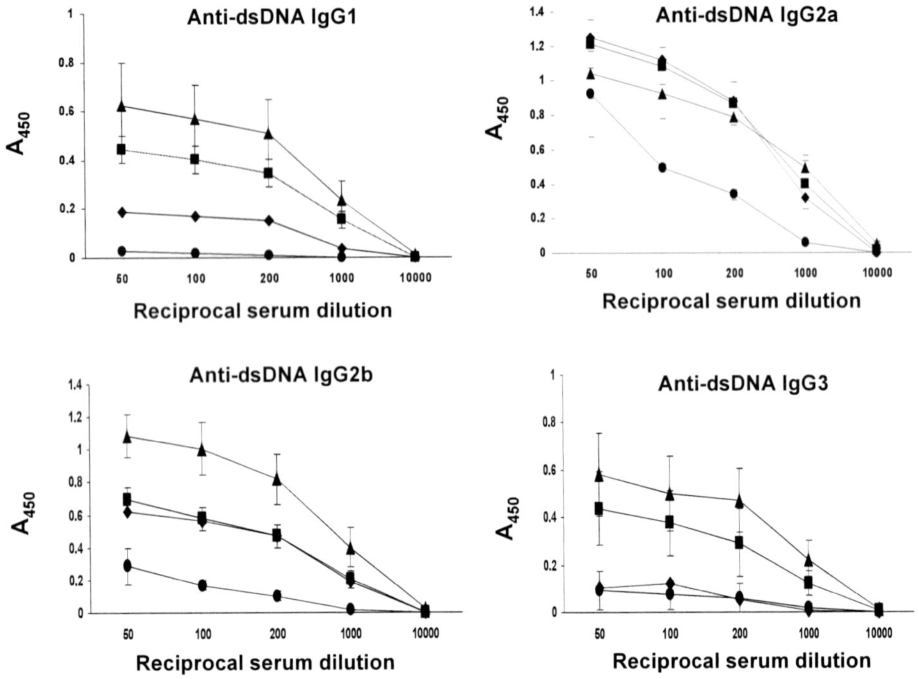

Figure 4. Serum anti-dsDNA antibody titer levels of different IgG subclasses between burn injured MRL/MpJ mice (● 1-2 weeks post burn; ■1-2 months post burn; ▲ 3-6 months post burn) and sham-treated MRL/MpJ mice (♦ 6 months). Reactivity of diluted serum with calf thymus DNA was determined by ELISA. Values are the mean $\pm$ SD absorbance values at 450nm (4-8 serum samples per time point).

Glomeruli from sham-treated or burn injured BALB/c mice showed no evidence of glomerular disease. Consistent with this observation, immunofluorescence staining against total Ig showed intense positive staining of the peripheral capillary loops of the glomeruli from wounded MRL/MpJ mice. Immunostaining against C3 showed comparable immune complex deposition. Such deposits were found mainly within the affected glomeruli. In sharp contrast, immunofluorescence and immunostaining analysis of sham-treated MRL/MpJ kidneys demonstrated minimal Ig and C3 deposition. Together these findings suggest that wound trauma promotes glomerulonephritis in lupus-prone mice.

Expression of Cytokine mRNA in Skin Post Burn Injury

Abnormalties in cytokine production have been shown to contribute to the development of autoimmune disease in lupus-prone mice.

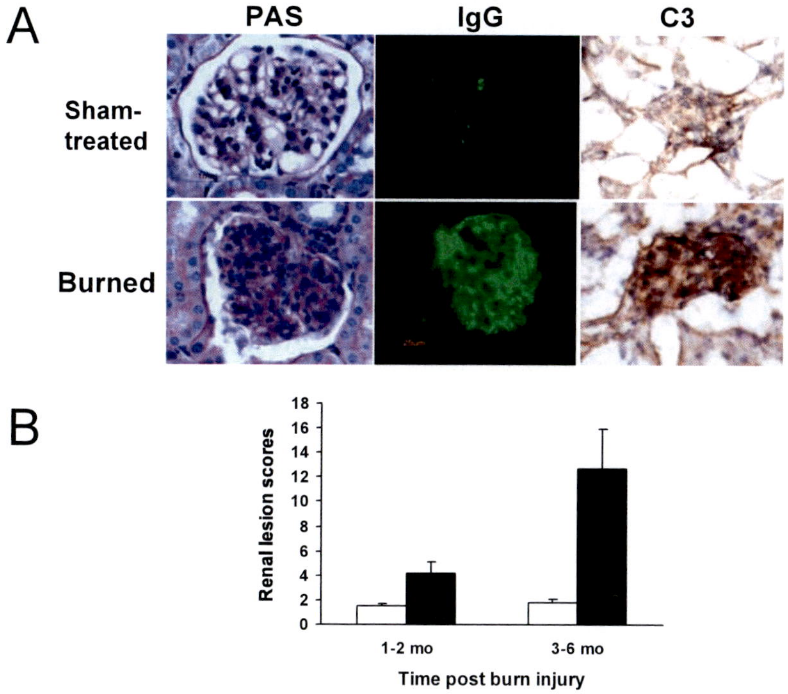

Figure 5. Accelerated glomerulonephritis and immune complex deposition in lupus-prone MRL/MpJ mice following burn injury trauma. (A) At the time of sacrifice, the kidneys were removed and then sectioned before staining with PAS, FITC-conjugated anti-mouse IgG, or anti-mouse C3. Representative photomicrographs of glomeruli from burn injured and sham-treated MRL/MpJ mice are shown (400x magnification; scale bars = 25 μm). In burn injured mice immunofluorescence for IgG was diffusely, globally and strongly present as intraglomerular deposits in the mesangium and capillary wall. C3 staining was present multifocally or globally as intraglomerular deposits in the cytoplasm of the mesangium and capillary wall. C3 deposits resulted in a thick appearance of the glomerular capillary loops. These IgG and C3 deposits resulted in a thick appearance of glomerular capillary loops. The level of Ig and C3 immunostaining was strong in comparison to age-matched sham-treated mice. (B) Kidney sections were graded for glomerular inflammation, cellular infiltration, proliferation, crescent formation, and necrosis. Scores from 0 to 3+ were assigned to each of these elements and then added together to yield a mean renal score (n= 5 mice; 10-15 glomeruli per kidney section were counted, 2-3 sections per mouse).

To determine whether accelerated lupus onset in burn injured MRL/MpJ mice is related to aberrant expression of mediators that play a role in the early inflammatory response, we measured the transcript levels of 184 genes (cytokines, chemokines, growth factors, wound repair response mediators) using custom made taqman cDNA arrays. We identified that transcripts for IL-1β, TNF-α and PGE2 were elevated in burned MRL/MpJ mice skin for the first 7 days (Figure 5) when compared to the expression levels of these mediators in the wound margins of burned BALB/c mice, which fail to develop cutaneous and renal autoimmunity. There was no significant difference in the expression of both Th1 and Th2 cytokine and other inflammatory gene transcripts between MRL/MpJ and BALB/c mice (data not shown).

Skin Isograft Rejection

To determine whether injured MRL/MpJ mice developed T-cell mediated autoimmunity following severe burn injury, we evaluated whether these mice could mount an isograft rejection response. We transplanted syngeneic naïve skin onto the dorsum of MRL/MpJ mice 30-40 days post burn injury. Graft survival was determined and compared with that of non-injured age-matched control MRL/MpJ mice. As shown in Figure 6, MRL/MpJ mice that were previously subjected to severe wound trauma promptly rejected the naïve MRL/MpJ syngeneic skin, with a mean survival time of 8 days (n = 5). Histological analysis of the isografts revealed heavy lymphocytic infiltration and extensive tissue damage (data not shown).

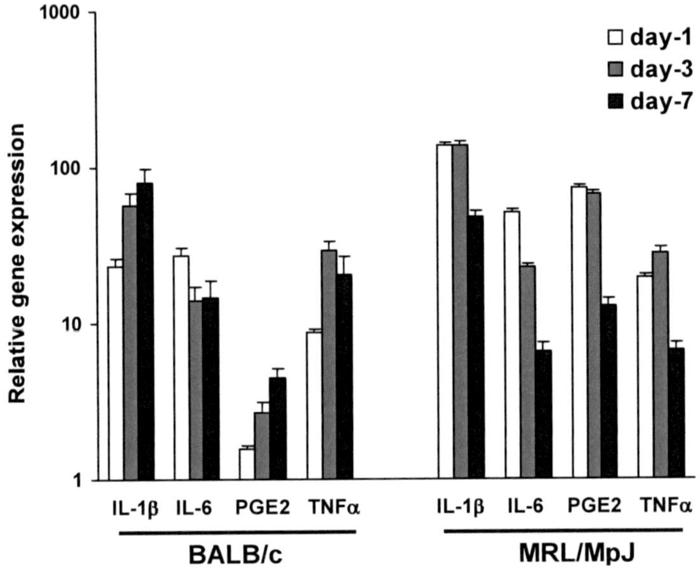

Figure 6. Quantitative analysis of IL-1β, IL-6, TNF-α and PGE-2 transcripts in MRL/MpJ and BALB/c wound margin skin tissue at days 1, 3, and 7 days post burn injury. The results represent the mean ± SD (n= 6) relative gene expression level of transcripts in comparison to those levels present in naïve skin.

In contrast, skin graft sites (n = 5) on sham-treated MRL/MPJ mice were uniformly healed by 2-weeks post transplantation. The graft integrity remained intact throughout the 30-day observation period without any gross visible evidence of rejection. Microscopic evaluations of these grafts failed to identify any inflammatory lesions and revealed normal epidermis and dermis architecture.

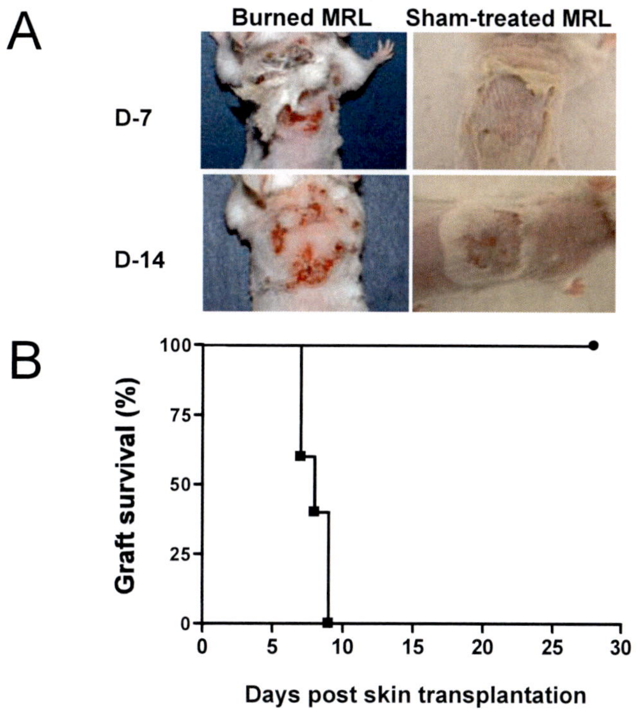

Figure 7. Burn injury in lupus-prone MRL/MpJ mice results in the loss of tolerance to self. Severely injured MRL/MpJ mice reject skin isografts from naïve MRL/MpJ donors whereas skin grafts were uniformly healed within 2-weeks and accepted for more than 30 days after transplantation in sham treated age-matched control MRL/MpJ recipient mice (n= 5). (A) Photographs of skin isografts at day 7 and 14 post transplantation. (B) Graft survival was determined and presented as a Kaplan-Meier plot (n= 5 per group, $p < 0.05$). Burn injured MRL/MpJ mice (■) and sham-treated MRL/MpJ mice [●].

Conclusion

SLE is an autoimmune disease with a complex etiology and is characterized by multiorgan autoreactivity leading to the production of autoantibodies [2, 3, 6]. In this study, we directly demonstrate that severe trauma can be added to the list of triggering events that promote the manifestation of SLE autoimmune disease in lupus-prone MRL/MpJ mice. Unlike wounded BALB/c mice (non-lupus prone), wounded MRL/MpJ mice show accelerated lethality, or had to be euthanized, within 2-6 months post-wounding due to complications associated with spontaneous development of severe vasculitis, lymphoadenopathy, or renal injury. Wounded MRL/MpJ mice (18 of 20 mice; 90%), unlike sham-treated mice or wounded BALB/c control non-lupus mice, developed severe skin lesions, hypergammaglobulinemia, increased circulating levels of anti-dsDNA antibodies, proteinuria, and renal pathologies. Light, immunohistochemical and immunofluorescent microscopic examination of glomeruli showed mesanglial proliferation, diffuse thickening of the basement membrane, inflammatory cell infiltration, and marked Ig and C3 deposition in glomeruli. Even more striking, we observed that MRL/MpJ mice, at 30-40 days after injury recovery, rejected syngeneic skin grafts at a time when disease onset was first evident at the macroscopic level. In contrast, sham-treated mice differ in their incidence of autoimmune disease progression, anti-dsDNA antibodies, immune complex glomerulonephritis and survival (1 out of 20 mice died < 6 months post burn injury) rate.

Severe injury has been shown to lead to pronounced defects in immune function, including increased proinflammatory cytokine production, decreased antigen recognition, increased Th2 cytokine production, and altered antibody production [30, 33, 36, 44-48]. Among other factors, imbalances in pro and anti-inflammatory cytokine production is thought to play a major role in the progression of autoimmune SLE disease [49-54]. Despite strain differences in expression, we found that IL-1β, IL-6, TNFα, and PGE2 transcripts were consistently elevated in MRL/MpJ wounds compared to BALB/c wounds. However, the degree of over expression differed greatly with IL-1β and PGE2 most markedly elevated. These factors are produced primarily by activated macrophages during an inflammatory insult and have potent stimulatory effects on T and B lymphocytes, NK cells and neutrophils, increasing PGE2 synthesis and acute phase protein production by these cells [55-59]. In major burns there is an abundant release of proinflammatory mediators that contribute to macrophage hyperstimulation [57]. After several days the hyperstimulated macrophages become globally inhibitory and induce elevated production of IL-10, which enhances Th2 responses [56-58, 60]. Our findings are consistent with studies suggesting potent local and systemic roles for proinflammatory mediators (IL-1β, IL-6, TNFα) in promoting the differentiation of Th2 autoimmune responses in both SLE patients and lupus-prone mice [38, 52-54, 61-67] . On the other hand, we found no evidence for increased expression of IL-1α, IL-2, IL-4, IL-5, IL-10, and TGF-β, transcripts in MRL/MpJ wounds when compared to BALB/c wounds. Furthermore, Voronov et al [68] and Liang et al [69] reported that IL-1β deficient mice and anti-IL-6 antibody treated mice are resistant to SLE induction, respectively. In our study, despite the marked increase in cytokine levels in the adjacent wound tissue at days 1-7 post burn injury the absolute levels of IL-1, IL-2, IL-4, IL-5, IL-6, IL-8, IL-10, IL-12, TNFα, and IFNγ in the serum were unaltered when compared to sham-treated control mice (data not shown). On the other hand, we did not monitor circulating and tissue levels of cytokines throughout disease progression. Therefore, the systemic kinetics of early Th1 versus Th2 responses following burn injury in MRL/MpJ mice and their correlation link with increasing autoimmune disease severity remains unclear.

The over expression (hyperstimulation) of IL-1 in MRL/MpJ wounds is intriguing given that marrow derived and peritoneal macrophages from SLE-prone mice have been shown to under express IL-1β and other multiple cytokines in response to LPS stimulation, apoptotic cells, other macrophage activators and danger signals due to a cell membrane signaling defect [70-73]. IL-1β can stimulate Ig production directly or synergize with other B-cell stimulatory factors [61,74]. Post severe burn injury, macrophage overstimulation has been shown to lead to global down modulation of inflammatory cytokine production and elevated anti-inflammatory IL-10 and PGE2 synthesis, which have been shown to augment Th2 immune responses. Elevated production of Th2-dependent Ig autoantibody subclasses in the serum of wounded MRL mice strongly suggests a skewing of the Th1/Th2 balance toward a Th2 response. MRL/MpJ wounded mice had significantly elevated serum levels of anti-dsDNA antibodies of the IgG1, IgG2b, and IgG3 isotypes, isotype switching which is known to be dependent on Th2 cytokines [64, 65]. Our results are consistent with the model that glomerulonephritis in autoimmune kidney disease is predominantly dependent upon IgG2b and IgG3 Th2-dependent nephritogenic autoantibodies, deposition [75, 76]. Recently, Shimizu et al [77] reported that the nature of Th1/Th2 response is critical in determining the type and severity of glomerulonephritis that develops in lupus prone mice.

Mice from the MRL strain are prone to develop systemic lupus erythematosus and have demonstrated accelerated wound healing and scarless tissue regeneration, however many of the mechanisms involved in these clinically relevant pathologies are unclear [78-80]. Notably, the nature of the antigen may be important in driving autoimmune pathology in lupus-prone mice. In burn wounds, clearing a plethora of self-antigens in necrotic tissue is an essential role of the macrophage and contributes to their hyperstimulated state [31, 60]. Macrophages from lupus-prone strains have been shown to have an apoptotic-dependent autoimmune phenotype which includes aberrant cytokine expression [73]. Importantly, non-autoimmune mice do not demonstrate this defect. Dysregulated functional activity (decreased phagocytosis, errors in self-Ag recognition and processing) and aberrant signaling events (cytokines, apoptotic ligands and receptors) involved with the clearance of apoptotic cells are thought to predispose an individual to autoimmune disease [15, 73, 81-85]. Rapid clearance of apoptotic cells is essential to prevent intracellular leakage of toxic cell contents, additional inflammatory cascades and the shift from tolerance to immunity [86-88].Thus, effective clearance of apoptotic cells might be an active process of immune tolerance following a traumatic injury or “danger signal” minimizing exposure to self antigens and the expansion of self-reactive effector T cells.

Autoimmunity coincides with the loss of tolerance to the self [1, 20]; it is thought of as a persistent failure of an integrated fabric of components rather than the adverse consequence of a specific "forbidden clone" [89, 90]. In comparison to uninjured MRL/MpJ mice, where skin acceptance and healing in the gross appeared to be complete at 14 days with a full pelt of hair by day 21, syngeneic skin grafts in previously wounded MRL/MpJ mice were uniformly rejected in 7-10 days. Thus, isografts were accepted in tolerant mice and rejected in mice exhibiting immunological reactivity against self (autoimmune). At this time, it is unclear whether the antigen-driven isograft rejection response is primarily T-cell or B-cell (humoral) mediated or both, although we detected high serum levels of autoimmune antibodies. No doubt, specific factors associated with severe trauma and the subsequent wound healing processes in lupus-prone mice play a role in triggering latent autoimmune responses. The relationship between the factors that trigger the early onset and development of autoimmune disease following traumatic injury remain to be defined. Our central hypothesis is that “the activation of specific cell types and the expression of genes, cytokines, and other mediators affecting wound healing and repair processes may be critical in the breakdown of self versus non-self recognition triggering autoimmune diseases following traumatic tissue injury”.

In summary, our research shows that traumatic injury can activate the SLE disease processes. The link between traumatic injury and the manifestation of SLE, along with the increasing numbers of female U.S. military personnel deployed to theatre, make autoimmune diseases, like SLE, highly relevant to military populations. Improved understanding of the mechanisms triggering SLE and disease progression could lead to diagnostic and prevention strategies that would reduce the negative impact of SLE not only on individual Warfighters, but the hundreds of thousands of civilians stricken with this debilitating (and potentially life-threatening) disease.

Acknowledgements

This work was supported by ONR work unit 601153N.4508.519.A0508.

The authors are employees of the U.S. Government. This work was prepared as part of their official duties. Title 17 U.S.C. §105 provides that 'Copyright protection under this title is not available for any work of the United States Government.' Title 17 U.S.C §101 defined a U.S. Government work as a work prepared by a military service member or employees of the U.S. Government as part of that person's official duties. The opinions or assertions contained in this paper are the private views of the authors and are not to be construed as reflecting the views, policy or positions of the Department of the Navy, Department of the Army, Department of Defense nor the U.S. Government. The experiments reported herein were conducted in compliance with the Animal welfare Act and in accordance with the principles set forth in the current edition of the *Guide for Care and Use of Laboratory Animals*, Institute for Laboratory Animal Resources, National Research Council, National Academy Press, 1996.

References

[1] Kyewski, B. and Klein, L. (2006) A CENTRAL ROLE FOR CENTRAL TOLERANCE. *Annual Review of Immunology* 24 (1), 571-606.

[2] Klinman, D.M. and Steinberg, A.D. (1995) Inquiry into murine and human lupus. *Immunol Rev.* 144, 157-193.

[3] McAlindon, T. (2000) Update on the epidemiology of systemic lupus erythematosus: New spins on old ideas. *Current Opinion in Rheumatology* 12 (2), 104-112.

[4] Ward, M.M. and Studenski, S. (1990) Age associated clinical manifestations of systemic lupus erythematosus: a multivariate regression analysis. *J. Rheumatol.* 17 (4), 476-481.

[5] Kotzin, B.L. (1996) Systemic lupus erythematosus. *Cell* 85 (3), 303-306.

[6] Mok, C.C. and Lau, C.S. (2003) Pathogenesis of systemic lupus erythematosus. *J. Clin. Pathol.* 56 (7), 481-490.

[7] Ward, M.M. et al. (1996) Mortality risks associated with specific clinical manifestations of systemic lupus erythematosus. *Arch. Intern. Med.* 156 (12), 1337-1344.

[8] Wallace, D.J. (1987) The role of stress and trauma in rheumatoid arthritis and systemic lupus erythematosus. *Semin Arthritis Rheum.* 16 (3), 153-157.

[9] Blanchard, M.S. et al. (2006) Chronic multisymptom illness complex in Gulf War I veterans 10 years later. *Am. J. Epidemiol.* 163 (1), 66-75.

[10] Eisen, S.A. et al. (2005) Gulf War veterans' health: medical evaluation of a U.S. cohort. *Ann. Intern. Med.* 142 (11), 881-890.

[11] Rook, G.A.W. and Zumla, A. (1997) Gulf War syndrome: is it due to a systemic shift in cytokine balance towards a Th2 profile? *The Lancet* 349 (9068), 1831-1833.

[12] Black, D.W. et al. (2000) Multiple Chemical Sensitivity Syndrome: Symptom Prevalence and Risk Factors in a Military Population. *Arch. Intern Med.* 160 (8), 1169-1176.

[13] Payne, D.C. et al. (2006) Development of the Vaccine Analytic Unit's research agenda for investigating potential adverse events associated with anthrax vaccine adsorbed. *Pharmacoepidemiol Drug Saf* 16 (1), 45-54.

[14] Hyams, K.C. (2005) Commentary: Adding to our comprehension of Gulf War health questions. *Int. J. Epidemiol.* 34 (4), 808-809.

[15] Drosera, M. et al. (2006) Role of soluble and cell surface molecules in the pathogenesis of autoimmune skin diseases. *Clin. Exp. Rheumatol.* 24 (1 Suppl 40), S7-13.

[16] Sarzi-Puttini, P. et al. (2005) Drug-induced lupus erythematosus. *Autoimmunity* 38 (7), 507-518.

[17] Sarzi-Puttini, P. et al. (2005) Environment and systemic lupus erythematosus: an overview. *Autoimmunity* 38 (7), 465-472.

[18] Parks, C.G. and Cooper, G.S. (2005) Occupational exposures and risk of systemic lupus erythematosus. *Autoimmunity* 38 (7), 497-506.

[19] Ravel, G. et al. (2004) Autoimmunity, environmental exposure and vaccination: is there a link? *Toxicology* 196 (3), 211-216.

[20] McClain, M.T. et al. (2005) Early events in lupus humoral autoimmunity suggest initiation through molecular mimicry. *Nat. Med.* 11 (1), 85-89.

[21] Cooper, G.S. et al. (2002) Risk factors for development of systemic lupus erythematosus: allergies, infections, and family history. *J. Clin. Epidemiol.* 55 (10), 982-989.

[22] Pope, J.E. et al. (2004) Close association of herpes zoster reactivation and systemic lupus erythematosus (SLE) diagnosis: case-control study of patients with SLE or noninflammatory nusculoskeletal disorders. *J. Rheumatol* .31 (2), 274-279.

[23] Murphy, F. et al. (1997) Women in the Persian Gulf War: health care implications for active duty troops and veterans. *Mil. Med.* 162 (10), 656-660.

[24] Martin, P. (1997) Wound healing--aiming for perfect skin regeneration. *Science* 276 (5309), 75-81.

[25] Hunt, T.K. et al. (1999). Wound healing. *Science* 284 (5421), 1775.

[26] Thornton, F.J. et al. (1997) Wound healing in sepsis and trauma. *Shock* 8 (6), 391-401.

[27] Menke, N.B. et al. (2007) Impaired wound healing. *Clinics in Dermatology* 25 (1), 19-25.

[28] Mast, B.A. and Schultz, G.S. (1996) Interactions of cytokines, growth factors, and proteases in acute and chronic wounds. *Wound Repair Regen* 4 (4), 411-420.

[29] Trengove, N.J. et al. (1999) Analysis of the acute and chronic wound environments: the role of proteases and their inhibitors. *Wound Repair Regen* 7 (6), 442-452.

[30] O'Sullivan, S.T. and O'Connor, T.P. (1997) Immunosuppression following thermal injury: the pathogenesis of immunodysfunction. *Br. J. Plast. Surg.* 50 (8), 615-623.

[31] Foex, B.A. (1999) Systemic responses to trauma. *Br. Med. Bull.* 55 (4), 726-743.

[32] Schlag, G. and Redl, H. (1996) Mediators of injury and inflammation. *World J. Surg.* 20 (4), 406-410.

[33] Lederer, J.A. et al. (1999) The effects of injury on the adaptive immune response. *Shock* 11 (3), 153-159.

[34] Rennie, M.J. (1985) Muscle protein turnover and the wasting due to injury and disease. *Br. Med. Bull.* 41 (3), 257-264.

[35] Sauaia, A. et al. (1996) Early risk factors for postinjury multiple organ failure. *World J. Surg.* 20 (4), 392-400.

[36] O'Sullivan, S.T. et al. (1995) Major injury leads to predominance of the T helper-2 lymphocyte phenotype and diminished interleukin-12 production associated with decreased resistance to infection. *Ann. Surg.* 222 (4), 482-490; discussion 490-482.

[37] Akahoshi, M. et al. (1999) Th1/Th2 balance of peripheral T helper cells in systemic lupus erythematosus. *Arthritis Rheum.* 42 (8), 1644-1648.

[38] Funauchi, M. et al. (1998) Decreased Th1-like and increased Th2-like cells in systemic lupus erythematosus. *Scandinavian Journal of Rheumatology* 27 (3), 219-224.

[39] Liu, T.F. and Jones, B.M. (1998) Impaired production of IL-12 in systemic lupus erythematosus: IL-12 production in vitro is correlarted negatively with serum IL-10, positively with serum IFN-gamma and negatively with disease activity in SLE. *Cytokine* 10 (2), 148-153.

[40] Theofilopoulos, A.N. and Dixon, F.J. (1985) Murine models of systemic lupus erythematosus. *Adv. Immunol* .37, 269-390.

[41] Liu, K. and Mohan, C. (2006) What do mouse models teach us about human SLE? *Clin. Immunol.* 119 (2), 123-130.

[42] Hoffmann, S.C. et al. (2003) Immune profiling: molecular monitoring in renal transplantation. *Front Biosci.* 8, e444-462.

[43] Livak, K.J. and Schmittgen, T.D. (2001) Analysis of relative gene expression data using real-time quantitative PCR and the 2(-Delta Delta C(T)) Method. *Methods* 25 (4), 402-408.

[44] Decker, D. et al. (1996) Surgical stress induces a shift in the type-1/type-2 T-helper cell balance, suggesting down-regulation of cell-mediated and up-regulation of antibody-mediated immunity commensurate to the trauma. *Surgery* 119 (3), 316-325.

[45] Mack, V.E. et al. (1996) Dominance of T-helper 2-type cytokines after severe injury. *Arch. Surg.* 131 (12), 1303-1308; discussion 1308-1309.

[46] Goebel, A. et al. (2000) Injury induces deficient interleukin-12 production, but interleukin-12 therapy after injury restores resistance to infection. *Ann Surg* 231 (2), 253-261.

[47] Kelly, J.L. et al. (1999) Severe injury triggers antigen-specific T-helper cell dysfunction. *Shock* 12 (1), 39-45.

[48] Miyara, M. et al. (2005) Global natural regulatory T cell depletion in active systemic lupus erythematosus. *J. Immunol.* 175 (12), 8392-8400.

[49] Mosmann, T.R. and Sad, S. (1996) The expanding universe of T-cell subsets: Th1, Th2 and more. *Immunol. Today* 17 (3), 138-146.

[50] Takahashi, S. et al. (1996) Imbalance towards Th1 predominance is associated with acceleration of lupus-like autoimmune syndrome in MRL mice. *J. Clin. Invest.* 97 (7), 1597-1604.

[51] Kelley, V.R. and Wuthrich, R.P. (1999) Cytokines in the pathogenesis of systemic lupus erythematosus. *Semin. Nephrol.* 19 (1), 57-66.

[52] Boswell, J.M. et al. (1988) Increased tumor necrosis factor and IL-1 beta gene expression in the kidneys of mice with lupus nephritis. *J. Immunol.* 141 (9), 3050-3054.

[53] Boswell, J.M. et al. (1988) Novel and enhanced IL-1 gene expression in autoimmune mice with lupus. *J. Immunol.* 141 (1), 118-124.

[54] Finck, B.K. et al. (1994) Interleukin 6 promotes murine lupus in NZB/NZW F1 mice. *J. Clin. Invest.* 94 (2), 585-591.

[55] Faunce, D.E. et al. (2003) A role for CD1d-restricted NKT cells in injury-associated T cell suppression. *J. Leukoc. Biol.* 73 (6), 747-755.

[56] Schwacha, M.G. et al. (1998) Thermal injury alters macrophage responses to prostaglandin E2: contribution to the enhancement of inducible nitric oxide synthase activity. *J. Leukoc. Biol.* 64 (6), 740-746.

[57] Schwacha, M.G. and Somers, S.D. (1998) Thermal injury induces macrophage hyperactivity through pertussis toxin-sensitive and -insensitive pathways. *Shock* 9 (4), 249-255.

[58] Schwacha, M.G. and Somers, S.D. (1998) Thermal injury-induced immunosuppression in mice: the role of macrophage-derived reactive nitrogen intermediates. *J. Leukoc. Biol.* 63 (1), 51-58.

[59] Gillitzer, R. and Goebeler, M. (2001) Chemokines in cutaneous wound healing. *J. Leukoc. Biol.* 69 (4), 513-521.

[60] Faist, E. et al. (1988) Alteration of monocyte function following major injury. *Arch. Surg.* 123 (3), 287-292.

[61] Dinarello, C.A. and Savage, N. (1989) Interleukin-1 and its receptor. *Crit. Rev. Immunol.* 9 (1), 1-20.

[62] Prud'homme, G.J. et al. (1995) Quantitative polymerase chain reaction analysis reveals marked overexpression of interleukin-1 beta, interleukin-1 and interferon-gamma mRNA in the lymph nodes of lupus-prone mice. *Mol. Immunol* .32 (7), 495-503.

[63] Jandl, R.C. et al. (1987) The effect of interleukin 1 on IgG synthesis in systemic lupus erythematosus. *Clin. Immunol. Immunopathol* 45 (3), 384-394.

[64] Haas, M. (1994) IgG subclass deposits in glomeruli of lupus and nonlupus membranous nephropathies. *Am. J. Kidney Dis* 23 (3), 358-364.

[65] Imai, H. et al. (1997) IgG subclasses in patients with membranoproliferative glomerulonephritis, membranous nephropathy, and lupus nephritis. *Kidney Int.* 51 (1), 270-276.

[66] Bijl, M. et al. (2002) IgG subclass distribution of autoantibodies differs between renal and extra-renal relapses in patients with systemic lupus erythematosus. *Rheumatology (Oxford)* 41 (1), 62-67.

[67] Steward, M.W. and Hay, F.C. (1976) Changes in immunoglobulin class and subclass of anti-DNA antibodies with increasing age in N/ZBW F1 hybrid mice. *Clin. Exp. Immunol.* 26 (2), 363-370.

[68] Voronov, E. et al. (2006) IL-1 beta-deficient mice are resistant to induction of experimental SLE. *Eur. Cytokine Netw*. 17 (2), 109-116.

[69] Liang, B. et al. (2006) Anti-interleukin-6 monoclonal antibody inhibits autoimmune responses in a murine model of systemic lupus erythematosus. *Immunology* 119 (3), 296-305.

[70] Donnelly, R.P. et al. (1990) Aberrant regulation of IL-1 expression in macrophages from young autoimmune-prone mice. *J. Immunol.* 145 (10), 3231-3239.

[71] Levine, J.S. et al. (1993) Interleukin-1 dysregulation is an intrinsic defect in macrophages from MRL autoimmune-prone mice. *Eur. J. Immunol*. 23 (11), 2951-2958.

[72] Fitzpatrick, J.M. et al. (1996) Dysregulated cytokine expression in vivo in prediseased and diseased autoimmune-prone MRL mice. *Autoimmunity* 23 (4), 217-229.

[73] Koh, J.S. et al. (2000) Cytokine dysregulation induced by apoptotic cells is a shared characteristic of murine lupus. *J. Immunol.* 165 (8), 4190-4201.

[74] Armitage, R.J. et al. (1993) Human B cell proliferation and Ig secretion induced by recombinant CD40 ligand are modulated by soluble cytokines. *J. Immunol.* 150 (9), 3671-3680.

[75] Takahashi, S. et al. (1991) IgG3 production in MRL/lpr mice is responsible for development of lupus nephritis. *J. Immunol.* 147 (2), 515-519.

[76] Lemoine, R. et al. (1992) Induction of "wire-loop" lesions by murine monoclonal IgG3 cryoglobulins. *Kidney Int.* 41 (1), 65-72.

[77] Shimizu, S. et al. (2005) Membranous glomerulonephritis development with Th2-type immune deviations in MRL/lpr mice deficient for IL-27 receptor (WSX-1). *J. Immunol.* 175 (11), 7185-7192.

[78] Davis, T.A. and Lennon, G. (2005) Mice with a regenerative wound healing capacity and an SLE autoimmune phenotype contain elevated numbers of circulating and marrow-derived macrophage progenitor cells. *Blood Cells Mol. Dis.* 34 (1), 17-25.

[79] Davis, T.A. et al. (2005) Prior injury accelerates subsequent wound closure in a mouse model of regeneration. *Cell Tissue Res.* 320 (3), 417-426.

[80] Clark, L.D. et al. (1998) A new murine model for mammalian wound repair and regeneration. *Clin. Immunol. Immunopathol.* 88 (1), 35-45.

[81] Herrmann, M. et al. (1998) Impaired phagocytosis of apoptotic cell material by monocyte-derived macrophages from patients with systemic lupus erythematosus. *Arthritis Rheum.* 41 (7), 1241-1250.

[82] Potter, P.K. et al. (2003) Lupus-prone mice have an abnormal response to thioglycolate and an impaired clearance of apoptotic cells. *J. Immunol.* 170 (6), 3223-3232.

[83] Alleva, D.G. et al. (1997) Aberrant cytokine expression and autocrine regulation characterize macrophages from young MRL+/+ and NZB/W F1 lupus-prone mice. *J. Immunol.* 159 (11), 5610-5619.

[84] Alleva, D.G. et al. (1998) Intrinsic defects in macrophage IL-12 production associated with immune dysfunction in the MRL/++ and New Zealand Black/White F1 lupus-prone mice and the Leishmania major-susceptible BALB/c strain. *J. Immunol.* 161 (12), 6878-6884.

[85] Segal, R. et al. (1997) Kinetics of cytokine production in experimental systemic lupus erythematosus: involvement of T helper cell 1/T helper cell 2-type cytokines in disease. *J. Immunol.* 158 (6), 3009-3016.

[86] Savill, J. et al. (2002) A blast from the past: clearance of apoptotic cells regulates immune responses. *Nat. Rev. Immunol.* 2 (12), 965-975.

[87] Fadok, V.A. et al. (1998) Macrophages that have ingested apoptotic cells in vitro inhibit proinflammatory cytokine production through autocrine/paracrine mechanisms involving TGF-beta, PGE2, and PAF. *J. Clin. Invest.* 101 (4), 890-898.

[88] Aderem, A. and Underhill, D.M. (1999) Mechanisms of phagocytosis in macrophages. *Annu. Rev. Immunol.* 17, 593-623.

[89] Klinman, D.M. and Steinberg, A.D. (1987) Systemic autoimmune disease arises from polyclonal B cell activation. *J. Exp. Med.* 165 (6), 1755-1760.

[90] Peng, S.L. et al. (1996) Propagation and regulation of systemic autoimmunity by gammadelta T cells. *J. Immunol.* 157 (12), 5689-5698.

In: Progress in Systemic Lupus Erythematosus Research
Editor: Tomas I. Seward, pp. 131-153
ISBN 978-1-60021-861-3

Chapter 4

Immunotherapy with Ig-Derived Peptides in SLE: Current Status and Directions

Antonio La Cava** and Bevra H. Hahn
Division of Rheumatology, Department of Medicine,
David Geffen School of Medicine at the University of California Los Angeles,
Los Angeles, California 90095-1670

Abstract

Understanding the mechanisms that control autoimmune reactivity is an essential step to improve management of autoimmune diseases including systemic lupus erythematosus (SLE). In SLE, the interaction between hyperactive T cells and B cells causes dysregulated production of autoantibodies that by themselves or in immune complexes fix to tissue and cause organ damage. The immune cell subsets that take part in this process have come under intense scrutiny in the past few years, and new information has been acquired on how they interact to induce and/or modulate disease. This information has also led to the development of autoantibody-derived peptide therapies that can effectively influence murine SLE. This chapter describes the rationale, current experimental evidence, preclinical models, and future directions for the use of autoantigen- and Ig-derived peptides in SLE. Considering that autoantibodies in lupus patients have amino acid sequences similar to those of murine antibodies, and at similar locations, it is likely that some of those strategies will be potentially useful in the therapy of human SLE.

* Corresponding author. Tel.: (310) 267 4975; Fax: (310) 206 8606; E-mail: alacava@mednet.ucla.edu

Introduction

The functionality of the immune system relies upon an intricate network of interactions among soluble mediators and lymphocyte subpopulations that have both regulatory and effector functions. The fine balance among the components of this network constitutes what is known as immune homeostasis, which is the ability of the immune system to maintain a condition of internal equilibrium even when faced with (mostly external) challenges. If one or more of the mechanisms of immune homeostasis become impaired and unable to control lymphocytes that are autoreactive (reactive to self), autoimmunity can ensue [1-2].

Although autoreactivity is an intrinsic feature of the immune system and is the result of a diverse repertoire protecting individuals from most pathogens, it carries nonetheless the potential risk to harm the host. To prevent such a possibility, several mechanisms are in place to limit the number and/or activity of autoreactive clones. During ontogeny, most of the self-reactive T cells are eliminated in the thymus, and B cells that react against self-determinants are deleted in the bone marrow. However, a large number of autoreactive lymphocytes escape those "central" processes of selection and form a peripheral pool of potentially autoimmunity-inducing lymphocytes (which could become activated in the presence of self-antigens released after destruction of tissue, injury, or inflammation). To avoid the pathological consequences of autoimmune reactivity, several "peripheral" tolerance mechanisms operate throughout life.

Schematically, those mechanisms can be divided into the following: 1) hyporesponsiveness (anergy) to antigenic stimulation; 2) activation-induced cell death (apoptosis), when lymphocytes receive strong activating signals that lead to a cascade of events resulting in cell death; 3) ignorance to antigens that are sequestered in locations not directly exposed to immune surveillance; 4) phenotypic skewing of cytokine production; 5) suppression. The last category includes the action of specialized regulatory/suppressor T lymphocytes that keep autoimmunity at bay via functional or physical inactivation of autoreactive cells. As seen later, those lymphocyte subsets may represent a major target of immune modulation by peptide therapy.

Rationale for Using Peptide-Based Immunotherapy in Autoimmune Disease

Autoimmunity is highly influenced by genetic and environmental factors. A widely accepted view of the pathogenesis of autoimmune diseases is that an abnormal immune response of genetically susceptible individuals to environmental agents can lead to development of autoimmune reactivity, which then is ineffectively controlled by immunoregulatory mechanisms [5]. Once established, the dysregulated activity, function and signaling of immune cells can promote tissue and organ damage concomitantly with an ongoing poorly regulated production of pro-inflammatory soluble mediators [6].

T cells need two signals to become activated. Signal one is given by the engagement of the T cell receptor on the T cell and the major histocompatibility complex (MHC)/peptide complex on the antigen presenting cell (APC). Signal two involves the binding of a costimulatory molecule on the T cell with its ligand on the APC. Increased costimulation in conjunction with a lowered threshold for T-cell activation is common in autoimmunity and contributes to abnormal regulatory and effector immune cell functions [7].

Preclinical studies using various animal models of autoimmune diseases have demonstrated that blocking costimulation (e.g. CTLA-4/CD80/CD86, CD40/CD40 ligand) [8-9] and/or effector $CD4^{+}$ T cells may help to control autoreactivity [10]. Considering that this approach blocks T cell activation in general, it lacks specificity. Therefore, dose and duration of treatment need to be balanced against the risk of side effects. Other therapeutic targets and alternative options that have emerged include soluble receptors, monoclonal antibodies and molecular mimetics or biologicals that can target defined disease pathways [11]. In SLE, candidate molecules for therapies have included antagonists of B-cell-activating molecules such as B lymphocyte stimulator (BLyS), of pro-inflammatory cytokines such as interferon (IFN)-α, and of receptors such as FcγRIIB receptor or the toll-like receptors [12-14]. Selective targeting of selected immune cell subsets (i.e. dendritic cells, $CD20^{+}$ B cells) has also been evaluated with encouraging preliminary results, particularly for B-cell depletion [15-16] (Figure 1).

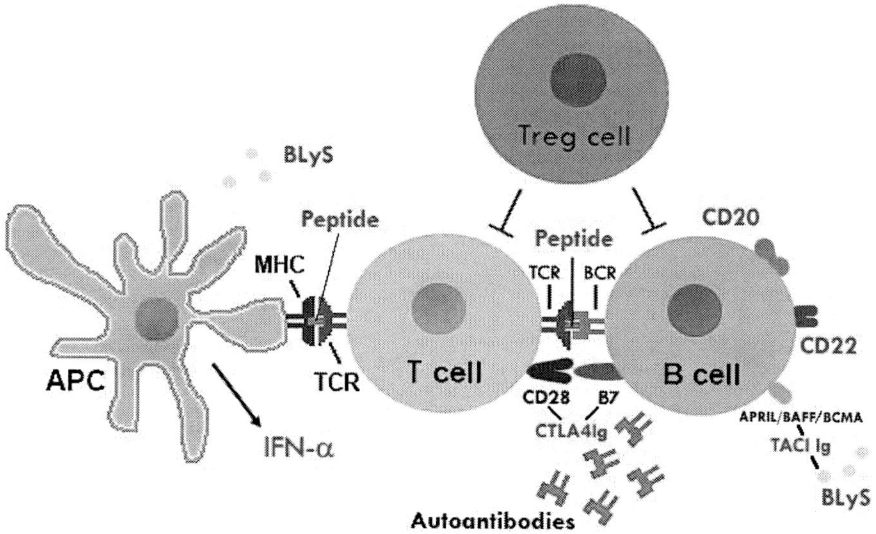

Figure 1. Schematic representation of the current targets of immunotherapy in SLE. After presentation of autoantigen by APC, T cells can provide help to B cells for the production of autoantibodies that cause tissue and organ damage. The targets of immunotherapy are indicated in red and include – in addition to the autoantigen- or Ig-derived peptides described in the chapter – soluble molecules such as IFN-α (targeted by anti-IFN-α antibodies), and BLyS (and/or its receptor(s), targeted by anti-BlyS antibodies or by TACI Ig). Target surface molecules include CD20 (targeted by anti-CD20 antibody), CD22 (targeted by anti-CD22 antibody), and CD28/B7 (targeted by CTLA4 Ig). Other immunotherapeutics not included in the figure are mycophenolate mofetil (which targets intracellular pathways common to T and B cells), and LJP 394 (abetimus sodium), an oligonucleotide of four dsDNA epitopes coupled to an inert platform. The term Tregs refers to regulatory/suppressor T cell subsets with different phenotypes.

The benefits of those approaches vary in degree depending on the disease status, the heterogeneous clinical characteristics of patients, and concomitant therapies. Some of these novel approaches are constrained either by their limited specificity or by concomitant side effects caused by the broad targeting of disparate immune cell subsets and pathways.

To induce immune tolerance with a more specific, selective targeting of antigen-reactive cells (including helper T cells, regulatory t cells and B cells), another approach uses peptides to eliminate only deleterious cells while sparing the host from adverse side effects. The rationale behind this approach is that if a peptide is immunogenic – i.e. it can help to provoke disease – it is then possible that it can also prevent disease when administered at certain "tolerogenic" doses and under defined routes and circumstances [17]. In other words, immunogenic peptides derived from disease-associated antigens that modulate cell functions and/or interactions might replace autoantigens for the modulation of T cell autoreactivity (and thus pathology).

Considerations for Using Peptides to Induce Tolerogenic Immune Responses

The form in which an antigen is administered has a crucial role in influencing the immune system and in inducing an immunogenic response or not, since antigen in aggregated form or mixed with adjuvant provoke immunogenic responses, while soluble monomeric antigens induce tolerance.

To inhibit T-cell activation, soluble synthetic peptides are typically administered using the oral, intravenous, intraperitoneal, or intranasal routes. The mechanisms underlying the induction of tolerance after administration of soluble peptides remain debated and may involve one or more of the mechanisms of peripheral tolerance, with different cells being anergised, killed, regulated, or being functionally diverted during the process of tolerisation. Bystander suppression may be an important additional feature of suppression to several antigens, capable of "spreading" tolerance to additional epitopes and thus helping compensate for the problem that responses to individual antigens may wax and wane over time, even in the same individual [18].

Peptide Selection

The selection of the most appropriate epitopes in the design of therapeutic peptides is crucial for success. An aspect to consider is that a peptide can bind to one or more MHC alleles and not to others. In mice, the use of inbred strains of animals provides major help in the identification and choice of peptides for therapy.

In humans, the polymorphism of the MHC genes represents an important challenge in peptide design. However, certain associations of defined HLA (the human MHC) with autoimmune diseases provide a natural platform for peptide design, once target antigens have been identified [19], to obtain theoretically maximal coverage for most disease-associated alleles in the general population [20].

Peptide Dosage

It may often be difficult to identify the ideal dose of peptide for induction of immune tolerance, considering that both high and low doses may be effective yet responsible for significantly different protective mechanisms. In mice, doses used to induce immune tolerance have ranged from a few micrograms [21] to milligrams [22]. In general, high dose regimens seem to cause substantial deletion of antigen-specific cells [23] and/or T cell anergy [24-25], while both high- and low-dose models seem to induce populations of T cells with immunoregulatory activities [26-28].

Route of Administration

Another crucial aspect in determining the active dose and activity of a peptide is the route of administration, in addition to peptide solubility, half-life, vehicle of administration, and structural characteristics.

The route of administration is central in the activity of a peptide because it can either determine tolerogenicity or immunogenicity (also depending on dosage, as mentioned above). Although intradermal or intravenous administration may require the lowest doses of peptide to achieve tolerogenicity, the inconvenience of injection may favor in some cases the choice of highly effective high-dose regimens - i.e. via intranasal delivery [29]. For example, nasal instillation of lupus-prone SNF1 female mice with a histone-derived peptide $H4_{71\text{-}93}$ induced a dose-dependent nasal tolerance to the peptide before or after peptide sensitization of those mice. The effect was associated with increased production of interleukin (IL)-10 and the suppression of T helper (Th)1-type cytokines by lymph node cells. Chronic nasal instillation of mice with the $H4_{71\text{-}93}$ peptide not only suppressed the development of autoantibodies, but also altered the severity of glomerulonephritis in lupus-prone (SWR x NZB)F_1 (SNF1) mice [30].

Duration of Tolerance

The duration of tolerance has considerable therapeutic implications in the clinical use of peptides. In general, peptide immunotherapy is more effective in preventing rather than reversing or halting disease.

For example, intranasal [31] or intraperitoneal [32] administration of a single dose of a soluble form of a myelin basic protein (MBP) peptide corresponding to the dominant epitope of autoimmune encephalomyelitis is effective in preventing disease for 1–6 weeks [33]. However, from 8 weeks onward, autoreactive responsiveness slowly recovers in euthymic, but not adult, thymectomised mice, suggesting that peptide-induced tolerance is a peripheral phenomenon which can be reversed by new effector T cells exported from the thymus. A consequence of this phenomenon is that sustained suppression by peptide therapy may require repeated administration of peptide, as suggested by many studies [34].

Mechanisms of Peptide-Induced Tolerisation: The Role of APCs

The binding of a peptide to the MHC has to mimic the naturally processed epitope of the autoantigen and also has to lack an associated inflammatory innate immune response [35]. In normal conditions, APC encounter antigens in a proinflammatory environment of cytokines and innate immune responses that are triggered by pathogen-derived molecules. After encounter, APC differentiate and migrate to draining lymph nodes where they stimulate Th1 or Th2 responses. If an antigen is given in the form of peptide – which means in the absence of proinflammatory cytokines and innate triggers – when APC migrate to the draining lymphatics, they will generate immunoregulatory responses.

The APC that seem to best induce tolerance after soluble peptide administration are the dendritic cells (DC), to which cells soluble peptides are known to bind directly [36-38], following which the DC activate regulatory T cells. Indeed, repeated injections of self-peptide–loaded immature DC can protect from autoimmune disease through the generation of IL-10–producing $CD4^+$ T cells [39].

Types of Immunotherapeutic Peptides

A limited knowledge of the T-cell epitopes that are critical to the pathogenesis of an autoimmune disorder is the most significant obstacle for using peptides as surrogate native antigens capable of inducing immune tolerance.

For certain diseases, target autoantigens are relatively well defined, such as the acetylcholine receptor (AchR) in myasthenia gravis [40] and thyroglobulin in autoimmune thyroid disease [41]. For other diseases, the knowledge of the role of candidate autoantigens in the disease pathogenesis is a necessary prerequisite before embarking in the design of any therapeutic approach aimed at modulating immune responses to those autoantigens. Only once these premises are met, the synthesis of peptides can possibly target pathogenic T-cell autoreactivity.

Peptides can be synthesized to be structurally similar to their native form or they can be designed as altered peptide ligands [42-44] (APL – which are analogue peptides with defined substitutions at individual residues causing lack of stimulation of antigen-specific T cells but retaining ability to bind the MHC). Peptides can also be prepared as multiple antigenic peptides [45] (MAP – which are multiple, usually identical, peptide sequences attached to a core of branching lysine residues to yield a multivalent construct). In SLE, MAP have only been used as immunogens capable of inducing lupus-like disease in non-autoimmune mice [46] and will therefore not described further. For APL, different subtypes exist. The APL that give equivalent responses are referred to as agonist peptides; those capable of stimulating at reduced doses are called superagonists; and those that do not stimulate T-cell clones but inhibit antigen-specific activation are called antagonist peptides.

In general, APL-based vaccination is complicated by factors including the broadness of the T-cell repertoire and their often unpredictable effects (i.e. hyperreactivity), yet several groups have investigated – often with success – the use of APL antagonists as potential vaccines for autoimmune disease [47].

A recent, unconventional approach to inactivate autoreactive T cells that drive pathology using peptide delivery is represented by gene therapy with minigenes that encode self antigen-derived peptides [48]. This strategy seems to promote tolerance by inducing cytotoxic/suppressive T $CD8^+$ cells after endogenous expression of peptide in the context of MHC class I molecules [49-50]. With gene therapy, however, the possible release of cytokines or apoptotic bodies associated with cell lysis should be pondered in view of possible (even if temporary) exacerbation of disease [51].

Peptide-Based Therapy in Autoimmunity

Several studies in mice have provided useful insights into the therapeutic use of immunogenic peptides to delay onset and/or progression of autoimmune disease. These approaches have enabled the evolution from the traditional pharmacologic strategies of immune suppression to therapies that attack the pathologic process at a different level, arguably more directly, via selective control of certain aspects of the inflammatory process accompanying the autoimmune response. While these studies have given impetus to the development of alternative strategies of disease management, they have shown in the meantime significant limitations, e.g. inability to restore long-term immune homeostasis and superiority in preventing rather than curing inflammation. The new challenge is to overcome those difficulties by improving current protocols for longer-lasting, possibly curative effects.

Overview of Peptide Immunotherapy in Autoimmunity

To increase the chances of clinically relevant treatment of autoimmunity, it may be preferable, at least theoretically, to focus on antigens that participate in the mechanisms that control and sustain inflammation.

In the case of multiple sclerosis, desensitization of T cells specific for the autoantigen myelin basic protein (MBP) can be achieved via the therapeutic use of a random amino acid copolymer (glatiramer acetate or Copaxone) – which competes with MBP epitopes for presentation to T cells, and induces Th2 responses [52].

In experimental autoimmune encephalomyelitis (EAE), an animal model of multiple sclerosis caused primarily by Th1 cells, glatiramer acetate effectively suppressed the disease. Copaxone has been approved by health agencies for treatment of multiple sclerosis in humans, and it has measurable but limited benefits in some patients [53].

However, while bias toward Th2 responses is beneficial in EAE - and possibly in multiple sclerosis - the same may not be said for SLE, a disease in which both the Th1 and Th2 arms of the adaptive immune system are hyperactive and affected by the disease [54]. In the case of SLE, experimental evidence in animal models has revealed the potential of self antigen-based peptide therapies using mechanisms that in addition to modulation of cytokine profiles also involve the functional activity of T cells that regulate/suppress production of autoantibodies [55-56].

Other explored therapies in systemic autoimmune diseases include the neutralization of pathogenic autoantibodies (anti-β2GP1 antibodies) with peptides in the treatment of the antiphospholipid syndrome [57].

In organ-specific autoimmunity, different routes of peptide administration have been tested with encouraging results [58]. Effectiveness of mucosal tolerance induced by peptides of the AChR in autoimmune myasthenia gravis is under consideration as a therapeutic modality for patients with myasthenia gravis [59], and intraperitoneal injections of a peptide derived from glutamic acid decarboxylase in one trial delayed the onset and incidence of type-1 diabetes in mice [60].

Two studies with peptides derived from heat-shock proteins for the treatment of diabetes and rheumatoid arthritis have also provided encouraging results. Individuals with newly diagnosed type-1 diabetes treated by subcutaneous injections at three time points (at study entry and after 1 month and 6 months) with 1 mg of a peptide derived from the heat-shock protein hsp60 maintained islet cell function ten months after the first injection, in association with a modulation toward Th2-type responses [61].

In individuals with rheumatoid arthritis, a peptide derived from the bacterial heat-shock protein *dnaJ* administered orally resulted in an increased percentage of T cells producing IL-4 and IL-10 as well as reduced production of interferon (IFN)-γ and tumor necrosis factor (TNF)-α, also suggesting an induction of regulatory T cells after therapy [62].

Last but not least, the activation of suppressive $CD8^+$ T cells may represent an additional way to regulate autoantibody production. Administration of plasmid DNA encoding MHC class I-binding peptide T-cell epitopes from the V_H regions of anti-DNA antibodies induced specific $CD8^+$ T cells that killed anti-DNA-producing B cells in lupus-prone (NZB x NZW)F_1 (BWF1) mice [49]. The vaccination with those CTL-activating epitopes inhibited anti-DNA antibody production, delayed development of nephritis, and prolonged survival of the treated lupus-prone mice [49].

Rationale for Using Immunotherapeutic Peptides in SLE

The current pharmacologic treatment of SLE is not curative and may often result in nonspecific immune suppression, with complications including infection and the disruption of natural immune regulation. In general, to suppress the autoimmune response in SLE, treatments use drugs such as corticosteroids, cyclophosphamide and mycophenolate mofetil – highly effective in reducing mortality, yet associated with several important adverse side effects, particularly infection. Alternative approaches of molecular intervention, using peptides, can interfere with the production of specific pathogenic autoantibodies and modulate the activity of autoreactive B and/or T cells, thus avoiding many of the effects of those classical non-specific therapeutic agents.

As for other autoimmune disease, the strategies used to develop peptide treatment in SLE have mostly consisted of identification of sequences that could stimulate autoreactive T cells *ex vivo,* followed by the synthesis of the corresponding relevant peptides for administration to lupus mice. In general, different protocols have tested efficacy using different routes of delivery, doses and frequency of peptide administration in different spontaneous or induced murine lupus models. After that step, initial translational studies in humans have used either T cell clones or peripheral blood mononuclear cells *in vitro* or *ex vivo* for tests of peptide validity before embarking into clinical trials. At the time of this writing, one such peptide (Edratide – a peptide from a CDR region in an antibody to DNA) has been studied in patients with SLE, with phase II/III trials near completion.

CONSIDERATIONS FOR PEPTIDE-BASED IMMUNOTHERAPY OF SLE

The ability to modify pathogenic responses via tolerisation with synthetic peptides is currently under evaluation in SLE. The approach typically follows the validation from mechanistic studies that have confirmed the value of targeting certain defined antigenic specificities rather than others. Subsequently, tolerogenic regimens are designed in accordance with the concept discussed above that if tolerisation to an antigen in an animal models leads to clinical control of autoimmunity, this control could possibly be translated to humans using the same approach. However, for SLE there are several limitations in this assumption. First, the antigens that trigger the autoimmune process in SLE probably include a series of antigens that are temporally, quantitatively and qualitatively involved in different ways and/or in the diverse phases of the pathogenesis of the disease (for example histones associated with nucleosomes induce ANA and anti-DNA antibodies, mimotopes in Epstein-Barr virus may induce anti-Sm antibodies, β2GP1 can induce anti-cardiolipin antibodies; immunization with one of these may induce responses that spread to include the others). Second, even if identified in murine or human SLE, antigens might differ in the two species. Third, by the time of immunotherapeutic intervention, an initiating antigen may be less relevant in a process that is self-sustaining through other mechanisms. Despite these important limitations, peptide-based therapy holds great promise in SLE, and significant progress has been made. On the other hand, given the above premises, immunotherapy with peptides in SLE should not rely on a single peptide because of the multiple autoantigens involved in the pathogenesis of the disease and because of the diversity of patients and their clinical status. Since we cannot tolerise T cells against all known and unknown epitopes involved in the pathogenesis of SLE, the suppression of responses to multiple epitopes after administration of a single peptide would be particularly appealing. In practice, the current situation seems to lead toward that possibility, considering that often the peptides derived from self-epitopes can be promiscuously presented and recognized by lupus T cells in the context of diverse MHC alleles. These findings have opened up practical new possibilities to develop tolerogenic peptides for the therapy of human SLE.

Many of the experiments in SLE have been performed using high doses of peptides administered to lupus mice in the absence of adjuvant, to minimize the development of an immune response. One reason for the requirement of high doses of peptide has been the limited stability of peptides, an aspect that might possibly be partly overcome using peptide analogues of higher stability [63].

Table I. Prevention of lupus-like disease manifestations following administration of Ig-based peptides in murine SLE*

Mouse	Peptide	Autoantigen	Dose	Route	Ref.
BWF1	p34+p58+p84	V_H from anti-DNA Ig	5 x 300 g	i.v.	67
BWF1	pCDR3	anti-DNA Ig (16/6 Id)	4 x 50 g	i.p.	96
BWF1	pCDR3	anti-DNA Ig (16/6 Id)	10 x 100-500 g	i.v., s.c.	80
BWF1	pCons	(artificial, Ig consensus)	1 mg monthly	i.v.	79
BWF1	pCD.III (minigene)	V_H from anti-DNA Ig	3 x 50 g	i.d.	49
BWF1	pIgCons (minigene)	(artificial, Ig consensus)	6x10*5 transfected B cells	i.v.	50

*The Ig-derived peptide was given to premorbid mice at the doses indicated. The protective effects consisted of delayed onset of proteinuria and/or prolonged survival of the mice.

Table II. Therapy of murine lupus-like disease using Ig-based peptides*

Mouse	Peptide	Autoantigen	Dose	Route	Ref.
BWF1	pCons	(artificial, Ig consensus)	1 mg monthly	i.v.	79
BWF1	pCDR3	anti-DNA Ig (16/6 Id)	10 x 100-500 g	i.v., s.c.	81

*The Ig-derived peptide was given to nephritic mice at the doses indicated. The therapeutic effects were represented by prolonged survival of the mice and/or delayed progression of renal disease.

Procedures of Peptide Selection in SLE

Peptides Eluted from MHC Molecules

To identify T cell epitopes in autoimmune mice and patients, a strategy has been to elute and sequence self peptides bound to MHC class II molecules on the APC.

This approach has allowed characterization of I-A^k and I-E^k-associated self-peptides from lymph nodes of lupus-prone MRL/lpr mice, including peptides from histone H2A, the RNA splicing factor SRp20, and different ribosomal proteins that were absent in similar preparations from non-autoimmune C3H mice (which have the same MHC haplotype of MRL/lpr mice) (64). Among a set of eleven peptides that stimulated proliferation of T cells from both lupus and normal peptide-immunized mice, only four peptides (i.e. peptides 4–23 of SRp20, 84–103 of H2A, 42–59 of β2-microglobulin, and 110–129 of the MHC class II molecule I-$A^k\beta$) induced proliferation of T cells from I MRL/lpr mice (65). Using a similar approach, Datta and coworkers identified a peptide eluted from MHC class II molecules of a murine APC line (fed with chicken chromatin) that corresponded to residues 22–42 of the chicken histone H5 (homologous to H1′) [66]. This naturally-processed peptide was recognized by B and T cells of SNF1 mice, stimulated helper functions of several nucleosome-specific pathogenic T helper clones, and the antibodies against the peptide cross-reacted with DNA and nucleosomes and accelerated nephritis in SNF1 mice [66].

Peptides Derived from the V_H Region of Anti-DNA Antibodies

Using more than 400 overlapping peptides representing the entire V_H region of four anti-DNA antibodies, Singh, Hahn and coworkers isolated four Ig peptides that induced proliferation of splenocytes from young BWF1 mice and that were able to stimulate IgG anti-dsDNA Ab production, when cultured in the presence of spleen B and T cells from BWF1 lupus mice [67-68].

Peptides Recognized by T Cells from Both Lupus Mice and Patients

Datta and coworkers identified dominant nucleosomal epitopes involved in cognate interactions between autoimmune SLE T helper cells and anti-DNA Ig-producing B cells. By scanning overlapping synthetic peptides, and by mass spectrometry of naturally processed peptides, five major epitopes in nucleosomal histones were localized, namely $H1'_{22\text{-}42}$, $H2B_{10\text{-}33}$, $H3_{85\text{-}105}$, $H4_{16\text{-}39}$, and $H4_{71\text{-}94}$ [69-70, 66]. Mice and patients with SLE had in their peripheral blood T cells as well as B cells which recognized these epitopes, and with age, autoantibodies against those epitopes reacted with nuclear autoantigens. Tolerogenic therapy with a single histone peptide epitope could stop the progression of established glomerulonephritis in lupus-prone mice which by tolerance spreading inactivated autoimmune T and B cells. Importantly, those histone peptides could bind multiple human HLA-DR motifs and behaved as promiscuous epitopes [71].

Another peptide of interest is the aminoacid sequence 83–119 of the spliceosomal SmD1 protein (a D1 protein of the Smith (Sm) antigen, part of the small nuclear ribonucleoprotein), which encompasses a B cell epitope in lupus mice and patients [72-73] and is capable of binding dsDNA and nucleosomes [74]. This peptide provides $CD4^+$ T cell help to anti-dsDNA antibodies in BWF1 mice and in one third of lupus patients [75].

High-dose intravenous tolerance to $SmD1_{183\text{-}119}$ (0.6-1 mg/month) delayed production of autoantibodies, postponed onset of nephritis, and prolonged survival of BWF1 lupus-prone mice [76]. Of note, one week after $SmD1_{183\text{-}119}$ tolerance induction in prenephritic mice, a decrease of IFN-γ and IL-4 expression were observed concomitantly with an increased expression of transforming growth factor (TGF)-β1 [76]. The immune tolerance to $SmD1_{183\text{-}119}$ could be adoptively transferred by $CD90^+$ T cells, which were capable of reducing T-cell help for autoreactive B cells *in vitro*. The increased frequency of regulatory $CD4^+$ type-1 regulatory T cells in this system associated with the prevention of autoantibody generation [76].

Finally, Muller and coworkers identified an epitope located within the peptide 131–151 of the spliceosomal U1-70 K protein that stimulated proliferation of and IL-2 release by $CD4^+$ T cells from MRL/lpr and BWF1 lupus mice [77]. These authors showed that a phosphorylated analogue of peptide 131–151 (called P140) was a promiscuous epitope recognized by $CD4^+$ T cells and antibodies from MRL/lpr mice as well as antibodies from SLE patients [78].

PEPTIDE-BASED IMMUNOTHERAPY OF SLE

Unlike animal models, it is not yet feasible in humans to begin prophylactic treatment at the early stages of an autoimmune process (i.e. before it manifests clinically). This aspect may represent a problem for peptide immunotherapy, considering that it has been frequently shown that peptide-based therapies in animal models are less effective at inhibiting or reversing an established disease rather than at preventing it.

Only a few studies were successful in mice that have already developed disease. In one of those studies, administration of $H4_{16-39}$ peptide to SNF1 mice with established glomerulonephritis prolonged survival and halted the progression of renal disease [18]. A similar result was obtained after monthly intravenous administration into 20-week-old BWF1 mice of the peptide pCons, an artificial consensus peptide based on the V_H regions of several BWF1 IgG anti-DNA antibodies that had T-cell stimulatory activity [79]. Last, a peptide derived from the sequence of the complementary-determining region 3 (pCDR3) of an anti-DNA monoclonal antibody that expressed the 16/6 Id was used successfully in the therapy of 20–28-week-old BWF1 mice [80-81].

ANTI-DNA IG-DERIVED PEPTIDE FOR THE IMMUNOTHERAPY OF SLE

pCons Peptide

Several autoantibodies to DNA – the hallmark antibodies of SLE – contain amino acid sequences that induce *in vitro* T cell proliferation and cytokine secretion [82-83]. Identification of several such T cell epitopes encoded within the V_H regions of murine autoantibodies to DNA indicated that these immunogenic sequences have similar location and amino acid content in several anti-DNA antibodies [79].

An algorithm was derived to design a 15-mer synthetic consensus peptide (pCons) which described most of the self-Ig-derived stimulatory sequences in the CDR1/FR2 region of V_H regions from several murine anti-DNA antibodies, for possible use as tolerogen in BWF1 mice. A non-stimulatory peptide with analogous $I\text{-}E^d$ binding motifs, yet violating the consensus motif, was synthesized as a negative control and was called pNeg [79]. Monthly intravenous injection of 1 mg of pCons was effective in delaying appearance of multiple autoantibodies and nephritis and in prolonging the survival of treated BWF1 mice beginning at 10 weeks of age (healthy) or at 20 weeks of age (diseased)[79]. Tolerance was induced by pCons but not by pNeg, in spite of their strikingly similar molecular structure (Figure 2).

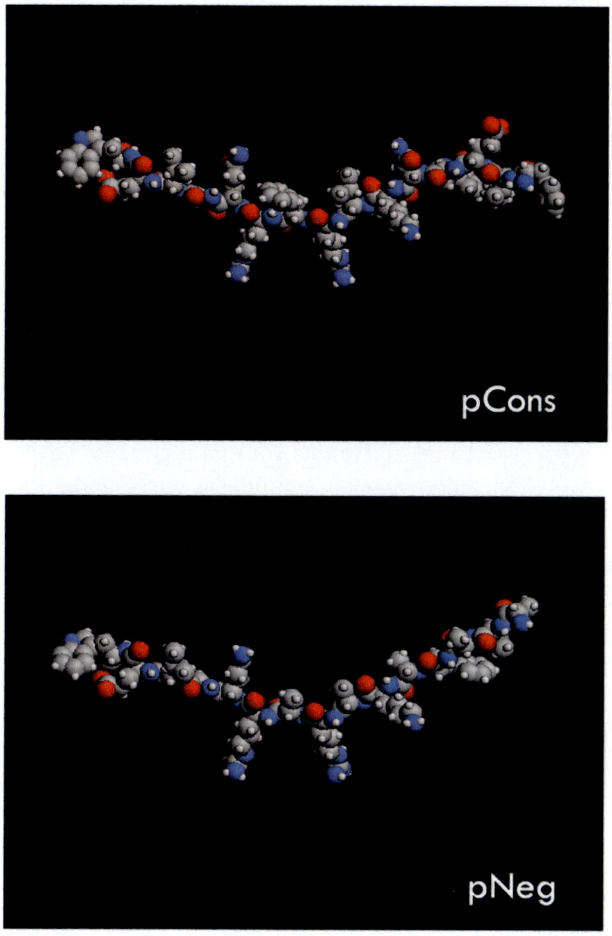

Figure 2. Molecular structure of pCons and pNeg peptides. Despite the similarity, only the Ig-based peptide pCons can protect BWF1 mice from lupus-like disease, whereas pNeg has virtually no effects on disease (see text for details).

Since pCons contained amino acid sequences that bound both the MHC class II molecule and the MHC class I molecules, tolerisation by pCons affected both $CD4^+$ and $CD8^+$ T cell compartments. Both $CD8^+$ T suppressors (Ts) and $CD4^+CD25^+$ regulatory T cells (Tregs) expanded *in vivo* in pCons-treated mice, and were fully capable of suppressing anti-DNA production from B cells [84-85].

$CD8^+$ suppressor T (Ts) cells mainly operated via soluble factors such as cytokines (as indicated by transwell experiments) to block B cell-mediated production of anti-DNA antibodies [84].

Previous data had suggested that $CD8^+$ Ts became physiologically defective in aging BWF1 mice that developed SLE [86]. Therefore, the data seemed to indicate that it could still be possible to call up these cells and have them be functionally active under appropriate conditions. Studies aimed at defining the mechanisms by which pCons-induced $CD8^+$ Ts blocked anti-DNA antibody production and nephritis suggested that the protection exerted by these cells both *in vitro* and *in vivo* depended in part on the upregulation of TGF-β and *Foxp3* molecules, and on an increased resistance to apoptosis of the Ts (as compared to similar cells from naïve mice) [84].

Importantly, tolerisation with pCons not only affected $CD8^+$ Ts, but also the number and function of peptide-reactive $CD4^+CD25^+$ Tregs (85). Although the protocol of tolerisation did not associate with significant expansion of $CD4^+CD25^+$ Tregs when considered *in toto*, the relative percent and absolute number of Tregs specific for pCons expanded considerably after tolerisation [85]. The pCons-induced peptide-reactive *Foxp3*-expressing Tregs suppressed anti-DNA antibody production via cell contact mechanisms that included engagement of membrane-bound TGF-β and glucocorticoid-induced TNF-receptor (TNF-R) family member 18 (GITR), since blockade of these surface molecules on Tregs partly abrogated their *in vitro* suppressive capability on the B cells [85].

Overall, the suppressor and regulatory T cells raised by tolerisation with the anti-DNA-based peptide pCons appeared to use different yet complementary mechanisms to skew the hyperactive state of lupus B cells towards a reduced production of autoantibodies. One mechanism was a direct suppression on B cells, and another was an interference with the help provided by $CD4^+$ T cells to the B cells [87].

Another consideration is that since the pCons-reactive Tregs mainly required cell contact while the Ts needed soluble factors to operate, the Ts were likely influenced by the local milieu to suppress in a broader fashion than the Tregs, for which antigen specificity was necessary [88].

hCDR1 Peptide

The peptide hCDR1 – which is based on the complementarity-determining region (CDR)1 of a human monoclonal anti-DNA autoantibody that bears the 16/6 idiotype (common to mice and humans) – also ameliorates the serological and clinical manifestations of lupus in both spontaneous (BWF1 mice) and induced (BALB/c mice) SLE models [89].

Ten subcutaneous weekly injections of hCDR1 (50 or 200 μg/mouse) mitigated proteinuria and kidney damage, reduced anti-dsDNA antibody titers and proinflammatory cytokines, and upregulated production of TGF-β [89]. The therapeutic potential of hCDR1 was also tested in a model of lupus of severe combined immunodeficient (SCID) mice engrafted intraperitoneally with peripheral blood lymphocytes from patients with SLE. SCID mice that were treated with hCDR1 (50 μg/mouse) once a week for 8 weeks developed lower quantities of human dsDNA antibodies than mice treated with a control peptide. Furthermore, treatment with hCDR1 resulted in reduced proteinuria, and reduced glomerular deposition of human IgG immune complexes, and of murine complement C3 than in controls [90].

One molecular mechanism that associated with the amelioration of SLE after hCDR1 therapy was a diminished expression of phosphorylated JNK kinase in the T cells, which also exhibited a reduced rate of apoptosis (most likely because of the down-regulation of the activity of the pro-apoptotic JNK kinase) [91]. Another mechanism induced by hCDR1 was the down-regulation of the cell adhesion receptors LFA-1 and CD44 [92]. Since these receptors operate as accessory molecules in mediating APC-T cell interactions, the reduced proliferation of autoreactive T cells could be possibly ascribed, at least in part, to this specific action of hCDR1 on the T cells. Importantly, the beneficial effects induced by hCDR1 could be transferred to diseased lupus BWF1 mice, in which the adoptive transfer of hCDR1-treated cells downregulated the disease manifestations [93]. The beneficial effects observed included an increase in the number of regulatory $CD4^{+}CD25^{+}$ T cells expressing cytotoxic T lymphocyte antigen 4 (CTLA-4) and *Foxp3* (93). The central role of Tregs in the mechanisms of protection were confirmed by experiments in which the depletion of the $CD25^{+}$ cells diminished significantly the therapeutic effects of hCDR1, whereas administration of enriched $CD4^{+}CD25^{+}$ T cells was highly beneficial in diseased mice [93]. Finally, the amelioration of disease manifestations was associated with a down-regulation of the cytokines IFN-γ and IL-10 and an upregulation of TGF-β, a molecule that substantially contributed to the suppression of T-cell autoreactivity [93].

Safety Considerations in the Use of Immunotherapeutic Peptides

In the use of immunotherapeutic peptides, at least in the early stages of clinical development (phase I/II clinical trials), relevant information on the efficacy and safety of the treatment should be recorded together with the use of biomarkers of immunological relevance (helpful in defining response patterns, thus identifying surrogate markers of efficacy). These approaches are in place in studies with the only Ig-based peptide currently in phase II/III clinical trials in SLE patients, the peptide developed in the Mozes' laboratory called Edratide.

Tolerisation of humans with nucleosomal-associated histone peptides might offer an advantage over the Ig-derived peptides, in that histone peptides are widely conserved in ontogeny and thus unlikely to provoke allergic reactions. The Ig-based peptides currently under study are either artificial or present in some but not all human anti-DNA antibodies, and therefore could be foreign to some patients. However, these possibilities are theoretical and remain to be tested in human trials.

Conclusion

Despite our growing understanding of the immune mechanisms elicited by Ig-derived peptide immunotherapy in SLE, there are still many obstacles in fully exploiting the potential of these therapeutic agents in clinical practice. The data available in the mouse are encouraging because similar peptide sequences exist in murine and human anti-DNA antibodies, and, as mentioned before, insights into the mechanisms of immune dysfunction in lupus mice may have the potential for rapid translational therapeutic use in human SLE [94-95].

Our current knowledge seems to indicate that many, if not most, of the beneficial effects of peptide immunotherapy may result from specific elimination or modulation of autoreactive T cells and/or the expansion of regulatory immune responses. Despite this information, additional work is required to establish peptide sequences with optimal effects in most patients, such as peptides based on promiscuous epitopes with broad specificity, capable of providing long-lasting immune tolerance, and peptides likely to tolerise against more than one antigenic specificity. In any case, combination with standard therapeutic agents will most likely be still needed to obtain maximal benefits in the clinical use of peptides in SLE.

ACKNOWLEDGMENTS

A.L.C. and B.H.H. are supported in part by grants from the National Institutes of Health (AR53239 and AI63515 to A.L.C., and AI/AR46776 to B.H.H.), the Arthritis Foundation Southern California Chapter, and gifts from the Dorough Foundation, the Horchow Family Foundation, and Jeanne Rappaport.

REFERENCES

[1] Reinherz, E. L. and Schlossman, S. F. 1980. Current concepts in immunology: Regulation of the immune response - inducer and suppressor T-lymphocyte subsets in human beings. *N. Engl. J. Med. 303:* 370-373.

[2] Kumar, V. 2004. Homeostatic control of immunity by TCR peptide-specific Tregs. *J. Clin. Invest. 114:* 1222-1226.

[3] La Cava, A. and Shi, F.-D. 2006. Natural and adaptive immune cell-based therapies in autoimmunity. *Curr. Med. Chem. 13:* 1557-1566.

[4] O'Garra, A. and Vieira P. 2004. Regulatory T cells and mechanisms of immune system control. *Nat. Med. 10:* 801-805.

[5] Arbuckle, M. R.; McClain, M. T.; Rubertone, M. V.; Scofield, R. H.; Dennis, G. J.; James, J. A.; Harley, J. B. 2003. Development of autoantibodies before the clinical onset of systemic lupus erythematosus. *N. Engl. J. Med. 349:* 1526-1533.

[6] La Cava, A. and Sarvetnick, N. 1999. The role of cytokines in autoimmune diseases. *Curr. Dir. Autoimmun. 1:* 56-71.

[7] Rubin, R. L. and Kretz-Rommel, A. 1999. Linkage of immune self-tolerance with the positive selection of T cells. *Crit. Rev. Immunol.19:* 199-218.

[8] Daikh, D. I. and Wofsy, D. 2001. Reversal of murine lupus nephritis with CTLA4Ig and cyclophosphamide. *J. Immunol. 166:* 2913-2916.

[9] Boumpas, D. T.; Furie, R.; Manzi, S.; Illei, G. G.; Wallace, D. J.; Balow, J. E.; Vaishnaw, A.; BG9588 Lupus Nephritis Trial Group. 2003. A short course of BG9588 (anti-CD40 ligand antibody) improves serologic activity and decreases hematuria in patients with proliferative lupus glomerulonephritis. *Arthritis Rheum. 48:* 719-727.

[10] Stuart, R. W. and Racke, M. K. 2002. Targeting T cell costimulation in autoimmune disease. *Expert Opin. Ther. Targets. 6:* 275-289.

[11] Mouzaki, A.; Deraos, S.; Chatzantoni, K. 2005. Advances in the treatment of autoimmune diseases; cellular activity, type-1/type-2 cytokine secretion patterns and their modulation by therapeutic peptides. *Curr. Med. Chem. 12:* 1537-1550.

[12] Stohl W. 2005. BlySfulness does not equal blissfulness in systemic lupus erythematosus: a therapeutic role for BlyS antagonists. *Curr. Dir. Autoimmun. 8:* 289-304.

[13] Crow, M. K. and Kirou, K. A. 2004. Interferon-α in systemic lupus erythematosus. *Curr. Opin. Rheumatol. 16:* 541-547.

[14] Anders, H. J.; Banas, B.; Schlondorff, D. 2004. Signaling danger: Toll-like receptors and their potential roles in kidney disease. *J. Am. Soc. Nephrol. 15:* 854-867.

[15] Ng, K. P.; Cambridge, G; Leandro, M. J.; Edwards, J. C.; Ehrenstein, M.; Isenberg, D. 2004. B cell depletion therapy in systemic lupus erythematosus: Long term follow up and predictors of response. *Ann. Rheum. Dis.* In press.

[16] Looney, R. J.; Anolik, J.; Sanz, I. 2005. Treatment of SLE with anti-CD20 monoclonal antibody. *Curr. Dir. Autoimmun. 8:* 193-205.

[17] Anderton, S. M. 2001. Peptide-based immunotherapy of autoimmunity: A path of puzzles, paradoxes and possibilities. *Immunology 104:* 367-376.

[18] Kaliyaperumal, A.; Michaels, M. A.; Datta, S. K. 1999. Antigen-specific therapy of murine lupus nephritis using nucleosomal peptides: Tolerance spreading impairs pathogenic function of autoimmune T and B cells. *J. Immunol. 162:* 5775-5783.

[19] Martin, R.; McFarland, H. F.; McFarlin, D. E. 1992. Immunological aspects of demyelinating diseases. *Annu. Rev. Immunol. 10:* 153-187.

[20] Texier, C.; Pouvelle, S.; Busson, M.; Herve, M.; Charron, D.; Menez, A.; Maillere, B. 2000. HLA-DR restricted peptide candidates for bee venom immunotherapy. *J. Immunol.* 164:3177-3184.

[21] Chai, J. G.; James, E.; Dewchand, H.; Simpson, E.; Scott, D. 2004. Transplantation tolerance induced by intranasal administration of HY peptides. *Blood 103:* 3951-3959.

[22] Karin, N.; Mitchell, D. J.; Brocke, S.; Ling, N.; Steinman, L. 1994. Reversal of experimental autoimmune encephalomyelitis by a soluble peptide variant of a myelin basic protein epitope: T cell receptor antagonism and reduction of interferon-γ and tumor necrosis factor-α production. *J. Exp. Med. 180:* 2227-3227.

[23] Kearney, E. R.; Pape, K. A.; Loh, D. Y.; Jenkins, M. K. 1994. Visualization of peptide-specific T cell immunity and peripheral tolerance induction *in vivo*. *Immunity 1:* 327-339.

[24] Wu, H. Y.; Monsonego, A.; Weiner, H. L. 2006. The mechanism of nasal tolerance in lupus prone mice is T-cell anergy induced by immature B cells that lack B7 expression. *J. Autoimmun.* 26: 116-126.

[25] Paas-Rozner, M.; Sela, M.; Mozes, E. 2001. The nature of the active suppression of responses associated with experimental autoimmune myasthenia gravis by a dual altered peptide ligand administered by different routes. *Proc. Natl. Acad. Sci. USA 98:* 12642-12647.

[26] Wraith, D. C.; Nicolson, K. S.; Whitley, N. T. 2004. Regulatory CD4$^+$ T cells and the control of autoimmune disease. *Curr. Opin. Immunol. 16:* 695-701.

[27] Apostolou, I. and von Boehmer, H. 2004. *In vivo* instruction of suppressor commitment in naïve T cells. *J. Exp. Med. 199:* 1401-1408.

[28] Verhoef, A.; Alexander, C.; Kay, A. B.; Larché, M. 2005. T cell epitope immunotherapy induces a CD4$^+$ T cell population with regulatory activity. *PloS Med. 2:* e78.

[29] Metzler, B.; Anderton, S. M.; Manickasingham, S. P.; Wraith, D. C. 2000. Kinetics of peptide uptake and tissue distribution following a single intranasal dose of peptide. *Immunol. Invest. 29:* 61-70.

[30] Wu, H. Y.; Ward, F. J.; Staines, N. A. 2002. Histone peptide-induced nasal tolerance: suppression of murine lupus. *J. Immunol. 169:* 1126-1134.

[31] Metzler, B. and Wraith, D. C. 1993. Inhibition of experimental autoimmune encephalomyelitis by inhalation but not oral administration of the encephalitogenic peptide: influence of MHC binding affinity. *Int. Immunol. 5:* 1159-1165.

[32] Liu, G. Y. and Wraith, D. C. 1995. Affinity for class II MHC determines the extent to which soluble peptides tolerize autoreactive T cells in I and primed adult mice– implications for autoimmunity. *Int. Immunol. 7:* 1255-1263.

[33] Metzler, B. and Wraith, D. C. 1999. Inhibition of T-cell responsiveness by nasal peptide administration: influence of the thymus and differential recovery of T-cell-dependent functions. *Immunology 97:* 257-263.

[34] Monneaux, F. and Muller, S. 2004. Peptide-based immunotherapy of systemic lupus erythematosus. *Autoimm. Rev. 3:* 16-24.

[35] Larché, M. and Wraith, D. C. 2005. Peptide-based therapeutic vaccines for allergic and autoimmune diseases. *Nat. Med. 11:* S69-76.

[36] Metzler, B.; Anderton, S. M.; Manickasingham, S. P.; Wraith, D. C. 2000. Kinetics of peptide uptake and tissue distribution following a single intranasal dose of peptide. *Immunol. Invest. 29:* 61-70.

[37] Santambrogio, L.; Sato, A. K.; Carven, G. J.; Belyanskaya, S. L.; Strominger, J. L.; Stern, L. J. 1999. Extracellular antigen processing and presentation by immature dendritic cells. *Proc. Natl. Acad. Sci. USA 96:* 15056-15061.

[38] Santambrogio, L.; Sato, A. K.; Fischer, F. R.; Dorf, M. E.; Stern, L. J. 1999. Abundant empty class II MHC molecules on the surface of immature dendritic cells. *Proc. Natl. Acad. Sci. USA 96:* 15050-15055.

[39] Menges, M.; Rossner, S.; Voigtlander, C.; Schindler, H.; Kukutsch, N. A.; Bogdan, C.; Erb, K.; Schuler, G.; Lutz, M. B. 2002. Repetitive injections of dendritic cells matured with tumor necrosis factor-α induce antigen-specific protection of mice from autoimmunity. *J. Exp. Med. 195:* 15-21.

[40] Vincent, A. 2002. Unravelling the pathogenesis of myasthenia gravis. *Nat. Rev. Immunol. 2:* 797-804.

[41] Weetman, A. P. 2004. Autoimmune thyroid disease. *Autoimmunity 37:* 337-340.

[42] Dressel, A.; Chin, J. L.; Sette, A.; Gausling, R.; Hollsberg, P.; Hafler, D. A. 1997. Autoantigen recognition by human CD8 T cell clones: enhanced agonist response induced by altered peptide ligands. *J. Immunol. 159:* 4943-4951.

[43] Pfeiffer, C.; Stein, J.; Southwood, S.; Ketelaar, H.; Sette, A.; Bottomly, K. 1995. Altered peptide ligands can control CD4 T lymphocyte differentiation *in vivo*. *J. Exp. Med. 181:* 1569-1574.

[44] Windhagen, A.; Scholz, C.; Hollsberg, P.; Fukaura, H.; Sette, A.; Hafler, D. A. 1995. Modulation of cytokine patterns of human autoreactive T cell clones by a single amino acid substitution of their peptide ligand. *Immunity 2:* 373-380.

[45] Sakarellos-Daitsiotis, M.; Krikorian, D.; Panou-Pomonis, E.; Sakarellos, C. 2006. Artificial carriers: A strategy for constructing antigenic/immunogenic conjugates. *Curr. Top. Med. Chem. 6:* 1715-1735.

[46] Khalil, M.; Inaba, K.; Steinman, R.; Ravetch, J.; Diamond, B. 2001. T cell studies in a peptide-induced model of systemic lupus erythematosus. *J. Immunol. 166:* 1667-1674.

[47] Sloan-Lancaster, J. and Allen, P. M. 1996. Altered peptide ligand-induced partial T cell activation: molecular mechanisms and role in T cell biology. *Annu. Rev. Immunol. 14:* 1-27.

[48] Choi, E. W.; Shin, I. S.; Youn, H. Y.; Kim, D. Y.; Lee, H.; Chae, Y. J.; Lee, C. W. 2005. Gene therapy using non-viral peptide vector in a canine systemic lupus erythematosus model. *Vet. Immunol. Immunopathol. 103:* 223-233.

[49] Fan, G. C. and Singh, R. R. 2002. Vaccination with minigenes encoding V_H-derived major histocompatibility complex class I-binding epitopes activates cytotoxic T cells that ablate autoantibody-producing B cells and inhibit lupus. *J. Exp. Med.* 196:731-741.

[50] Ferrera, F.; Hahn, B. H.; Rizzi, M.; Anderson, M.; FitzGerald, J.; Millo, E.; Indiveri, F.; Shi, F.-D.; Filaci, G.; La Cava, A. 2007. Protection against renal disease in (NZB x NZW)F_1 lupus-prone after somatic B-cell gene vaccination with anti-DNA immunoglobulin consensus peptide. *Arthritis Rheum. In press.*

[51] Levine, J. S.; Subang, R.; Nasr, S. H.; Fournier, S.; Lajoie, G.; Wither, J.; Rauch, J. 2006. Immunization with an apoptotic cell-binding protein recapitulates the nephritis and sequential autoantibody emergence of systemic lupus erythematosus. *J. Immunol. 177:* 6504-6516.

[52] Duda, P. W.; Schmied, M. C.; Cook, S. L.; Krieger, J. I.; Hafler, D. A. 2000. Glatiramer acetate (Copaxone) induces degenerate, Th2-polarized immune responses in patients with multiple sclerosis. *J. Clin. Invest. 105:* 967-976.

[53] Steinman, L. and Zamvil, S. S. 2006. How to successfully apply animal studies in experimental allergic encephalomyelitis to research on multiple sclerosis. *Ann. Neurol. 60:* 12-21.

[54] La Cava, A. 2003. Cytokines and autoimmune rheumatic diseases. *Int. J. Adv. Rheumatol. 1:* 10-19.

[55] La Cava, A.; Fang, C. J.; Singh, R. P.; Ebling, F.; Hahn, B. H. 2005. Manipulation of immune regulation in systemic lupus erythematosus. *Autoimmun. Rev.* 4: 515-519.

[56] Hahn, B. H.; Ebling, F.; Singh, R. R.; Singh, R. P.; Karpouzas, G.; La Cava, A. 2005. Cellular and molecular mechanisms of regulation of autoantibody production in lupus. *Ann. N. Y. Acad. Sci. 1051:* 433-441.

[57] Blank, M. and Shoenfeld, Y. 2004. β-2-glycoprotein-I, infections, antiphospholipid syndrome and therapeutic considerations. *Clin. Immunol. 112:* 190-199.

[58] Krause, I.; Blank, M.; Shoenfeld, Y. 2000. Peptide immunotherapy in autoimmune diseases. *Drug News Perspect.* 13: 78-84.

[59] Souroujon, M. C.; Maiti, P. K.; Feferman, T.; Im, S. H.; Raveh, L.; Fuchs, S. 2003. Suppression of myasthenia gravis by antigen-specific mucosal tolerance and modulation of cytokines and costimulatory factors. *Ann. N. Y. Acad. Sci. 998:* 533-536.

[60] Tisch, R.; Wang, B.; Serreze, D. V. 1999. Induction of glutamic acid decarboxylase 65-specific Th2 cells and suppression of autoimmune diabetes at late stages of disease is epitope dependent. *J. Immunol.* 163:1178-1187.

[61] Raz, I.; Elias, D.; Avron, A.; Tamir, M.; Metzger, M.; Cohen, I. R. 2001. β-cell function in new-onset type 1 diabetes and immunomodulation with a heat-shock protein peptide (DiaPep277): a randomized, double-blind, phase II trial. *Lancet 358:* 1749-1753.

[62] Prakken, B. J.; Samodal, R.; Le, T. D.; Giannoni, F.; Yung, G. P.; Scavulli, J.; Amox, D.; Roord, S.; de Kleer, I.; Bonnin, D.; Lanza, P.; Berry, C.; Massa, M.; Billetta, R.; Albani, S. 2004. Epitope-specific immunotherapy induces immune deviation of proinflammatory T cells in rheumatoid arthritis. *Proc. Natl. Acad. Sci. USA 101:* 4228-4233.

[63] Meziere, C.; Viguier, M.; Dumortier, H.; Lo-Man, R.; Leclerc, C.; Guillet, J. G.; Briand, J. P.; Muller, S. 1997. *In vivo* T helper cell response to retro-inverso peptidomimetics. *J. Immunol. 159:* 3230-3237.

[64] Freed, J. H.; Marrs, A.; VanderWall, J.; Cohen, P. L.; Eisenberg, R. A. 2000. MHC class II-bound self peptides from autoimmune MRL/lpr mice reveal potential T cell epitopes for autoantibody production in murine systemic lupus erythematosus. *J. Immunol.* 164: 4697-4705.

[65] Suh, C. H.; Freed, J. H.; Cohen, P. L. 2003. T cell reactivity to MHC class II-bound self peptides in systemic lupus erythematosus-prone MRL/lpr mice. *J. Immunol. 170:* 2229-2235.

[66] Kaliyaperumal, A.; Michaels, M. A.; Datta, S. K. 2002. Naturally processed chromatin peptides reveal a major autoepitope that primes pathogenic T and B cells of lupus. *J. Immunol. 168:* 2530-2537.

[67] Singh, R. R.; Ebling, F. M.; Sercarz, E. E.; Hahn, B. H. 1995. Immune tolerance to autoantibody-derived peptides delays development of autoimmunity in murine lupus. *J. Clin. Invest. 96:* 2990-2996.

[68] Singh, R. R.; Hahn, B. H.; Tsao, B. P.; Ebling, F. M. 1998. Evidence for multiple mechanisms of polyclonal T cell activation in murine lupus. *J. Clin. Invest. 102:* 1841-1849.

[69] Kaliyaperumal, A.; Mohan, C.; Wu, W.; Datta, S. K. 1996. Nucleosomal peptide epitopes for nephritis-inducing T helper cells of murine lupus. *J. Exp. Med. 183:* 2459-2469.

[70] Lu, L.; Kaliyaperumal, A.; Boumpas, D. T.; Datta, S. K. 1999. Major peptide autoepitopes for nucleosome-specific T cells of human lupus. *J. Clin. Invest. 104:* 345-355.

[71] Datta, S. K. 2003. Major peptide autoepitopes for nucleosome-centered T and B cell interaction in human and murine lupus. *Ann. N. Y. Acad. Sci. 987:* 79-90.

[72] Riemekasten, G.; Marell, J.; Trebeljahr, G.; Klein R.; Hausdorf G.; Haupl, T.; Schneider-Mergener, J.; Burmester, G. R.; Hiepe, F. 1998. A novel epitope on the C-terminus of SmD1 is recognized by the majority of sera from patients with systemic lupus erythematosus. *J. Clin. Invest. 102:* 754-763.

[73] Monneaux, F.; Dumortier, H.; Steiner, G.; Briand, J. P.; Muller, S. 2001. Murine models of systemic lupus erythematosus: B and T cell responses to spliceosomal ribonucleoproteins in MRL/Fas(lpr) and (NZB x NZW)F_1 lupus mice. *Int. Immunol. 13:* 1155-1163.

[74] Dieker, J. W.; Van Bavel, C. C.; Riemekasten, G.; Berden, J. H.; van der Vlag, J. 2006. The binding of lupus-derived autoantibodies to the C-terminal peptide (83-119) of the major SmD1 autoantigen can be mediated by double-stranded DNA and nucleosomes. *Ann. Rheum. Dis. 65:* 1525-1528.

[75] Riemekasten, G.; Weiss, C.; Schneider, S.; Thiel, A.; Bruns, A.; Schumann, F.; Blass, S.; Burmester, G. R.; Hiepe, F. 2002. T cell reactivity against the $SmD_{183-119}$ C terminal peptide in patients with systemic lupus erythematosus. *Ann. Rheum. Dis. 61:* 779-785.

[76] Riemekasten, G.; Langnickel, D.; Enghard, P.; Undeutsch, R.; Humrich, J.; Ebling, F. M.; Hocher, B.; Humaljoki, T.; Neumayer, H.; Burmester, G. R.; Hahn, B. H.; Radbruch, A.; Hiepe, F. 2004. Intravenous injection of a D1 protein of the Smith proteins postpones murine lupus and induces type 1 regulatory T cells. *J. Immunol. 173:* 5835-5842.

[77] Monneaux, F.; Briand, J. P.; Muller, S. 2000. B and T cell immune response to small nuclear ribonucleoprotein particles in lupus mice: autoreactive $CD4^+$ T cells recognize a T cell epitope located within the RNP80 motif of the 70K protein. *Eur. J. Immunol. 30:* 2191-2200.

[78] Monneaux, F.; Lozano, J. M.; Patarroyo, M. E.; Briand, J. P.; Muller, S. 2003. T cell recognition and therapeutic effect of a phosphorylated synthetic peptide of the 70K snRNP protein administered in MR/lpr mice. *Eur. J. Immunol. 33:* 287-296.

[79] Hahn, B. H.; Singh, R. R.; Wong, W. K.; Tsao, B. P.; Bulpitt, K.; Ebling, F. M. 2001. Treatment with a consensus peptide based on amino acid sequences in autoantibodies prevents T cell activation by autoantigens and delays disease onset in murine lupus. *Arthritis Rheum. 44:* 432-441.

[80] Eilat, E.; Zinger, H.; Nyska, A.; Mozes, E. 2000. Prevention of systemic lupus erythematosus-like disease in (NZB x NZW)F_1 mice by treating with CDR1- and CDR3-based peptides of a pathogenic autoantibody. *J. Clin. Immunol. 20:* 268-278.

[81] Zinger, H.; Eilat, E.; Meshorer, A.; Mozes, E. 2003. Peptides based on the complementarity-determining regions of a pathogenic autoantibody mitigate lupus manifestations of (NZB x NZW)F_1 mice via active suppression. *Int. Immunol. 15:* 205-214.

[82] Waisman, A.; Ruiz, P. J.; Israeli, E.; Eilat, E.; Konen-Waisman, S.; Zinger, H.; Dayan, M.; Mozes, E. 1997. Modulation of murine systemic lupus erythematosus with peptides based on complementarity determining regions of a pathogenic anti-DNA monoclonal antibody. *Proc. Natl. Acad. Sci. USA 94:* 4620-4625.

[83] Kalsi, J. K.; Grossman, J.; Kim, J.; Sieling, P.; Gjertson, D. W.; Reed, E. F.; Ebling, F. M.; Linker-Israeli, M.; Hahn, B. H. 2004. Self-peptides from autoantibody molecules elicit different cytokines from lymphocytes of patients with SLE depending on peptide concentration and duration of disease. *Lupus 13:* 490-500.

[84] Hahn, B. H.; Singh, R. P.; La Cava, A.; Ebling, F. M. 2005. Tolerogenic treatment of lupus mice with consensus peptide induces *Foxp3*-expressing, apoptosis-resistant, TGF-β-secreting $CD8^+$ T cell suppressors. *J. Immunol.* 175: 7728-7737.

[85] La Cava, A.; Ebling, F. M.; Hahn, B. H. 2004. Ig-reactive $CD4^+CD25^+$ T cells from tolerized (New Zealand Black x New Zealand White)F_1 mice suppress *in vitro* production of antibodies to DNA. J. Immunol. 173: 3542-3548.

[86] Karpouzas, G. A.; Singh, R. R.; Ebling, F. M.; La Cava, A.; Hahn, B. H. 2004. Defects in $CD8^+$ cell inhibitory function characterize lupus prone but not non-autoimmune mice. *Eur. J. Immunol. 34:* 2489-2499.

[87] Singh, R. R. and Hahn, B. H. 1998. Reciprocal T-B determinant spreading develops spontaneously in murine lupus: implications for pathogenesis. *Immunol. Rev. 164:* 201-208.

[88] Singh, R. P., La Cava, A., Wong, M.; Ebling, F.; Hahn, B. H. 2007. $CD8^+$ T cell-mediated suppression of autoimmunity in a murine lupus model of peptide-induced immune tolerance depends on *Foxp3* expression. *J. Immunol. In press.*

[89] Luger, D.; Dayan, M.; Zinger, H.; Liu, J. P.; Mozes, E. 2004. A peptide based on the complementarity determining region 1 of a human monoclonal autoantibody ameliorates spontaneous and induced lupus manifestations in correlation with cytokine immunomodulation. *J. Clin. Immunol. 24:* 579-590.

[90] Mauermann, N.; Sthoeger, Z.; Zinger, H.; Mozes, E. 2004. Amelioration of lupus manifestations by a peptide based on the complementarity determining region 1 of an autoantibody in severe combined immunodeficient (SCID) mice engrafted with peripheral blood lymphocytes of systemic lupus erythematosus (SLE) patients. *Clin. Exp. Immunol. 137:* 513-520.

[91] Rapoport, M. J.; Sharabi, A.; Aharoni, D.; Bloch, O.; Zinger, H.; Dayan, M.; Mozes, E. 2005. Amelioration of SLE-like manifestations in (NZB x NZW)F_1 mice following treatment with a peptide based on the complementarity determining region 1 of an autoantibody is associated with a down-regulation of apoptosis and of the pro-apoptotic factor JNK kinase. *Clin. Immunol. 117:* 262-270.

[92] Sela, U.; Mauermann, N.; Hershkoviz, R.; Zinger, H.; Dayan, M.; Cahalon, L.; Liu, J. P.; Mozes, E.; Lider, O. 2005. The inhibition of autoreactive T cell functions by a peptide based on the CDR1 of an anti-DNA autoantibody is via TGF-β-mediated suppression of LFA-1 and CD44 expression and function. *J. Immunol. 175:* 7255-7263.

[93] Sharabi, A.; Zinger, H.; Zborowsky, M.; Sthoeger, Z. M.; Mozes, E. 2006. A peptide based on the complementarity-determining region 1 of an autoantibody ameliorates

lupus by up-regulating $CD4^+CD25^+$ cells and TGF-β. *Proc. Natl. Acad. Sci. USA 103:* 8810-8815.

[94] Monneaux, F.; Hoebeke, J.; Sordet, C.; Nonn, C.; Briand, J. P.; Maillere, B.; Sibillia, J.; Muller, S. 2005. Selective modulation of $CD4^+$ T cells from lupus patients by a promiscuous, protective peptide analog. *J. Immunol. 175:* 5839-5847.

[95] Kang, H. K.; Michaels, M. A.; Berner, B. R.; Datta, S. K. 2005. Very low-dose tolerance with nucleosomal peptides controls lupus and induces potent regulatory T cell subsets. *J. Immunol. 174:* 3247-3255.

[96] Jouanne, C.; Avrameas, S.; Payelle-Brogard, B. 1999. A peptide derived from a apolyreactive monoclonal anti-DNA natural antibody can modulate lupus development in (NZB x NZW)F_1 mice. *Immunology 96:* 333-339.

In: Progress in Systemic Lupus Erythematosus Research
Editor: Tomas I. Seward, pp. 155-175
ISBN 978-1-60021-861-3

Chapter 5

AUTOANTIBODIES AS PROGNOSTIC OR DIAGNOSTIC MARKERS OF PSYCHIATRIC MANIFESTATIONS IN SLE

Paola Margutti, Federica Delunardo, Tania Colasanti, Ettore Piro and Elena Ortona [*]
Dipartimento di Malattie Infettive, Parassitarie e Immunomediate,
Istituto Superiore di Sanità, Rome, Italy.

ABSTRACT

In the course of Systemic Lupus Erythematosus (SLE), a variety of psychiatric disturbances are reported, including mood disorders (depressive symptoms), psychosis and anxiety. The reported prevalence of psychiatric disorders in SLE varies widely, ranging from 17% to 75%, but the diagnosis of these syndromes is difficult and depends on the exclusion of complications due to an iatrogenic effect of drugs, to metabolic abnormalities or to infections. Moreover, the diagnosis requires a careful psychiatric evaluation to exclude merely reactive psychological disturbances.

It has been suggested that several autoantibody specificities play a role in the pathogenesis of neuropsychiatric SLE. Potential pathogenic relevance has been attributed to, among others, antineuronal, antiphospholipid, antiganglioside, anti-DNA, anti-ribosomal P protein and anti-endothelial cell antibodies. However, particularly regarding psychiatric syndromes, conflicting results have been reported on the association between serum autoantibodies and symptoms.

The diagnostic and/or prognostic role of autoantibodies associated to psychiatric disorders in SLE is discussed.

[*] Address correspondence to: Elena Ortona, Department of Infectious, Parasitic and Immune-Mediated Diseases; Section of Immune-Mediated Diseases; Istituto Superiore di Sanità, V.le Regina Elena 299, 00161 Rome Italy. Phone: +39.06.49902760; Fax.+39.06.49387112; E-mail elena.ortona@iss.it

INTRODUCTION

Neuropsychiatric involvement in patients with Systemic Lupus Erythematosus (SLE), first mentioned by Kaposi more than 100 years ago, still remains one of the main challenge facing rheumatologists and other physicians [1]. The American College of Rheumatology recently proposed a classification of 19 different neurological and psychiatric syndromes of SLE [2, 3]. These case definitions encompass neurological syndromes, involving the central and peripheral nervous system as well as psychiatric disorders, cognitive deficits and acute confusional states (Table). However, major problems are still related to low specificity of some of these syndromes such as headache, cognitive impairment or mood disorders [4].The diagnosis of neuropsychiatric SLE (NPSLE) is complex not only because of the considerable prevalence variation (14-80%) but also because of the wide spectrum of neuropsychiatric manifestations. Different neuropsychiatric manifestations result from a variety of mechanisms including antibodies, vasculitis, thrombosis, hemorrhages and cytokine-mediated damages.

Table 1. American College of Rheumatology Classification of Neuropsychiatric Manifestations in SLE

Neurological manifestations
Myasthenia gravis
Acute inflammatory demyelinating polyradiculoneuropathy (Guillan-Barrè syndrome)
Demyelinating syndrome
Myelopathy
Headache
Neuropathy, cranial
Aseptic meningitis
Mononeuropathy (single/mutiplex)
Plexopathy
Autonomic disorder
Polyneuropathy
Cerebrovascular disease
Movement disorder (chorea)
Seizure and seizure disorders
Psychiatric manifestations
Acute confusional state
Cognitive dysfunction
Anxiety disorder
Mood disorder
Psychosis

Of note, despite the dramatic clinical manifestations, too often changes at the morphological neuroimaging techniques are minimal and non specific. The diagnosis of NPSLE remains largely one of exclusion and is approached in individual patients by thorough clinical evaluation, supported when necessary by autoantibody profiles, diagnostic imaging, electrophysiologic studies and objective assessment of cognitive performance [5]. Autoantibodies associated to NPSLE may have a diagnostic and/or prognostic role. This chapter describes and discusses the role of the autoantibodies reported to be associate to NPSLE.

Autoantibodies in NPSLE

Anti-Neuronal Antibodies

Anti-neuronal antibodies are a group of antibodies that react to neuronal components. Several studies, using different techniques to detect antibodies, demonstrated that anti-neuronal antibodies are detected predominantly in sera of patients with neuropsychiatric SLE than in patients without neuropsychiatric manifestations [6-13]. Competition assays showed that the binding of anti-neuronal antibodies was blocked by mycobacterial glycolipids, suggesting a link between mycobacterial infection and neuropsychiatric SLE [9]. Hanson and coworkers showed that a 50-kDa protein may be an important target for these autoantibodies, preponderantly found in NPSLE patients and that the antigen may play a role in the pathogenesis of some neurological manifestations in SLE [8]. To validate the hypothesis that some neuropsychiatric manifestations of SLE are mediated by the direct effect of antibody binding to neuronal membranes, one study of Bluestein and coworkers showed that anti-neuronal antibodies were significantly more concentrated in cerebrospinal fluid (CSF) of patients with SLE and central nervous system diseases than in CSF of SLE patients without neurological involvement [13].

Brain Reactive Antibodies

Brain reactive antibodies (BRA) are a subgroup of anti-neuronal antibodies that bind to integral membrane proteins of the brain. BRA correlates with psychosis and/or seizures in SLE patients [14].

Anti-Microtubule-Associated Protein 2 Antibodies

Microtubule-associated proteins (MAPs) interact with the microtubules of the cellular cytoskeleton. Other specific immunological markers of neuropsychiatric SLE are the autoantibodies to microtubule-associated protein 2. This cellular protein is restricted to neurons and is important in the control of cytoskeletal integrity and other neuronal functions [15].

Anti-Neurofilament Antibodies

Antibodies to cytoskeletal neurofilament protein antigens (ANFA) had an increased incidence in patients with neuropsychiatric SLE compared with SLE patients without neuropsychiatric symptoms. ANFA were found to be directed against the 205 and 160 kDa proteins of the neurofilament triplet [16].

Anti-Ganglioside Antibodies

Ganglioside is a compound composed of a glycosphingolipid with one or more sialic acids linked on a hydrophilic sugar chain that contains antigenic determinants. It is a component of the cell plasma membrane which modulates cell signal transduction events. The gangliosides most commonly recognized by neuropathy-associated autoantibodies are GM1, asialo-GM1, GD1a, GD1b, GM2 and GQ1b. Persistent high titer of anti-ganglioside (AGA) IgM is associated with several diseases, particularly neuropathies. The role of AGA IgM is to eliminate the immunosuppressive gangliosides shed from tissues during ageing, degeneration of neural and extraneural tissues and tumor growth and necrosis. In addition, *in vitro* observations with human and murine monoclonal antibodies suggest that they are capable of complement dependent cytotoxicity and apoptosis. AGA IgM can cause leakage of the blood brain barrier (BBB) in a concentration-dependent and complement-independent manner, bind to neuronal gangliosides to create a neuromuscular block and serve as a marker of axonal damage in neuropathies such as multiple sclerosis [17]. Several studies demonstrated the association between AGA and neuropsychiatric SLE and one study demonstrated that AGA may have predictive value [18], but these autoantibodies are not specific of NPSLE and are present also in sera of patients with different neuropathies. In a study, Pereira and coworkers showed a significant correlation between IgG AGA in the CSF and IgM AGA in the serum of NPSLE patients. Some NPSLE patients had AGA in the CSF but not in the sera, suggesting that intrathecal antibody production can result in the development of this manifestations [19]. Galeazzi and coworkers, in a study of a large cohort of European patients with SLE, showed an association between AGA IgG and migraine, dementia and peripheral neuropathy and an association between AGA IgM and depression [20]. In another study, Chen and coworkers demonstrated the presence of AGA in the CSF of children with NPSLE, and showed a clear association between AGA and brain computerized tomography scan. This study suggested that the detection of AGA in the CSF have a predictive value for the onset of a neuropsychiatric flare [21].

Anti-Triosephosphate Isomerase Antibodies

Sera from patients with NPSLE were screened for antibodies to mouse choroid plexus cell line ECPC-4 by Western blotting. A 29-kDa protein band detected in NPSLE sera was identified as triosephosphate isomerase (TPI). TPI plays an important role in glycolysis and is essential for efficient energy production. Using western blotting technique, Watanabe and coworkers demonstrated IgG specific to TPI in sera and CSF of patients with NPSLE. The serum anti-TPI IgG index was higher in the NPSLE than in other autoimmune diseases, demonstrating a high specificity for the diagnosis of NPSLE [22]. In CSF anti-TPI IgG form immunocomplexes and contribute to the pathogenesis of NPSLE by activating the complement system [23].

Anti-Glial Fibrillary Acidic Protein Antibodies

Glial fibrillary acidic protein (GFAP) is expressed in the central nervous system in astrocyte cells. It is involved in cell structure and movement, in cell communication and in the functioning of the BBB. A high positive predictive value of anti-GFAP antibodies for NPSLE has been described [24]. Recently, Trysberg and coworkers showed increased levels of GFAP in the cerebrospinal fluid of patients with NPSLE. Moreover, successful therapy with cyclophosphamide in NPSLE patients resulted in significantly decreased CSF levels of GFAP [25]. On the contrary, Conti and coworkers found no correlation between anti-GFAP antibodies and psychiatric morbidity [26].

Serum Lymphocytotoxic Antibodies

An important place in the immune network is reserved for specific interactions between regulatory antibodies and their ligands on T and B lymphocytes. Lymphocytotoxic antibodies (LCA) are detected in a great majority of patients with SLE. Several studies show or claim a relationship between the presence of LCA and neurological manifestations in SLE patients; the results, however, remain questionable due to the difference in detection methods as well as in definition of central nervous system (CNS) involvement [27]. Analysing frequency of HLA class II antigens (DR and DQ) and LCA in patients with NPSLE, Silva and Donadi showed that HLA-DR4 may have a protective role for the development of NPSLE whereas HLA-DR9, in addition to HLA-DR3 and to LCA, may predispose to neuropsychiatric abnormalities [28]. Analysis of LCA serially in SLE patients revealed fluctuations in LCA associated with NPSLE relapses or remissions [29].

Anti-CD4 Antibodies

Several lines of evidence indicate that the CD4 glycoprotein may be recognized by autoantibodies. Lenert and coworkers evaluated the presence of serum anti-CD4 antibodies in patients with SLE. The antibody reactivity has been analyzed both on native CD4 (by immunofluorescence) and on recombinant CD4 (by ELISA and Western blot). The results of this study showed that the anti-CD4 reactivity occurred in SLE patients with active disease and, as measured by the SLEDAI, was associated with particular clinical manifestations, including neuropsychiatric disease [30].

Anti-SSA/Ro Antibodies

The SSA/Ro antigens are nuclear and cytoplasmic polypeptides which serve as autoantigens in SLE and Sjögren's syndrome. They contain two major isoforms of 60 and 52 kDa. Initially, these antibodies were thought to be an epiphenomenon of autoimmune diseases. Recent studies have shown that they are associated with specific clinical manifestations and disease subsets [31]. To identify factors predictive of NPSLE, a large cohort of SLE patients was followed over 11 years. The presence of anti-SSA/Ro antibodies was demonstrated to be one independent predictor of significant neuropsychiatric damage [32]. Anti-SSA/Ro antibodies were detected also in CSF of patients with NPSLE [33]. In a clinical observation regarding suicide attempts in NPSLE patients, all harbored elevated titers of anti-SSA/Ro antibodies [34]. On the other hand, Shimojima and coworkers investigating the predictive value of distinct clinical factors in patients with NPSLE, demonstrated that anti-SSA/Ro antibodies were not significant for NPSLE and they did not predict the development of NPSLE [35]. In accordance with the previous study, Conti and coworkers did not find any significant correlation between the presence of anti-SSA/Ro autoantibodies and psychiatric involvement [26].

Anti-Sm Antibodies

Anti-Sm antibodies are directed against 7 proteins (B/B', D1, D2, D3, E, F, G) that constitute the common core of U1, U2, U4 and U5 small nuclear ribonucleoprotein (snRNP) particles [36]. Winfield and coworkers, in a serologic study on patients with NPSLE, found a higher incidence of anti-Sm antibodies in the patients with CNS dysfunction compared with a large group of patients without neuropsychiatric disease, suggesting an association of anti-Sm with CNS disease in SLE [37]. On the contrary, results of another study found no association between anti-Sm antibodies and neuropsychiatric features [38].

Anti-DNA Antibodies Cross-Reactive with NMDA Receptor

Many clinical manifestations of SLE are mediated by anti-DNA antibodies that in particular correlate with disease activity and cause kidney damage [39]. The anti-DNA antibodies may react directly with DNA or cross-react with non-DNA tissue antigens. In a study to determine the distinct antigens that anti-DNA antibodies recognize, a phage display library was screened with a monoclonal antibody specific to double stranded DNA and a pentapeptide consensus sequence (DWEYS) was revealed [40]. This consensus sequence is contained in *N*-methyl-D-aspartate (NMDA) receptors NR2A and NR2B (residues 283-287). NR2A and 2B are polypeptide chains that associate with the NR1 polypeptide to form NMDA receptors. NR2 receptors bind the neurotransmitter glutamate and play a role in learning and memory [41]. DeGiorgio and coworkers demonstrated that a subset of anti-DNA antibodies cross-react with NMDA receptors and, through an excitotoxic mechanism, can induce neuronal apoptosis both *in vitro* than inoculated directly in mouse brain [42]. These anti-DNA antibodies are present in CSF of patients with SLE who experienced cognitive decline, but it is not yet known whether they are produced *in situ* in the brain or cross the BBB.

BALB/c mice are a strain of mice which not present spontaneous brain pathology, permitting the analysis of antibody-mediated brain pathology and cognitive dysfunction. To study whether the anti-dsDNA/NR2 antibodies could cause brain damage when present in systemic circulation, BALB/c mice were immunized with the peptide to develop cross-reactive anti-DNA and anti-NR2 antibodies [43]. The administration of LPS to mice breaking the integrity of BBB, allowed to antibodies to pass from circulation to the brain. In fact, neuropathology requires a breach in the integrity of BBB and bacterial infection leads to a loss of the BBB function. The anti-NR2 antibodies showed a preferential binding in the hippocampus and consequent loss of hippocampal neurons. The loss of neurons in hippocampus leaded to an impairment in memory function. Mice receiving LPS and intravenously human antibodies specific to DNA and NMDA receptors extracted from sera of patients with SLE, elicited cognitive impairment [44]. To determine whether anti-NR2 antibodies exist in the brain of patients with SLE, IgG was eluted from patients' brain. The eluted IgG showed binding to DNA and NR and induced neuronal apoptosis when injected into mouse brain.

The breakdown of BBB may occur not only as infection, but also as cerebral vasculitis, stress, nicotine exposure, etc. The rise of epinephrine induced by stress is known to increase cerebral blood flow and to break the integrity of BBB, preferentially in the amygdale. In the mouse model immunized with the pentapeptide, the administration of epinephrine leaded to apoptosis of neurons of the lateral amygdale, resulting in behavioral disorders [45]. So the same antibody specificity can cause either a cognitive or an emotional disorder depending on the agent used to break the BBB. The presence of anti-DNA, anti-NR2 antibodies are found in 25-50% of patients with SLE [46]. Several studies yielded conflicting data about the correlation between the neuropsychological function and serum anti-NR2 antibody levels, but brain dysfunctions seem clearly correlate to the presence of antibody to the pentapeptide in CSF and symptom severity correlate with antibody titer [47]. An emerging quantitative magnetic resonance imaging technique offers the promise of a quantitative physiological measure of cellular integrity. A recent study using this technique showed that a small group of patients with SLE and anti-NR2 antibodies presented alteration in amygdale compared with patients without anti-NR2 antibodies [48].

Non-competitive inhibitors of NMDA receptors, such as MK801 and memantine, are promising therapeutic tools to protect mice from neuronal injury caused by the direct injection of anti-NR2 antibodies into the mouse brain. The use of the D-isoform of the consensus peptide could also lead to neuronal sparing binding to anti-NR2 antibodies and so preventing their binding to NR2 [45].

Anti-Ribosomal P Antibodies

Anti-ribosomal P antibodies recognize 3 specific ribosomal proteins P0, P1 and P2 [49]. One of the major points of interest of anti-ribosomal P antibodies derives from their high specificity for NPSLE [50,51]. Elevated titers of anti-ribosomal P antibodies are mainly detected in SLE patients immediately before and during active disease [52] and may be associated with particular clinical manifestations, including lupus nephritis, hepatitis [53-55] and neuropsychiatric involvement [5, 56-60].

In particular, the clinical association between elevated titers of anti-ribosomal P antibodies and psychosis was originally described by Bonfa and coworkers in patients with psychosis secondary to SLE [61]. Several studies showed a strong association between elevated titers of serum anti-P antibodies and NPSLE, predominantly psychosis and severe depression [54, 61-73]. One study of West and coworkers, examining a cohort of SLE patients with and without psychiatric manifestations over a period of 10 years, demonstrate the relationship between psychosis and depression and anti-ribosomal P antibodies [68]. On the contrary, some reports failed to find any relationship between anti-ribosomal P antibodies and NPSLE [26, 54, 74-78]. In particular, in a recent study the association between the presence of anti-ribosomal P antibodies and either lupus psychosis or depression, among a large cohort of patients with SLE, was not observed [79]. There are conflicting reports on the importance of anti-ribosomal P antibodies in the CSF. In a recent study, elevated titers of anti-ribosomal P antibodies were measured in the CSF and in the serum samples of a large cohort of patients with SLE. Patients were divided into 4 groups: patients with neurologic syndromes of the CNS; patients with diffuse psychiatric/neuropsychological syndromes; patients with complex presentations (neurologic syndromes of the CNS and diffuse psychiatric/neuropsychological syndromes); patients without NPSLE based on ACR diagnostic criteria [2]. In patients with NPSLE the frequency of CSF anti-ribosomal P antibodies was significantly higher than in patients without NPSLE. These results suggest that the presence of IgG anti-ribosomal P antibodies in CSF of SLE patients may be involved in the appearance of NPSLE, expecially in complex presentations [62].

Anti-ribosomal P antibodies bind and penetrate cells in culture. The cellular receptor appears to be a membrane form of the P0 38 kDa phosphoprotein, which mediates the binding and penetration of anti-ribosomal P antibodies. Following penetration, anti-ribosomal P antibodies were found to localize in the cytoplasm and in the nucleus [80]. Anti-ribosomal P antibodies are potent inhibitors of protein synthesis and *via* this pathway mediate cellular dysfunction. The ability of anti-ribosomal P antibodies to bind and penetrate into living cells was shown to induce the production of pro-inflammatory cytokines and to increase apoptosis of penetrated cells. This raises the possibility that these antibodies are of importance in the pathogenesis of NPSLE [52].

Anti-Endothelial Cells Antibodies

Anti-endothelial cells antibodies (AECA) are a heterogeneous group of autoantibodies directed against antigens in the membrane of endothelial cells. Originally described in 1971, a number of targets have now been identified for these autoantibodies [81]. They have been detected in several autoimmune diseases and have been associated with nephritis and vasculitis in SLE patients [82]. Recent data suggest their implication in endothelial dysfunction and a pathogenic role of AECA in SLE [82, 83]. AECA are capable of causing up-regulation of pro-inflammatory markers and apoptosis in endothelial cells [84]. Song and coworkers showed a clinical association of AECA with disease activity and neuropsychiatric manifestations in SLE [85]. Meroni and coworkers found AECA positivity in a high percentage of SLE patients with involvement of the CNS [86]. In a recent study Conti and coworkers, investigating the possible correlation of psychiatric manifestations in SLE and the reactivity of autoantibodies to different autoantigens (endothelial cells, cardiolipin, beta2 glycoproteinI (beta2-GPI), SSA/Ro, La, glial fibrillary acidic protein, ribosomal P protein, dsDNA and nucleosomes), demonstrated a significant association between AECA and psychiatric involvement in SLE patients [26, 87]. In this study, patients were categorized as either with or without psychiatric disorders on the basis of the clinical psychiatric examination. Patients were considered with psychiatric manifestations only when presented a severe psychopathology such as psychosis and mood disorders (recurrent major depressive disorders, dysthymic disorder, and depressive disorder not otherwise specified). Anxiety and mild depression were not included since these disorders are frequently detected in SLE patients and are predominantly psychoreactive [3, 88].

Identifying endothelial autoantigens involved in the autoimmune processes during neuropsychiatric SLE could help to explain the pathogenetic mechanisms involved in the initiation and progression of psychiatric symptoms.

Anti-Nedd5 Antibodies

With the aim of seeking and characterizing molecules that behave as autoantigens in NPSLE, Margutti and coworkers provided evidence that the C-terminal region of Nedd5 (Nedd5 C-ter) is a novel autoantigen with a role in neuropsychiatric manifestations [89]. In fact, the percentage of patients with anti-Nedd5 C-ter serum IgG was higher in group of patients with neuropsychiatric manifestations than in patients without these disorders. Nedd5 is a mammalian septin known to associate with actin-based structures, such as the contractile ring and stress fibers [90, 91]. The septins are a family of cytoskeletal GTPases that play an essential role in cytokinesis, in yeast and mammalian cells [92]. Interestingly, Nedd5 is predominantly expressed in the nervous system and may contribute to the formation of neurofibrillary tangles as integral constituent of paired helical filaments in Alzheimer's disease [93, 94]. Margutti and coworkers demonstrated that Nedd5 presented an intracellular redistribution on the cell surface during apoptosis, which may be in part responsible for its immunogenicity. Indeed, apoptosis may play an important role in by-passing tolerance to intracellular autoantigens. The specific modification of autoantigens and their redistribution into blebs at the surface of apoptotic cells may contribute to the induction of autoimmune responses [95, 96]. Moreover, apoptotic defects and impaired removal of apoptotic cells could contribute to an overload of autoantigens in the circulation or in target tissues that could become available to initiate an autoimmune response [97]. In susceptible individuals, this can lead to autoantibody-mediated tissue damage. Interestingly, the C-terminal region of Nedd-5 displays a coiled-coil domain. Several autoimmune autoantigens are characterized by the presence of such domain [98]. Coiled-coil proteins may be exposed to the immune system as surface structures in aberrant disease states associated with unregulated cell death and could become autoimmune targets [98]. The unanswered question is whether anti-Nedd5 C-ter antibodies can cause direct damage, thus contributing to the pathogenesis of psychiatric manifestations, or whether they are an epiphenomenon of these disorders.

Anti-Phospholipid Antibodies

Anti-phospholipid (aPL) autoantibodies are directed against anionic phospholipids or protein-phospholipid complexes. The negatively charged phospholipid targets include phosphatidyl inositol, phosphatidyl glycerol, phosphatidyl serine, phosphatidyl acid, and cardiolipin. Neutrally charged autoantigen targets include phosphatidyl ethanolamine, phosphatidyl choline, platelet activating factor and sphyngomyelin. By far, aPL antibodies, in particular anti-cardiolipin (aCL) antibodies and lupus anti-coagulant (LAC), have been the most widely investigated antibodies in NPSLE. The association of aPL antibodies in NPSLE has been reviewed [99]. This class of antibodies are reported to associate with focal neurological disease such as stroke, transient ischaemic attacks and transverse myelitis [99]. In a study on a large cohort of SLE patients, elevated titers of aPL antibodies were an independent risk factor for the development of cerebrovascular disease, seizures, and headache [100].

Anti-Cardiolipin Antibodies

A strong correlation between aCL antibodies and the overall frequency of neuropsychiatric manifestations was reported in many studies [101-103], but refuted in others [104,105]. In pediatric SLE, elevated titers of aCL antibodies are also frequently encountered, and aCL IgG are often associated with CNS involvement [103]. The frequency of aCL antibodies (IgG isotype) was significant for patients with cognitive dysfunction, chorea and cranial neuropathy [32]. In an open pilot study of children with NPSLE manifested as encephalopathy with or without grand mal seizures, focal seizures with depression or hallucinations, optic neuritis with transverse myelitis and psychosis with audiovisual hallucinations, a high percentage of these patients had elevated aCL IgG [106]. Paired measurements of aCL antibodies, in the serum and CSF, were performed using the ELISA method in SLE patients and in controls with other diseases. High titers of CSF aCL IgG were detected in NPSLE patients with lupus headache, acute psychosis, cognitive impairment, high cortical dysfunction and altered consciousness. Intrathecal synthesis occurred in these NPSLE patients, rather than the diffusion of aCL IgG from serum to CNS compartments [107]. In another study, aCL antibodies were studied in the serum and CSF of patients with SLE admitted for the assessment of NP disease. Patients with active neuropsychiatric complaints had positive aCL antibodies in the CSF, some of these patients presented simultaneous presence of antibodies in their sera and in their CSF. The assessment of the Q-albumin index revealed abnormal values in a subset of patients with active neuropsychiatric changes who exhibited positive CSF aCL antibodies, suggesting that impairment of the BBB function may lead to a leakage of intrathecal aPL antibodies from the systemic circulation. Additionally, a few patients revealed normal Q-albumin values with a high IgG-CSF index, suggesting increased intrathecal synthesis of antibodies. The study of aCL antibodies in CSF was useful in detecting active NPSLE [108]. In another small study, aCL antibodies were not detected in any CSF samples [109].

Experimental models show direct evidence for the pathogenicity of aCL antibodies and cognitive dysfunction. In one study, BALB/c mice were immunized with a pathogenic monoclonal aCL antibody and developed clinical and neurological manifestations [110]. In another mouse model, polyclonal aCL antibodies purified from pooled serum samples of patients with SLE had inhibitory effects on cultured normal rat brain astrocytes (RBA-1 cells). These results suggest that aCL Abs have an inhibitory effect on brain cells and elicit thrombus formation in brain vessels, both of which play a role in NPSLE [111].

Lupus Anti-Coagulant

One study evaluated the relationship between LAC and cognitive dysfunction in SLE patients. LAC-positive patients were 2 to 3 times more likely than LAC-negative patients to be designated as cognitively impaired. This study suggests that LAC positivity is associated with subclinical nervous system compromise and a pattern of deficits compatible with subcortical involvement, perhaps related to microthrombotic events or vasculopathy [112]. In a large study, utilizing MEDLINE from 1966 to 1989 to evaluate the validity of LAC in SLE patients, LAC was significantly associated with neuropsychiatric manifestations[113]. The findings of an association between LAC with seizures, cerebrovascular accidents and cognitive dysfunction were also corroborated in another study [32]. The association between neuropsychiatric manifestations and LAC was reported in many other studies [100, 101], but refuted in others [105].

Chapman and coworkers in a study on the LAC mechanism, showed that these antibodies may be involved in the pathogenesis of NPSLE by nonischemic mechanisms, including the inhibition of astrocyte proliferation and the nonspecific permeabilization and depolarization of synaptoneurosomes [114].

Anti-Phosphatidyl Ethanolamine Antibodies

In one study, Kamorchkine and coworkers investigating the presence of anti-phosphatidyl ethanolamine (aPE) antibodies in a population of SLE patients, showed that neurological involvement was present in most of the patients with aPE antibodies [115].

Other Autoantibodies

The antigenic targets of other autoantibodies demonstrated associated to NPSLE are the microfilament protein L-fimbrin, the nuclear protein DA1, the galactocerebrosides and the serine proteinase 3 [24, 116-118]. Further studies are necessary to assign to these autoantibodies a role as immunological markers of NPSLE.

Conclusion

Several published data reported the association between neuropsychiatric manifestations in SLE and the presence of autoantibodies, although in some cases contrasting data are reported. The high variability among different studies is probably related to differences in the populations of patients studied and the laboratory tests used to detect serum antibodies. Some autoantibodies had specificity to brain constituents such as neurotransmitter receptors, raising the possibility that autoimmune mechanisms could interrupt or modulate the neurotransmission or could signal neuronal death through an excitotoxic mechanism (Figure 1). Other autoantibodies could react against self molecules that cross-react with brain components, with the above described pathological effect. Other autoantibodies reacted against endothelium. These antibodies could react with BBB, breaking down the barrier integrity by induction of apoptosis and expression of adhesion molecules (Figure 2). In conclusion, further studies are necessary to better characterize the specific antigens or epitopes recognized by autoantibodies associated with NPSLE and to evaluate their potential use in the diagnosis of NPSLE. The characterization of the target molecules might help defining the precise role that specific autoantibodies may play in the autoimmune mechanisms, underlying psychiatric manifestations, and might let us investigate new and more effective therapeutical strategies.

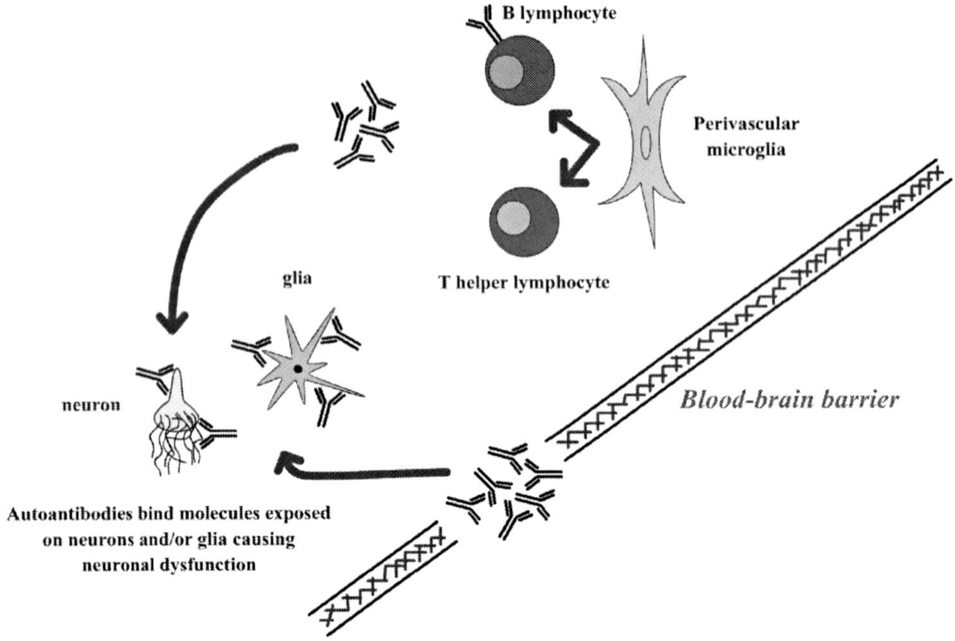

Figure 1. Access of antibodies to the central nervous system may occur through a disrupted blood-brain barrier or through *de novo* synthesis in nervous system. Autoantibodies, binding molecules exposed on the surfaces of neurons, lead to a neuro-toxic effect.

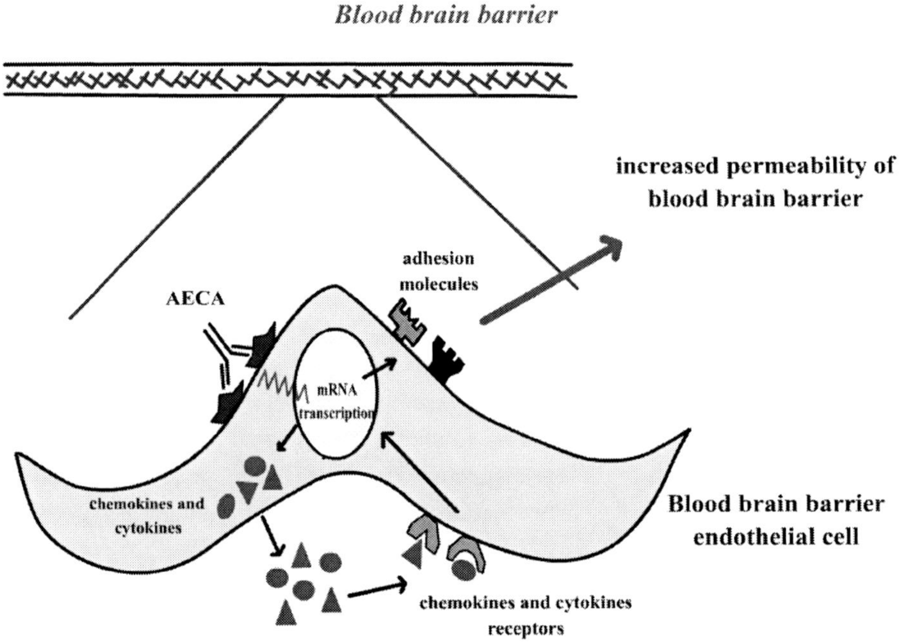

Figure 2. Effects of anti-endothelial cell antibodies. Anti-endothelial cell antibodies may activate the endothelium inducing the synthesis of pro-inflammatory cytokines and chemokines and expression of adhesion molecules, lead to the permeability of the blood-brain barrier.

References

[1] Kaposi, M. Neue beitrage zur kenntnis des lupus erythematosus. *Arch. Dermat. Syph.*, 1872 4, 36-79.

[2] ACR ad hoc committee on Neuropsychiatric Lupus Nomenclature: The American College of Rheumatology nomenclature and case definitions for neuropsychiatric lupus syndromes. *Arthritis Rheum.*, 1999 42, 599-608.

[3] Ainiala, H; Hietaharju, A; Loukkola, J; Peltola, J; Korpela, M; Metsanoja, R; Auvinen, A. Validity of the new American College of Rheumatology criteria for neuropsychiatric lupus syndromes: a population-based evaluation. *Arthritis Rheum.*, 2001 45, 419-423.

[4] Kozora, E; Ellison, MC; West, S. Depression, fatigue, and pain in systemic lupus erythematosus (SLE): relationship to the American College of Rheumatology SLE neuropsychological battery. *Arthritis Rheum.,* 2006 55, 628-35.

[5] Borchers, AT; Aoki, CA; Naguwa, SM; Keen, CL; Shoenfeld, Y; Gershwin, ME. Neuropsychiatric features of systemic lupus erythematosus. *Autoimmun. Rev.*, 2005 4, 329-44.

[6] Danon, YL; Garty, BZ. Autoantibodies to neuroblastoma cell surface antigens in neuropsychiatric lupus. *Neuropediatrics,* 1986 17, 23-7.

[7] Alosachie, IJ; Terryberry, JW; Mevorach, D; Chapman, Y; Lorber, M; Torre, D; Youinou, P; Peter, JB; Shoenfeld, Y. Central nervous system (CNS) involvement in SLE. The diagnostic role of antibodies to neuronal antigens. *Clin. Rev. Allergy Immunol.,* 1998 16, 275-84.

[8] Hanson, VG; Horowitz, M; Rosenbluth, D; Spiera, H; Puszkin, S. Systemic lupus erythematosus patients with central nervous system involvement show autoantibodies to a 50-kD neuronal membrane protein. *J. Exp. Med.*, 1992 176, 565-73.

[9] Avinoach, I; Amital-Teplizki, H; Kuperman, O; Isenberg, DA; Shoenfeld, Y. Characteristics of antineuronal antibodies in systemic lupus erythematosus patients with and without central nervous system involvement: the role of mycobacterial cross-reacting antigens. *Isr. J. Med. Sci.*, 1990 26, 367-73.

[10] Denburg, JA; Carbotte, RM; Denburg, SD. Neuronal antibodies and cognitive function in systemic lupus erythematosus. *Neurology*, 1987 37, 464-7.

[11] Hanly, JG; Behmann, S; Denburg, SD; Carbotte, RM; Denburg, JA. The association between sequential changes in serum antineuronal antibodies and neuropsychiatric systemic lupus erythematosus. *Postgrad. Med. J.*, 1989 65, 622-7.

[12] Bresnihan, B; Oliver, M; Williams, B; Hughes, GR. An antineuronal antibody cross-reacting with erythrocytes and lymphocytes in systemic lupus erythematosus. *Arthritis Rheum.*, 1979 22, 313-20.

[13] Bluestein, HG; Williams, GW; Steinberg, AD. Cerebrospinal fluid antibodies to neuronal cells: association with neuropsychiatric manifestations of systemic lupus erythematosus. *Am. J. Med.*, 1981 70, 240-6.

[14] Tin, SK; Xu, Q; Thumboo, J; Lee, LY; Tse, C; Fong, KY. Novel brain reactive autoantibodies: prevalence in systemic lupus erythematosus and association with psychoses and seizures. *J. Neuroimmunol.,* 2005 169, 153-60.

[15] Williams, RC Jr; Sugiura, K; Tan, EM. Antibodies to microtubule-associated protein 2 in patients with neuropsychiatric systemic lupus erythematosus. *Arthritis Rheum.*, 2004 50, 1239-47.

[16] Robbins, ML; Kornguth, SE; Bell, CL; Kalinke, T; England, D; Turski, P; Graziano, FM. Antineurofilament antibody evaluation in neuropsychiatric systemic lupus erythematosus. Combination with anticardiolipin antibody assay and magnetic resonance imaging. *Arthritis Rheum.*, 1988 31, 623-31.

[17] Ravindranath, MH; Muthugounder, S; Saravanan, TS; Presser, N; Morton, DL. Human antiganglioside autoantibodies: validation of ELISA. *An. NY Acad. Sci.*, n2005 1050, 229-42.

[18] Martinez, X; Tintore, M; Montalban, J; Ordi, J; Vilardell, M; Codina, A. Antibodies against gangliosides in patients with SLE and neurological manifestations. *Lupus,* 1992 1, 299-302.

[19] Pereira, RM; Yoshinari, NH; De Oliveira, RM; Cossermelli, W. Antiganglioside antibodies in patients with neuropsychiatric systemic lupus erythematosus. *Lupus*, 1992 1, 175-9.

[20] Galeazzi, M; Annunziata, P; Sebastiani, GD; Bellisai, F; Campanella, V; Ferrara, GB; Font, J; Houssiau, F; Passiu, G; De Ramon Garrido, E; Fernandez-Nebro, A; Bracci, L; Scorza, R; Puddu, P; Jedryka-Goral, A; Smolen, J; Tincani, A; Carcassi, C; Morozzi, G; Marcolongo, R. Anti-ganglioside antibodies in a large cohort of European patients with systemic lupus erythematosus: clinical, serological, and HLA class II gene associations. *J. Rheumatol.,* 2000 27, 135-41.

[21] Chen, Y; Wu, F; Hou, L; Ma, S; He, X. Antiganglioside antibodies in cerebrospinal fluid of children with neuropsychiatric lupus erythematosus. *Chin. Med. J. (Engl),* 1997 110, 594-7.

[22] Watanabe, H; Seino, T; Sato, Y. Antibodies to triosephosphate isomerase in patients with neuropsychiatric lupus. *Biochem. Biophys. Res. Commun.*, 2004 321, 949-53.

[23] Sasajima, T; Watanabe, H; Sato, S; Sato, Y; Ohira, H. Anti-triosephosphate isomerase antibodies in cerebrospinal fluid are associated with neuropsychiatric lupus. *J. Neuroimmuno*l., 2006 181, 150-6.

[24] Sanna, G; Piga, M; Terryberry, JW; Peltz, MT; Giagheddu, S; Satta, L; Ahmed, A; Cauli, A; Montaldo, C; Passiu, G; Peter, JB; Shoenfeld, Y; Mathieu, A. Central nervous system involvement in systemic lupus erythematosus: cerebralimaging and serological profile in patients with and without overt neuropsychiatric manifestations. *Lupus*, 2000 9, 573-83.

[25] Trysberg, E; Nylen, K; Rosengren, LE; Tarkowski, A. Neuronal and astrocytic damage in systemic lupus erythematosus patients with central nervous system involvement. *Arthritis Rheum.*, 2003 48, 2881-7.

[26] Conti, F; Alessandri, C; Bompane, D; Bombardieri, M; Spinelli, FR; Rusconi, AC; Valesini, G. Autoantibody profile in systemic lupus erythematosus with psychiatric manifestations: a role for anti-endothelial-cell antibodies. *Arthritis Res. Ther.*, 2004 6, R366-72.

[27] Osman, C; Swaak, AJ. Lymphocytotoxic antibodies in SLE: a review of the literature. *Clin. Rheumatol.*, 1994 13, 21-7.

[28] Silva, LM; Donadi, EA. Is immunogenetic susceptibility to neuropsychiatric systemic lupus erythematosus (SLE) different from non-neuropsychiatric SLE? *Ann. Rheum. Dis.*, 1996 55, 544-7.

[29] Temesvari, P; Denburg, J; Denburg, S; Carbotte, R; Bensen, W; Singal, D. Serum lymphocytotoxic antibodies in neuropsychiatric lupus: a serial study. CD4-reactive antibodies in systemic lupus erythematosus. *Clin. Immunol. Immunopathol.*, 1983 28, 243-51.

[30] Lenert, P; Lenert, G; Senecal, JL. CD4-reactive antibodies in systemic lupus erythematosus. *Hum. Immunol.*, 1996 49, 38-48.

[31] Ben-Chetrit, E. The molecular basis of the SSA/Ro antigens and the clinical significance of their autoantibodies. *Br. J. Rheumatol.*, 1993 32, 396-402.

[32] Mikdashi, J; Handwerger, B. Predictors of neuropsychiatric damage in systemic lupus erythematosus: data from the Maryland lupus cohort. *Rheumatology* (Oxford), 2004 43, 1555-60.

[33] Mevorach, D; Raz, E; Steiner, I. Evidence for intrathecal synthesis of autoantibodies in systemic lupus erythematosus with neurological involvement. *Lupus*, 1994 3, 117-21.

[34] Karassa, FB; Magliano, M; Isenberg, DA. Suicide attempts in patients with systemic lupus erythematosus. *Ann. Rheum. Dis.*, 2003 62, 58-60.

[35] Shimojima, Y; Matsuda, M; Gono, T; Ishii, W; Ikeda, S. Relationship between clinical factors and neuropsychiatric manifestations in systemic lupus erythematosus. *Clin. Rheumatol.*, 2005 24, 469-75.

[36] Migliorini, P; Baldini, C; Rocchi, V; Bombardieri, S. Anti-Sm and anti-RNP antibodies. *Autoimmunity*, 2005 38, 47-54.

[37] Winfield, JB; Brunner, CM; Koffler, D. Serologic studies in patients with systemic lupus erythematosus and central nervous system dysfunction. *Arthritis Rheum.*, 1978 21, 289-94.

[38] Singh, RR; Malaviya, AN; Kailash, S; Varghese, T. Clinical significance of anti-Sm antibody in systemic lupus erythematosus and related disorders. *Indian J. Med. Res.*, 1991 94, 206-10.

[39] Rahman, A; Hiepe, F. Anti-DNA antibodies--overview of assays and clinical correlations. *Lupus*, 2002 11, 770-3.

[40] Gaynor, B; Putterman, C; Valadon, P; Spatz, L; Scharff, MD; Diamond, B. Peptide inhibition of glomerular deposition of an anti-DNA antibody. *Proc. Natl. Acad. Sci. USA*, 1997 94, 1955-60.

[41] Morris, RG; Anderson, E; Lynch, GS; Baudry, M. Selective impairment of learning and blockade of long-term potentiation by an N-methyl-D-aspartate receptor antagonist, AP5. N*ature*, 1986 319, 774-6.

[42] DeGiorgio, LA; Konstantinov, KN; Lee, SC; Hardin, JA; Volpe, BT; Diamond, B. A subset of lupus anti-DNA antibodies cross-reacts with the NR2 glutamate receptor in systemic lupus erythematosus. *Nat. Med.,* 2001 7, 1189-93.

[43] Kowal, C; DeGiorgio, LA; Nakaoka, T; Hetherington, H; Huerta, PT; Diamond, B; Volpe, BT. Cognition and immunity; antibody impairs memory. *Immunity*, 2004 21, 179-88.

[44] Kowal, C; DeGiorgio, LA; Lee, JY; Edgar, MA; Huerta, PT; Volpe, BT; Diamond, B. Human lupus autoantibodies against NMDA receptors mediate cognitive impairment. *Proc. Natl. Acad. Sci. USA*, 2006 103, 19854-9.

[45] Huerta, PT; Kowal, C; DeGiorgio, LA; Volpe, BT; Diamond, B. Immunity and behavior: antibodies alter emotion. *Proc. Natl. Acad. Sci. USA*, 2006 103, 678-83.

[46] Sharma, A; Isenberg, D; Diamond, B. Studies of human polyclonal and monoclonal antibodies binding to lupus autoantigens and cross-reactive antigens. *Rheumatology* (Oxford), 2003 42, 453-63.

[47] Diamond, B; Kowal, C; Huerta, PT; Aranow, C; Mackay, M; DeGiorgio, LA; Lee, J; Triantafyllopoulou, A; Cohen-Solal, J; Volpe, BT. Immunity and acquired alterations in cognition and emotion: lessons from SLE. *Adv. Immunol.*, 2006 89, 289-320.

[48] Diamond, B; Volpe, BT. Antibodies and Brain Disease: A Convergence of Immunology and Physiology. *PLoS Med.*, 2006 3, e498.

[49] Elkon, KB; Parnassa, AP; Foster, CL. Lupus autoAbs target ribosomal P proteins. *J. Exp. Med.*, 1985 162, 459-71.

[50] Koffler, D; Miller, TE; Lahita, RG. Studies on the specificity and clinical correlation of antiribosomal Abs in systemic lupus erythematosus sera. *Arthritis Rheum.*, 1979 22, 463-70.

[51] Bonfa, E; Elkon, KB. Clinical and serologic associations of the antiribosomal P protein antibody. *Arthritis Rheum.,* 1986 29, 981-5.

[52] Toubi, E; Shoenfeld Y. Clinical and biological aspects of anti-P-ribosomal protein autoantibodies. *Autoimmun Rev.,* 2007 6, 119-25.

[53] Sato, T; Uchiumi, T; Ozawa, T; Kikuchi, M; Nakano, M; Kominami, R; Arakawa, M. AutoAbs against ribosomal proteins found with high frequency in patients with systemic lupus erythematosus with active disease. *J. Rheumatol.,* 1991 18, 1681-4.

[54] Reichlin, M; Wolfson-Reichlin, M. Evidence for the partecipation of anti-ribosomal P Abs in lupus nephritis. *Arthritis Rheum.*, 1999 42, 2728-9.

[55] Martin, AL; Reichlin, M. Fluctuations of antibody to ribosomal P proteins correlate with appearance and remission of nephritis in SLE. *Lupus*, 1996 5, 22-9.

[56] Greenwood, DL; Gitlits, VM; Alderuccio, F; Sentry, JW; Toh, BH. AutoAbs in neuropsychiatric lupus. *Autoimmunity,* 2002 35, 79-86.

[57] Ebert, T; Chapman, J; Shoenfeld, Y. Anti-ribosomal P protein and its role in psychiatric manifestations of systemic lupus erythematosus: myth or reality? *Lupus*, 2005 14, 571-5.

[58] Reichlin, M. Ribosomal P Abs and CNS lupus. *Lupus*, 2003 12, 916-8.

[59] Georgescu, L; Mevorach, D; Arnett, FC; Reveille, JD; Elkon, KB. Anti-P Abs and neuropsychiatric lupus erythematosus. *Ann. NY Acad. Sci.*, 1997 823, 263-9.

[60] McLaurin, EY; Holliday, SL; Williams, P; Brey, RL. Predictors of cognitive dysfunction in patients with systemic lupus erythematosus. *Neurology,* 2005 64, 297-303.

[61] Bonfa, E; Golombek, SJ; Kaufman, LD; Skelly, S; Weissbach, H; Brot, N; Elkon, KB. Association between lupus psychosis and anti-ribosomal P protein Abs. *N. Eng. J. Med.,* 1987 317, 265-71.

[62] Yoshio, T; Hirata, D; Onda, K; Nara, H; Minota, S. Anti-ribosomal P protein Abs in cerebrospinal fluid are associated with neuropsychiatric systemic lupus erythematosus. *J. Rheumatol.,* 2005 32, 34-9.

[63] Schneebaum, AB; Singleton, JD; West, SG; Blodgett, JK; Allen, LG; Cheronis, JC; Kotzin, BL. Association of psychiatric manifestations with Abs to ribosomal P proteins in systemic lupus erythematosus. *Am. J. Med.,* 1991 90, 54-62.

[64] Arnett, FC; Reveille, JD; Moutsopoulos, HM; Georgescu, L; Elkon, KB. Ribosomal P autoAbs in systemic lupus erythematosus. Frequencies in different ethnic groups and clinical and immunogenetic associations. *Arthritis Rheum*., 1996 39, 1833-1839.

[65] Gerli, R; Caponi, L; Tincani, A; Scorza, R; Sabbadini, MG; Danieli, MG; De Angelis, V; Cesarotti, M; Piccirilli, M; Quartesan, R; Moretti, P; Cantoni, C; Franceschini, F; Cavazzana, I; Origgi, L; Vanoli, M; Bozzolo, E; Ferrario, L; Padovani, A; Gambini, O; Vanzulli, L; Croce, D; Bombardieri, S. Clinical and serological associations of ribosomal P autoAbs in systemic lupus erythematosus: prospective evaluation in a large cohort of Italian patients. *Rheumatology* (Oxford), 2002 41, 1357-1366.

[66] Nojima, Y; Minota, S; Yamada, S; Takaku, F; Aotsuka, S; Yokohari, R. Correlation of Abs to ribosomal P protein with psychosis in patients with systemic lupus erythematosus. *Ann. Rheum. Dis*., 1992 51, 1053-1055.

[67] Massardo, L; Burgos, P; Martinez, ME; Perez, R; Calvo, M; Barros, J; Gonzales, A; Jacobelli, S. Antiribosomal P protein Abs in Chilean SLE patients: no association with renal disease. *Lupus*, 2002 11, 379-383.

[68] West, SG; Emlen, W; Wener, MH; Kotzin, BL. Neuropsychiatric lupus erythematosus: a 10-year prospective study on the value of diagnostic tests. *Am. J. Med.,* 1995 99, 153-163.

[69] Press, J; Palayew, K; Laxer, RM; Elkon, K; Eddy, A; Rakoff, D; Silverman, ED. Antiribosomal P Abs in pediatric patients with systemic lupus erythematosus and psychosis. *Arthritis Rheum.,* 1996 39, 671-676.

[70] Watanabe, T; Sato, T; Uchiumi, T; Arakawa, M. Neuropsychiatric manifestations in patients with systemic lupus erythematosus: diagnostic and predictive value of longitudinal examination of anti-ribosomal P antibody. *Lupus*, 1996 5, 178-183.

[71] Yoshio, T; Masuyama, J; Ikeda, M; Tamai, K; Hachiya T; Emori, T; Mimori, A; Takeda, A; Minota, S; Kano, S. Quantification of antiribosomal P0 protein Abs by ELISA with recombinant P0 fusion protein and their association with central nervous system disease in systemic lupus erythematosus. *J. Rheumatol*., 1995 22, 1681-1687.

[72] Isshi, K; Hirohata, S. Association of anti-ribosomal P protein Abs with neuropsychiatric systemic lupus erythematosus. *Arthritis Rheum.,* 1996 39, 1483-1490.

[73] Tzioufas, AG; Tzortzakis, NG; Panou-Pomonis, E; Boki, KA; Sakarellos-Daitsiotis, M; Sakarellos, C; Moutsopoulos, HM. The clinical relevance of Abs to ribosomal-P common epitope in two targeted systemic lupus erythematosus populations: a large cohort of consecutive patients and patients with active central nervous system disease. *Ann. Rheum Dis*., 2000 59, 99–104.

[74] Elkon, K. Ribosomal RNP. In: van Venrooij WJ, Maini RN, eds. *Manual of biological marker of diseases.* Dordrecht: Kluwer Academic Publishers, 1994 B2.5, 1-11.

[75] Derksen, RH; van Dam, P; Gmelig Meyling, FH; Bijlsma, JW; Smeenk, RJ. A prospective study on antiribosomal P proteins in two cases of familiar lupus and recurrent psychosis. *Ann. Rheum. Dis.*, 1990 49, 779-82.

[76] Teh, LS; Doherty, DG; Williams, BD. HLA-DRB genes and antiribosomal P Abs in systemic lupus erythematosus. *Br. J. Rheumatol.,* 1994 33, 1125-6.

[77] van Dam, A; Nossent, H; de Jong, J; Meilof, J; ter Borg, EJ; Swaak, T ; Smeenk, R. Diagnostic value of Abs against ribosomal phosphoproteins. A cross sectional and longitudinal study. *J. Rheumatol.,* 1991 18, 1026-34.

[78] Golombek, SJ; Graus, F; Elkon, KB. AutoAbs in the cerebrospinal fluid of patients with systemic lupus erythematosus. *Arthritis Rheum.*, 1986 29, 1090-7.

[79] Teh, LS; Bedwell, AE; Isenberg, DA; Gordon, C; Emery, P; Charles, PJ; Harper, M; Amos, N; Williams, BD. Antibodies to protein P in SLE. *Ann. Rheum. Dis.,* 1992 51, 489-94.

[80] Reichlin, M. Cellular dysfunction induced by penetration of autoantibodies into living cells: cellular damage and dysfunction mediated by antibodies to dsDNA and ribosomal P proteins. *J. Autoimmun.,* 1998 11, 557-61.

[81] Lindqvist, KJ; Osterland, CK. Human antibodies to vascolar endothelium. *Clin. Exp. Immunol.*, 1971 9, 753-60.

[82] D'Cruz, DP; Houssiau, FA; Ramirez, G; Baguley, Y; McCutcheon, J; Vianna, J; Haga, HJ; Swana, GT; Khamashta, MA; Taylor, JC; Davies, DR; Hughes, GRV. Antibodies to endothelial cells in systemic lupus erythematosus: a potential marker for nephritis and vasculitis. *Clin. Exp. Immunol.*, 1991 85, 254-61.

[83] Papa, ND; Raschi, E; Moroni, G; Panzeri, P; Borghi, MO; Ponticelli, C; Tincani, A; Balestrieri, G; Meroni, PL. Anti-endothelial cell IgG fractions from systemic lupus erythematosus patients bind to human endothelial cells and induce a pro-adhesive and a pro-inflammatory phenotype *in vitro*. *Lupus*, 1999 8, 423-9.

[84] Armitage, JD; Homer-Vanniasinkam, S; Lindsey, NJ. The role of endothelial cell reactive antibodies in peripheral vascular disease. *Autoimmun. Rev.*, 2004 3, 39-44.

[85] Song, J; Park, YB; Lee, WK; Lee, KH; Lee, SK. Clinical association of anti-endothelial cell antibodies in patients with systemic lupus erythematosus. *Rheumatol. Int.*, 2000 20, 1-7.

[86] Meroni, PL; Tincani, A; Sepp, N; Raschi, E; Testoni, C; Corsini, E; Cavazzana, I; Pellegrini, S; Salmaggi, A. Endothelium and the brain in CNS lupus. *Lupus*, 2003 129, 19-28.

[87] Valesini, G; Alessandri, C; Celestino, D; Conti, F. Anti-endothelial antibodies and neuropsychiatric systemic lupus erythematosus. *Ann. NY Acad. Sci.*, 2006 1069, 118-28.

[88] Shortall, E; Isenberg, D; Newman, SP. Factor associated with mood and mood disorders in SLE. *Lupus,* 1995 4, 272-9.

[89] Margutti, P; Sorice, M; Conti, F; Delunardo, F; Racaniello, M; Alessandri, C; Siracusano, A; Riganò, R; Profumo, E; Valesini, G; Ortona, E. Screening of an

endothelial cDNA library identifies the C-terminal region of Nedd5 as a novel autoantigen in systemic lupus erythematosus with psychiatric manifestations. *Arthritis Res. Ther.*, 2005 7, R896-R903.

[90] Vega, IE; Hsu, SC. The septin protein Nedd5 associates with both the exocyst complex and microtubules and disruption of its GTPase activity promotes aberrant neurite sprouting in PC12 cells. *Neuroreport*, 2003 14, 31-7.

[91] Surka, MC; Tsang, CW; Trimble, WS. The mammalian septin MSF localizes with microtubules and is required for completion of cytokinesis. *Mol. Biol. Cell*, 2002 13, 3532-45.

[92] Martinez, C; Ware J. Mammalian septin function in hemostasis and beyond. *Exp. Biol. Med.*, 2004 229, 1111-9.

[93] Peng, XR; Jia, Z; Zhang, Y; Ware, J; Trimble, WS. The septin CDCrel-1 is dispensable for normal development and neurotransmitter release. *Mol. Cell Biol.*, 2002 22, 378-87.

[94] Kinoshita, A; Kinoshita, M; Akiyama, H; Tomimoto, H; Akiguchi, I; Kumar, S; Noda, M; Kimura, J. Identification of septins in neurofibrillary tangles in Alzheimer's disease. *Am. J. Pathol.*, 1998 153, 1551-60.

[95] Cline, AM; Radic, MZ. Apoptosis, subcellular particles, and autoimmunity. *Clin. Immunol.*, 2004 112, 175-82.

[96] White, S; Rosen A. Apoptosis in systemic lupus erythematosus. *Curr. Opin. Rheumatol.*, 2003 15, 557-62.

[97] Pittoni, V; Valesini, G. The clearance of apoptotic cells: implications for autoimmunity. *Autoimmun. Rev.*, 2002 1, 154-61.

[98] Stinton, LM; Eystathioy, T; Selak, S; Chan, EK; Fritzler, MJ. Autoantibodies to protein transport and messenger RNA processing pathways: endosomes, lysosomes, Golgi complex, proteasomes, assemblyosomes, exosomes, and GW bodies. *Clinical Immunol.*, 2004 110, 30-44.

[99] Harris, EN, Pierangeli, S. Antiphospholipid antibodies and cerebral lupus. *Ann. NY Acad. Sci.*, 1997 823, 270-8.

[100] Sanna, G; Bertolaccini, ML; Cuadrado, MJ; Laing, H; Khamashta, MA; Mathieu, A; Hughes, GR. Neuropsychiatric manifestations in systemic lupus erythematosus: prevalence and association with antiphospholipid antibodies. *J. Rheumatol.*, 2003 30, 985-92.

[101] Mok, CC; Lau, CS; Wong, RW. Neuropsychiatric manifestations and their clinical associations in southern Chinese patients with systemic lupus erythematosus. *J. Rheumatol.*, 2001 28, 766-71.

[102] Afeltra, A; Garzia, P; Mitterhofer, AP; Vadacca, M; Galluzzo, S; Del Porto, F; Finamore, L; Pascucci, S; Gasparini, M; Lagana, B; Caccavo, D; Ferri, GM; Amoroso, A; Francia, A. Neuropsychiatric lupus syndromes: relationship with antiphospholipid antibodies. *Neurology*, 2003 61, 108-10.

[103] Ravelli, A; Caporali, R; Di Fuccia, G; Zonta, L; Montecucco, C; Martini, A. Anticardiolipin antibodies in pediatric systemic lupus erythematosus. *Arch. Pediatr. Adolesc. Med.*, 1994 148, 398-402.

[104] Emmi, L; Bramati, M; De Cristofaro, MT; Mascalchi, M; Dal Pozzo, G; Marconi, GP; Massai, G; Passaleva, A. MRI and SPECT investigations of the CNS in SLE patients. *Clin. Exp. Rheumatol.*, 1993 11, 13-20.

[105] Seaman, DE; Londino, AV Jr; Kwoh, CK; Medsger, TA Jr; Manzi, S. Antiphospholipid antibodies in pediatric systemic lupus erythematosus. *Pediatrics,* 1995 96, 1040-5.

[106] Reiff, A; Miller, J; Shaham, B; Bernstein, B; Szer, IS. Childhood central nervous system lupus; longitudinal assessment using single photon emission computed tomography. *J. Rheumatol.*, 1997 24, 2461-5.

[107] Lai, NS ; Lan, JL. Evaluation of cerebrospinal anticardiolipin antibodies in lupus patients with neuropsychiatric manifestations. *Lupus,* 2000 9, 353-7.

[108] Martinez-Cordero, E; Rivera Garcia, BE; Aguilar Leon, DE. Anticardiolipin antibodies in serum and cerebrospinal fluid from patients with systemic lupus erythematosus. *J. Investig. Allergol Clin. Immunol.*, 1997 7, 596-601.

[109] Fields, RA; Sibbitt, WL; Toubbeh, H; Bankhurst, AD. Neuropsychiatric lupus erythematosus, cerebral infarctions, and anticardiolipin antibodies. *Ann. Rheum. Dis.*, 1990 49, 114-7.

[110] Ziporen, L; Polak-Charcon, S; Korczyn, DA; Goldberg, I; Afek, A; Kopolovic, J; Chapman, J; Shoenfeld, Y. Neurological dysfunction associated with antiphospholipid syndrome:histopathological brain findings of thrombotic changes in a mouse model. *Clin. Dev. Immunol.*, 2004 11, 67-75.

[111] Sun, KH ; Liu, WT ; Tsai, CY; Liao, TS ; Lin, WM ; Yu, CL. Inhibition of astrocyte proliferation and binding to brain tissue of anticardiolipin antibodies purified from lupus serum. *Ann. Rheum. Dis.*, 1992 51, 707-12.

[112] Denburg, SD; Carbotte, RM; Ginsberg, JS; Denburg, JA. The relationship of antiphospholipid antibodies to cognitive function in patients with systemic lupus erythematosus. *J. Int. Neuropsychol. Soc.*, 1997 3, 377-86.

[113] Love, PE; Santoro, SA. Antiphospholipid antibodies: anticardiolipin and the lupus anticoagulant in systemic lupus erythematosus (SLE) and in non-SLE disorders. Prevalence and clinical significance. *Ann. Intern. Med.*, 1990 112, 682-98.

[114] Chapman, J; Cohen-Armon, M; Shoenfeld, Y; Korczyn, AD. Antiphospholipid antibodies permeabilize and depolarize brain synaptoneurosomes. *Lupus,* 1999 8, 127-33.

[115] Karmochkine, M; Berard, M; Piette, JC; Cacoub, P; Aillaud, MF; Harle, JR; Godeau, P; Boffa, MC; Harlet, JR. Antiphosphatidylethanolamine antibodies in systemic lupus erythematosus. *Lupus*, 1993 2, 157-60.

[116] De Mendonca Neto, EC ; Kumar, A ; Shadick, NA ; Michon, AM ; Matsudaira, P ; Eaton, RB ; Kumar, P ; Schur, PH. Antibodies to T- and L-isoforms of the cytoskeletal protein, fimbrin, in patients with systemic lupus erythematosus. *J. Clin. Invest.*, 1992 90, 1037-42.

[117] Asero, R; Origgi, L; Bertetti, E; D'Agostino, P; Riboldi, P. Detection of two associated precipitating autoantibodies (DA1 and DA2) in sera from patients with systemic lupus erythematosus. *J. Clin. Lab. Immunol.,* 1988 26, 63-6.

[118] Costallat, LT; de Oliveira, RM; Santiago, MB; Cossermelli, W; Samara, AM. Neuropsychiatric manifestations of systemic lupus erythematosus: the value of anticardiolipin, antigangliosides and antigalactocerebrosides antibodies. *Clin. Rheumatol.*, 1990 9, 489-97.of the blood-brain barrier.

In: Progress in Systemic Lupus Erythematosus Research ISBN 978-1-60021-861-3
Editor: Tomas I. Seward, pp. 177-192

Chapter 6

HIGH-DOSE IMMUNOSUPPRESSION WITH AUTOLOGOUS STEM CELL TRANSPLANTATION IN SEVERE REFRACTORY SYSTEMIC LUPUS ERYTHEMATOSUS

Igor A. Lisukov**, *Vera V. Sergeevicheva, Svetlana A. Sizikova, Alexander D. Kulagin*, Irina V. Kruchkova, Andrey V. Gilevich, Alexey E. Sizikov, Ludmila P. Konenkova, Elena R. Chernykh, Olga Y. Leplina and Vladimir A. Kozlov

Institute of Clinical Immunology RAMS SB, Novosibirsk, Russia
*Novosibirsk State Medical University

ABSTRACT

Carry out a prolonged studies to elucidate the role of high dose immunosupression therapy (HDIST) with autologous hematopoietic stem cells transplantation (SCT) in the treatment of severe and refractory autoimmune disease. In this study we analyzed single center experience of HDIST followed by SCT for refractory SLE.

The 13 patients with SLE, who had disease progression despite previously treatment with pulse Cy intravenous, prednisolone (standard doses and pulse therapy), oral Cy, azathioprine or metotrexate, were enrolled in the clinic of our Institution from 1998 to 2007. All patients were seriously ill, with SLE disease activity indices (SLEDAI) of 6-30, including cases with central nervous system lupus, lung vasculitis, carditis, nephritis with nephrotic syndrome and cytopenia. Autologous haemopoietic stem cells were collected from bone marrow (n=4) or mobilized from peripheral blood with Cy (3g/m2/once) and granulocyte colony-stimulating factor (G-CSF) (n=9). Pretransplant conditioning regimens included BEAM ± ATG (n=2), Melphalan 140 mg/m^2 + Etoposid

* Address correspondence to: Prof. Igor A. Lisukov, Institute of Clinical Immunology RAMS, Yadrintsevskaya str. 14, Novosibirsk 630099, Russia. Telefon 3832-28-59-56, fax 3832-25-05-22; E-mail: depsct@online.nsk.su

1600 mg/m^2 (n=2), Cy 200 mg/kg ± ATG (n=2) and Melphalan 120 mg/m^2 (n=1), Cy 140 mg/kg (n=6). Transplanted CD34+ MNC were more then 2x106/kg. Median time to an absolute neutrophil count (ANC) greater than $0{,}5x10^9$ /l and platelet count greater than $50x10^9$/l was 11 and 15 days, respectively. Three patients died on days 11, 22 and 63 due to transplant-related complications. All of the patients who died due to transplant-related complications had long history of the corticosteroids treatment, multiple and severe episodes of infections pre-SCT and received more then one anticytoststic drugs or ATG as conditioning regimen. All of the alive transplanted patients, who recovered hematopoiesis, showed improvement in disease activity: 8 (CR) and 2 (PR). The median follow up is now 14 month. One patient died due to lung vasculitis progression after 8 years after SCT. We conclude that HDIST followed by SCT for refractory SLE is feasible, effective and achievement of prolonged, corticosteroid-free remissions is a reality.

Keywords: stem cell transplantation, systemic lupus erythematosus.

Introduction

Some of the patients with SLE damaged severely or fatally from the uncontrolled disease progression, and conventional treatment are not effective. High-dose immunosuppression and SCT has been proposed as an investigational therapy for patients with severe refractory autoimmune diseases including SLE [1-5]. This approach is supported by hematopoietic SCT in animal autoimmune disorders [7-10] and in patients undergoing transplantation for hematologic disease who also had a coincidental autoimmune disease [11-12]. The rationale for using SCT to treat autoimmune disease is to maximally suppress or ablate the immune system and then rescue the patient from prolonged cytopenia by infusing autoulogous stem cells. Eradication of autoreactive cells by the conditioning regimen, redistribution of an altered cellular and humoral immunological network or thymic re-education are discussed as potential mechanisms for response ("reprogramming of the immune system") [13-17]. The EBMT/EULAR Registry has collected retrospective data on autoSCT from over 460 patient with autoimmune diseases [18]. Transplantation-related mortality (TRM) for all autoimmune disease has been reported to be 8,6% [17-19]. TRM was 12% for 51 patients undergoing transplantation for SLE [18]. Remission of disease activity was seen in 33/50 (66%) evaluable patients by six months, of which 10/31 (32%) subsequently relapsed after six months [18].

We describe 13 patients with primary severe SLE who received HDIST and auto-SCT in our Institution from 1998 to 2007 (Table 1). Six patients were registered in the EBMT/EULAR database.

Table 1. Results of autologous SCT in patients with SLE

	Sex/Age	Duration of SLE, years	Previous treatment	Organ involvement	Regimen	Number of infused cells	Results	Follow-up
Patient 1	F/21	3	oral corticosteroids, azathioprine, Cy pulse (1)	Lung, Renal	BEAM+ATG	2,4x10^8/kg (BM)	Complete remission	5 years
Patient 2	F/29	14	oral corticosteroids, azathioprine, Cy pulse (7), oral Cy (7g)	Renal, Serositis	BEAM	1,2x10^8/kg (BM)	Died on day 11 (sepsis)	
Patient 3	F/21	7	oral corticosteroids, azathioprine, Cy pulse (6)	CNS, Renal	Melphalan 120 mg/m^2 + etoposide 1600 mg/m^2	1,3x10^8/kg (BM)	Partial response	3,3 years
Patient 4	F/15	5	oral corticosteroids, azathioprine, Cy pulse (3), oral Cy (20,8g)	Renal	Melphalan 140 mg/m^2 + etoposide 1600 mg/m^2	1,3x10^8/kg (BM)	Died on day 22 (sepsis)	
Patient 5	F/19	9	oral corticosteroids, Cy pulse (9)	Renal, Cytopenia	Cy 200 mg/kg + ATG	20,6x10^6/kg (PBSC)	Died on day 63 (CMV)	
Patient 6	F/25	4	oral corticosteroids, azathioprine, Cy pulse (7)	Renal, CNS, Cytopenia	Cy 200 mg/kg	18x10^6/kg (PBSC)	Complete remission	3 years
Patient 7	F/42	7	oral corticosteroids, azathioprine, Cy pulse (9)	Lung, Heart (carditis) Renal	Cy 120 mg/kg	7x10^6/kg (CD34+ PBSC)	Complete remission	2.5 years

Table 1. (Continued)

	Sex/Age	Duration of SLE, years	Previous treatment	Organ involvement	Regimen	Number of infused cells	Results	Follow-up
Patient 8	F/34	8	oral corticosteroids, azathioprine, Cy+methylprednisolone pulse (6).	Renal, CNS	Melphalan 120 mg/m^2	$3.8x10^6$/kg (CD34+ PBSC)	Partial remission	1 year
Patient 9	F/24	1	oral corticosteroids, azathioprine, Cy+methylprednisolone pulse (6)	Renal	Cy 120 mg/kg	$4,3x10^8$/kg (CD34+ PBSC)	Complete remission	1 year
Patient 10	F/15	8	oral corticosteroids, Cy pulse (4), oral Cy (24g)	Renal, Lung, Heart (coronariitis)	Cy 120 mg/kg	$4.3x10^6$/kg (CD34+ PBSC)	Complete remission	6 months
Patient 11	F/25	2.5	oral corticosteroids, mtx, Cy+ methylprednisolone pulse pulse (4), cyclosporin A.	Renal, Lung, Heart (carditis)	Cy 130mg/kg	$5,9x10^6$/kg (CD34+ PBSC)	Complete remission	4 months
Patient 12	F/36	3	oral corticosteroids, Cy pulse (4), cyclosporin A	Renal cytopenia	Cy 120 mg/kg	$2,6x10^6$/kg (CD34+ PBSC)	Complete remission	3 months
Patient 13	F/34	4.5	oral corticosteroids, Cy pulse (9)	Renal, CNS	Cy 120 mg/kg	$3,6x10^6$/kg (PBSC)	Complete remission	3 months

Patient Selection

From April 1998 through February 2007 thirteen females aged between 15 and 41 years and suffered from SLE were enrolled in an high dose immunosupression (HDIST) with autologous hematopoietic stem cells transplantation (SCT) study at a single medical center.

Patient eligibility depended on a refractory to standard immunosupression therapies and either organ- or life-threatening visceral involvment. The inclusion criteria were: not controlled with pulse therapy Cy glomerulonephritis (World Health Organization (WHO) class III-IV), central nervous system (CNS) lupus, vasculitis involving the lung or heart, or transfusion-dependent autoimmune cytopenias. Evaluation of eligible patients by two independent rheumatologists and transplant physicians, informed consent and approval by the ethical committee were part of the protocol [13, 16].

Hematopoietic Stem Cell Procurement

Autologous hematopoietic stem cells were collected from bone marrow only for first four patients (n=4) under general anaestesia and all subsequent patients underwent peripheral blood hematopoietic stem cells collection (n=9). Three patients, whom bone marrow harvests was performed, has been achieved suboptimal MNC count ($<2x10^8$). PBSC mobilized from peripheral blood with Cy $4g/m^2$ and granulocyte colony-stimulating factor (G-CSF) (filgrastim) at 10 μg/kg subcutaneous daily with leukapheresis initiated when the white blood cells count reached $1x10^9/l$ (n=9). Apheresis was continued daily until the number of harvested progenitor cells reached a minimum of $2x10^6$ CD34+ cells/kg body weight. All of patients have successful collection after 2-3 leukapheresis session. The harvests were not manipulated. Stem cell products cryopreserved at the –80C for at least 2 week after collection.

Conditioning Regimen

The conditioning regimen was not started until at least 14 days after PBSC apheresis. Pretransplant conditioning regimens included BEAM (BCNU 300 mg/m^2 on day -7, Etoposid 800 mg/m^2 and Ara-C 800 mg/m^2 on days -6, -5, -4, -3, Melphalan 120 mg/m^2 on day -2) with antithimocyte globulin (ATG) in dose 30mg/kg infused over 10 hours on day 0 (n=1), BEAM (n=1), Etoposid 1600 mg/m^2 on day -2 with Melphalan 140 mg/m^2 on day -1 (n=2), Cy 200 mg/kg in divided doses of 50 mg/kg/day intravenously on days -6, -5, -4, -3 with ATG (total doses 60 mg/kg) infused over 10 hours in divided doses of 30 mg/kg/day on day +1, +2 (n=2), Melphalan 120 mg/m^2 (n=1), and Cy 200-140 mg/kg intravenously in divided doses for 4 days -6, -5, -4, -3 (n=6).

Supportive Care

Before, during and for 24 hours after treatment with high dose cyclophosphamide patient received hyperhydratation with forced diuresis and urometexan (Mesna) infusion for the prevention of haemorrhagic cystitis. Patients were treated in a single room without air filtration. All patients followed a standardized supportive care protocol including antiemetic therapy, analgesia for mucositis, transfusion support, and venoocclusive disease prophylaxis. A low microbial diet, oral daily fluoroquinolone (1 g/d) changed to intravenouse cefepime on neutropenic fever, fluconazole (400 mg/d) and acyclovir (10 mg/kg/d) and aerosolized amphotericin B (10 mg daily twice) were started upon admission and discontinued when the ANC rebounded to $0,5x10^9$ /l. All patients continued to receive prednisolone 15-30 mg/d. Methylprednisolone (1g) was administered intravenously 30 minutes before each dose of ATG. All of patient underwent BMT, received subcutaneous G-CSF (filgrastim) 5 μg/kg was started the day of hematopoietic stem cell infusion and continued untill the ANC was greater than $1x10^9$ /l for 3 consecutive days. Irradiated with 25 Gy platelets and red blood cells were given to maintain platelet count greater than 20 000/μL and hemoglobin level greater than 8.0 g/dL. For the first 6 months after transplantation, patients were treated with daily oral fluconazole and trimethoprim/sulfamethoxazole orally three times a week.

Table 2. Characteristics of the patients before SCT

	Anti-dsDNA, IU/ml[c]	C3 / C4, g/l[d]	ESR, mm/hr[e]	SLEDAI score
P1	580	0,42 / 0,1	58	18
P2	160	0,7 / 0,1	25	14
P3	740	0,74 /<0,1	65	30
P4	860	0,4 / 0,16	46	22
P5	107	0,66 /0,11	40	6
P6	1084	0,48 /<0,1	40	15
P7	13	0,3 / 0,1	27	2
P8	34	0,7 / 0,12	50	26
P9	260	0,7 /<0,1	29	12
P10	170	0,4 / 0,2	25	5
P11	50	0,55 /0,1	23	21
P12	18	0,9 /0,2	6	18
P13	98	0,72 /<0,1	25	14

Anti-dsDNA, antibodies to double stranded DNA were determined according to the manufacturer`s instructions (IMMCO Diagnostics Inc., USA) by enzyme linked immunosorbent assay (ELISA). Results were expressed in IU/ml, using Wo/80 as ultimate standard (negative result <50 IU/ml, positive result >60 IU/ml);

C3/C4, levels of the 3rd and 4th complement components were determined in immunoassay (BECKMAN Array[R] 360 system). The normal ranges were 0,8-2,0 g/l for C3 and 0,16-0,47 g/l for C4;

ESR, erythrocyte sedimentation rate, mm/hr

Assessment of Disease Status [18-22]

Patients returned for scheduled follow-up at 1, 3, 6 and 12 months and then yearly thereafter. If a patient was not able to return for follow-up, medical records and laboratory blood testing results were collected from local hospital.

Outcome was based on assessments before SCT (Table 2) and at 1, 3, and 6 months and yearly after transplantation. Early clinical response is evaluated using local interphysician vignettes, according the American College of Rheumatology Response criteria for SLE clinical trail: responder index for lupus erythematosis (RIFLE) criteria and improvement is revealed after mobilization regimen, including Cy [20].

Outcome was based on physical examination, serology (antibodies to double stranded DNA, antinuclear antibodies (ANA), anticardiolipin antibodies, C3 component level and lupus anticoagulant), lupus disease activity index (SLEDAI) [21], and response of pretransplant abnormalities in involved organ systems (eg, serum creatinine, 24-hour urine protein and creatinine clearance in nephritis, chest radiograph, and necessary imaging status, and pulmonary function tests in pneumonitis, evaluation of neurologic deficits in CNS lupus). Antibodies to double stranded DNA (anti-dsDNA) were determined according to the manufacturer`s instructions (IMMCO Diagnostics Inc., USA) by enzyme linked immunosorbent assay (ELISA). Results were expressed in IU/ml, using Wo/80 as ultimate standard (negative result <50 IU/ml, positive result >60 IU/ml). The presence of ANA was determined by the HEp-2000 indirect fluorescent antibody test system in accordance with the manufacturer`s instructions (IMMCO Diagnostics Inc., USA). Improvement was defined as a 50% improvement in any baseline parameter with no deterioration in any objective parameter. Criteria for complete remission requires that SLEDAI ≤ 3, prednisolone dose <10 mg daily and absence other immunosuppressive therapy.

Results

Patient data before SCT are summarized in Table 1. All patients had been treated unsuccessfully with Cy (intravenous pulse and oral) and other immunosupressive drugs. The reinfused bone marrow (n=4) contained median nucleated cell counts of $1,55x10^8$/kg (range $1,2\text{-}2,4x10^8$/kg). The reinfused peripheral blood stem cell harvest (n=9) contained median $4,34x10^6$/kg (range $2,6\text{-}20x10^6$/kg) CD34+ cells. Median time to an absolute neutrophil count (ANC) greater than $0,5x10^9$ /l and platelet count greater than $50x10^9$/l was 11 and 15 days, respectively. Three patients died on days 11, 22 and 63 due to transplant-related complications. All of the alive transplanted patients, who recovered hematopoiesis, showed improvement in disease activity: 8 (CR) and 2 (PR). The median follow up is now 15 month. One patient died due to SLE relapse: lung vasculitis progression after 8 years after SCT.

Transplant-Related Mortality (Toxity)

Main causes of death in patients with transplant related mortality before engrafment were infections (mucositis, pneumonia, sepsis) and hemorrhage (gastrointestinal bleeding) during the severe postchemotherapy cytopenia. All of the patients who died due to transplant-related complications had long history of the corticosteroids treatment, multiple and severe episodes of infections pre-SCT and received more then one anticytoststic drugs or ATG as conditioning regimen. One the patient developed secondary cytopenia due to virus-induced engrafment failure after hematopoiesis recovery. Lethal cases we presented in detail below.

Patient 1. The 29-year-old woman had a 14-year history of SLE, including arthritis, pericarditis, WHO class III glomerulonephritis, and elevated titers of ANA. The symptoms responded to corticosteroids, azathioprine and Cy. In November 1994 the patient developed nephrotic syndrome with proteinuria 3,3 g/l, acute renal failure (ARF), abdominal syndrome, ascite, anasarca and high titers of ANA (1:320). Pulse Cy intravenous (3 g in one month) in combination with pulse methylprednisolone intravenous was given with improvement. The disease was controlled by continuous therapy of oral prednisolone (minimum dose 20 mg daily) and azathioprine 150 mg/d and was complicated by frequent infections, including bacterial pneumonia, pyelonephritis, varicella zoster virus infection. In May 1998 relapse of the nephrotic syndrome with ARF has been diagnosed, and the remission of SLE was not achieved despite treatment with pulse Cy and methylprednisolone. The patient was not on dialysis. In November 1998 the patient underwent HDC (BEAM) followed by unmanipulated auto-BMT ($1,2x10^8$/kg of nucleated cells). Treatment was managed according to a standard supportive care protocol. The patient developed severe mucositis (grade 4), sepsis followed by multiorgan failure, severe hemorrhage (gastric bleeding) and died on day +11.

Patient 2. The 15-year-old female patient had suffered from SLE since 1995. SLE symptoms were arthritis, discoid rash, malar rash, photosensitivity, fever, elevated titers of ANA (1:160) and elevated titers of anticardiolipin antibodies. The treatment with 1 mg/kg/d prednisolone and 400 mg Cy weekly was started but did not induce complete response. Discoid rash, arthralgias and serological symptoms were uncontrolled. Eight months later, prednisolone was reduced to 20 mg/d because of side effects. In January 1998 lupus nephritis has been diagnosed. The treatment with oral Cy (at May 1998 total dose was 20,8g) with addition of penicillamine, azathioprine and increased corticosteroids was continued without significant improvement. Therefore three pulses of 1g Cy intravenous were given at monthly intervals. However, patients condition deteriorated, lupus nephritis progressed, disease activity remained high (SLEDAI 22). The option of HDC was discussed with the patient's parents and performed after approval by the ethics committee. In April 2000 unmanipulated non-cryopreserved autologous marrow ($1,32x10^8$/kg of nucleated cells) was reinfused after conditioning of the recipient with a combination of etoposide 1600 mg/m^2 on day -2 and melphalan 140 mg/m^2 on day -1. In the posttransplantation period the patient developed severe mucositis and enteropathy (day +5), sepsis followed by multiorgan failure (day +10), severe hemorrhage (gastrointestinal bleeding), pneumonia (day +12) and died on day +22. ANC reached $0,5x10^9$/l on day +15.

Patient 3. The 19-year-old woman had suffered from SLE (arthritis, malar rash, carditis, pneumonitis, immunologic disorder) since 1993. The treatment with 1 mg/kg/d prednisolone induced complete response that lasted till 1999. Relapse of SLE with lupus erythema and elevated titers of ANA was diagnosed in January 1999. In August 2000 the patient presented severe cutaneous vasculitis, cytopenia (platelets $45x10^9/l$, leukocytes $1,2x10^9/l$), fever, nephritis despite treatment with oral prednisolone 0,5 mg/kg/d. There was no sustained improvement with pulse intravenous Cy (7,4 g in 9 months) in combination with oral prednisolone (60-25 mg daily) and pulse intravenous methylprednisolone (total dose 5 g). The disease activity decreased, but cutaneous vasculitis, cytopenia and serological symptoms were uncontrolled. The functions of major organs were adequate. She was selected for high-dose immunosuppression and autologous SCT. Priming was with Cy 4 g/m^2 followed by G-CSF 480 μg/d subcutaneously. Significance regress of symptoms of cutaneous vasculitis and absence of cytopenia were achieved. Prednisolone was reduced to 10 mg/d. Two months later, conditioning with Cy 50 mg/kg daily for 4 days with ATG 30 mg/kg daily for 3 days was given. Transplantation of $20,8x10^6/kg$ CD34+ autologous stem cells was performed on October 2002. Engraftment occurred on day 10 (leukocytes $9,0x10^9/l$, platelets $80x10^9/l$). On day 20 the patient developed fever, abnormal liver function (ALT 4,1 mmol/l (normal<0,68), AST 2,0 mmol/l (normal<0,68), the total bilirubin level 6,08 mg/dl (normal<1,2)) and severe pancytopenia (leukocytes $0,2x10^9/l$, platelets $30x10^9/l$, haemoglobin 7 g/dl), on day 30 severe enteropathy. On the basis of clinical signs, positive results in polymerase chain reaction assay, detection of Cytomegalovirus (CMV) inclusions in bone marrow the CMV disease was diagnosed. We started treatment with intravenous ganciclovir 10 mg/kg daily in combination with intravenous immunoglobulin 0,5 g/kg for five consecutive days and thereafter once weekly maintenance was given. After two weeks, the liver function returned to normal and the symptoms of enterocolitis regressed. Unfortunately, the patient remained pancytopenic (despite the administration of G-CSF), developed sepsis, pneumonia and died on day 63 from multiorgan failure.

Overall and Disease-Free Survival

All of the transplanted patients, who recovered stabile hematopoiesis, showed rapid improvement in clinical disease activity. The median follow up is now 15 month. The probability of disease-free survival or complete remission defined as requiring no SLE-activity and immunosuppressive medication, except physiologic doses of prednisolone (<10 mg/day), however the time of entering remission was several month, often because of long-term high-dose pre-SCT corticosteroid therapy that had to be withdrawn gradually to avoid abstinent syndrom. Long time of achieving improvement or normalization of serology (ANA, anti-ds DNA) occurred in patient entering clinical remission (mean 6 month). We not exclude, there are because cyclophosphomaide-resistant specific memory B-cell prolong persistent.

The partial remission was defined in two patient, who suffered from CNS-lupus and mild symptoms are remain after SCT. One patients, admitted to our hospital in November 1999 was severely disabled (lower paraplegia, failure of the pelvic function due to myelitis) with

SLEDAI 30. The total observation time after transplantation is now 74 months. The functions of bladder and bowel returned to normal, but mild lower paraplegia and serology activity are remain, that require prolong immunosuppression therapy with steroid. Second SLE patient presented with organic encephaloneuropathies: abnormalities in neurocognitive function, such as memory, intellect; reflectory tetraplegia, sensitive ataxia in pretrasplantation period, present with mild neurological symptoms now (after 1 year after SCT): headache, depression and transitory psychosis. Patient need in symptomatic, antipsychotic treatment. Immunosupression by sreroid and cyclosporin is continuing.

The longest continuous duration of SLE remission has been 8 years. Disease progression-related mortality despite initial response was occurred once after long term stabile clinical and immunological remission. Case report is as followed.

Patient. The 21-year-old woman with SLE developed lung vasculitis in 1995. She was treated with corticosteroids 0,5 mg/kg over 10 weeks with some clinical improvement. Prednisolone was reduced to 10 mg/d. In 1997 lupus nephritis has been diagnosed, pulse Cy intravenous was given but withdrawn because of allergic dermatitis. The treatment with prednisolone 1 mg/kg and azathioprine was started but did not produce any effect. In March 1998 the patient was admitted to our hospital with dyspnea, progressive pulmonary hypertension (Doppler echo showed estimated sistolic pulmonary artery pressure (sPAP) of 49 mm Hg), arthritis, proteinuria (5,3 g/24 hour), renal failure (creatinine clearance 50 ml/min), elevated titres of ANA (1:160). In April 1998 HDC according to the BEAM protocol followed by unmanipulated autologous bone marrow transplantation (BMT) was applied. On day 0, ATG ("ATGAM" 30 mg/kg) was given for *in vivo* T cell-depletion. The patient developed moderate mucositis and enteropathy (grade 2), neutropenic fever (FUO) with response to the ceftriaxone 4 g/d + tobramycin 240 mg/d, genital herpes infection with response to the famciclovir 750 mg/d. Haemorrhage was mild. The time to achieve an ANC exceeded $0{,}5x10^9/l$ and platelet count exceeded $50x10^9/l$ was respectively 16 and 19 days. After six months complete remission of SLE has been established. The SLEDAI decreased from 18 to 0, pulmonary and renal function was recovered, ANA were negative. The oral prednisolone was withdrawn after 10 months of BMT. The follow up is now over five years. The patient was in stable clinical and immunologic remission and returned to work. At the November 2006 patient admitted in the hospital with symptoms of respiratory insufiency. Physical and laboratory examination was revealed progression of lung vasculitis (Doppler echo showed high sPAP, CT scanning revealed bullous pneumanitis) and 8 weeks of gestation. After therapeutic abortion, treatment with cyclosporine 150 mg and prednisolon 30 mg daily once was started with transitory clinical improvement, but patient died due to repeating spontaneously pneumothorax after 8 years after SCT.

The aim of high-doses immunosupression is to destroy self-reactive lymphocytes. We evaluate the efficacy and toxicity of ASCT with specific attention to long-term immune reconstitution. Immunological features were assessed before ASCT and at 1, 3, and 6 months and yearly after transplantation. HDIT induced profound lymphocytopenia. Mean absolute lymphocyte counts were back to baseline level at the 6 month. The CD4/CD8 ratio significantly decreased at 1 month after ASCT due to reduced proportions of CD4 T-cells and remained stable in 6 months. There were no significant changes from pretherapy in the proportions of CD4+DR+ and CD8+DR+ lymphocytes. At 1 month posttransplant the number of naïve CD4+45RA+ cell have been reduced significantly as well as CD8+45RA+ cells, but these subpopulations recovered at 6 month after ASCT completely. CD8+45RO+ cells decreased steadily during the posttransplant follow-up. Before conditioning in vitro T-cell mitogenic responses were decreased in most of all patients with a trend toward a baseline level at 3 month after ASCT.

Conclusion

Patients with refractory and active lupus involving multiple organ systems despite a relatively young age traditionally have a high disease related mortality rate. Continuing failing therapy for such patients is problematic but necessary to confirm that the increased risk HDIST with auto-SCT would be offset by better disease control and induced long-term remission or partial response with clinical improvement in all refractory alive SLE patients underwent SCT in our center.

Three patients died due to serious infections in the early posttransplantation period. Among them, the nucleated cell counts in the reinfused graft product in the two fatal cases (case1 and case 2) were less than $2x10^8$/kg recipient body weight, and probably it was not enough for stable hematopoiesis recovery. Although there are no universal agreement, recommended optimal CD 34+ cell dose ($2\text{-}5x10^8$ /kg) for successful engraftment after autologous myeloablative SCT for patient with malignancies has been accepted by most clinicians [23]. Non-myeloablative conditioning regimen used in most our patient carries virtually no risk of non-engraftment after SCT. However, our results (data no shown) demonstrated correlation between infused CD34+ cell dose and faster WBC and platelet engraftment supporting the role of autologous SC in shortening the period of neutropenia and critical trombocytopenia. Thus, for all patients in whom HSC collection was unsuccessful in achieving an adequate number of CD 34+ cells, repeat bone marrow harvest or mobilization should be performed [23, 24]. In our study, G-CSF in combination with CY did not cause a disease flare [25]. Most of patients showed an improvement in disease activity after high dose Cy and G-CSF for PBSC mobilization before pretransplant conditioning [5]. Only one patient, receiving Cy-mobilization, experienced severe complication and developed pneumonia and skin infection during pretransplantation period.

Culture negative neutropenic fever, although common during early posttransplantation regimen, was transient and easily controlled with empiric antibiotic therapy.

All of the patients who died due to transplant-related complications received more then one anticytostatic drugs in myeloablative doses or ATG as conditioning regimen. The conditioning regimen for autoimmune disease used to eliminate self-reactivity lymphocytes within the patient has been designed depending investigator to either specically target lymphocytes (lymphoablative i.e. non-myeloablative regimen) or to destroy the entire hematopoietic bone marrow compartment (myeloablative regimen). In cancers, autologous HSCT regimens are designed to be myeloablative as the rationale is to destroy leukemic cancer-causing stem cells. [1]. The goal of autologous HSCT for autoimmune diseases is to generate new self-tolerant lymphocytes after elimination of self- or auto-reactively lymphocytes (i.e. lymphoablation), rather than ablate and reconstitute the entire hematopoietic compartment myeloablation). Non-myeloablative regimens are often considered safer owing to lower organ toxicity, the more rapid engraftment following non-myeloablative HSCT demonstrated herein also supports of non-myeloablative regimens compared to myeloablative regimens. Therefore, in SLE, there are no reports comparing engraftment and responses after non-myeloablative compared to myeloablative regimens for autologous HSCT [1, 4].

Consistent with previously reports, we think that intensification of the chemotherapy is not a justified risk for SLE patients and we stoped to use myeloablative conditioning regimens specific for malignant disease. Now we used a dose-escalated Cy for conditionig, a standart lupus medication [4, 5]

One of the most important complications was cardiotoxicity, possibly related to direct CY toxicity and hyperhydration. The patient selection is important to reduce TRM and complete cardiological assessment before transplantation is highly recommended [26]. Careful patient selection, especially cardiac function evaluation, which is often underestimated in SLE-patient, may to avoid mortality [26].

A few patients developed CMV disease after AutoSCT [27]. We did not routinely monitor or of CMV viremia. One patient, who was severely immunosupressed owing to chronic use of high-dose steroids more then 9 years, was found to have fatal CMV-disease after ATG-including regimen, that more characterized postallotransplant complication. It may be cause for recommendation to use standart CMV pretrasplant prophylaxis and CMV-monitoring for SLE patients with long-term history of immunosuressive therapy. Positive CMV surveillance assay are the grounds for prompt treatment with ganciclovir [28]. Also, compared with patients with cancer, patients with lupus have a long history of chronic immunosuppression and appear unusually prone to infections during mobilization and after transplantation, mandating aggressive preemptive antimicrobial (i.e. antifungal and antiviral) prophylaxis [29].

Addition of ATG for SCT for SLE treatment further maximizes immunosupression, because specific target T-cells [30]. Equine ATG caused acute toxicities that mimicked active SLE flares and did not target memory B cells.[27,30] Because we obtained significant clinical response and low rate of severe infection, when treating with Cy along, ATG seem not to be necessary for the conditioning [5].

We did not found differences in T-cell recovery between patients with complete and partial response or between patients treated with different regimens. But we noted more rapid numerous and functional T-cell recovery in SLE patients treated with ASCT compared with lymphoma patients (data not shown).

Other method of immunoablation, such as anti-CD20 monoclonal antibody (Rituximab), may be an important therapeutic approach for the treatment of patients intolerant to HDIST with auto-SCT. Because Rituximab is generally well tolerated and selectively depletes B cells, its role in immune mediated diseases is now also being explored [31-34]. Future SLE transplant protocol should consider substitute ATG with rituximab, or alemtuzumab, targets both T and B-cells[35,36]. We did not incorporate ATG into the conditioning regimen from 2003 year.

Thus, the complication of autologous SCT is connected with patient selection, the choise of conditioning regimen, and supportive care during and after transplantation.

There are two of our groupe of patients, who developed symptoms of SLE during pregnancy (1 patient during fatal progression of the disease and 1 patient at the onset of the disease). Patients with SLE have normal fertility and should not be discouraged from having children. However, given the high frequency of SLE flares during pregnancy, SLE pregnancies should be regarded as high risk and close monitoring for disease activity is mandatory throughout the pregnancy. [37,38].

The involvement of the central nervous system (CNS) is one of the major causes of morbidity and mortality in systemic lupus erythematosus (SLE) patient [3,39]. Among the neurologic manifestations of SLE, the most common are the organic encephalopathies, which basically comprise all potential variations of acute confusion, lethargy, or coma; chronic dementias; depression, mania, or other affective disturbances; or psychosis; cranial nerve abnormalities (most prominently, optic neuritis), stroke, peripheral neuropathy et sta. Acute or subacute mental status changes may be secondary to diffuse cerebritis but should be differentiated from focal cortical dysfunction resulting from thromboembolic cerebrovascular accident (CVA) or from diffuse changes resulting from electrolyte or metabolic derangements (accentuated by concomitant renal failure) [39].

Spinal cord involvement in SLE patient is rare but devastating. Transverse myelitis, subacute-to-chronic demyelinating syndromes may caused severe invalidity [40,41]. Management of central nervous system (CNS) involvement still remains one of the most challenging and using of HDIST doesn't solve problems completely. Our two patient with CNS involvment did not achieved Cr after SCT but dramatically improved. Recently, the use of intrathecal methotrexate and dexamethasone has been reported in a small series of patients, with a good outcome in patients with severe CNS manifestations.

It should be mentioned that all of our patients had experienced multiple and severe episodes of infections pre-SCT and long-term history of corticosteroids therapy (3-14 years). The remissions were achieved despite a previous history of refractory or relapsing disease indicating the potential efficacy of this procedure. It was anticipated control of clinical lupus activity was reflected by marked falls of anti-ds DNA antibodies, normalization of complement levels and reduction or withdrawal of corticosteroids.

In concert with the consensus report from EULAR and EBMT [16], patients should be selected for autoSCT who have severe disease and are refractory to conventional therapy. In selecting patients, consideration should be given to the balance between disease severity and organ damage. For patients with SLE, in contrast with malignancies, since organ compromise is due to lupus, impaired visceral organ function is not a ultimately contraindication, but is one of the major indication for SCT. While this makes the transplant procedure more complicated, marked organ improvement, particularly of the lung, the kidney and the central nervous system has occurred following Cy-contained mobilization and SCT. Thus preexisting dysfunction of kidneys, liver, and lung is associated with increased mortality from transplant regimens. Treatment of such patients remains a difficult clinical problem. The presence of poor prognostic indicators would provide additional support in patient selection for future SCT studies. Recently, prognostic indicators suggesting a poor outcome in SLE have been proposed [43]. There are renal dysfunction, hypertension, anemia, low C3, central nervous system involvement and thrombocytopenia. Patients with these prognostic features have a considerably shortened life span. Thus, the 10-year survival of patients without features is estimated to be 86% compared with 60% of patients with these features. The quality of response to conventional therapy may be a useful criterion in selection of patients earlier in disease. Pulse Cy (500-1000 mg/m^2) is generally considered the standard of care. Eligible for SCT patients with nonrenal visceral involvement need only fail corticosteroids and 3 months of pulse Cy. For patients in whom the indication is nephritis, active disease must be present despite at least 6 cycles of monthly pulse Cy [17].

Judicious selection of patients earlier in disease or in remission, but with a high risk of relapse or further progression, will improved the results of treatment and transplantation-related complication.

References

[1] Burt R., Marmont A, Oyama Y, Slavin S. Randomized Controlled Trials of Autologous Hematopoietic Stem Cell Transplantation for Autoimmune Diseases The Evolution From Myeloablative to Lymphoablative Transplant Regimens. *ARTHRITIS and RHEUMATISM* 2006; Vol. 54, No. 12: pp 3750–3760.

[2] Marmont A, van Lint M, Gualandi F, Bacigalupo A. Autologous marrow stem cell transplantation for severe systemic lupus erythematosus of long duration. *Lupus* 1997; 6: 545-548.

[3] Trysberg E, Lindgren I, Tarkowski A. Autologous stem cell transplantation in case of treatment resistant central nervous system lupus. *Ann. Rheum. Dis.* 2000; 59: 236-238.

[4] Burt R and E Traynor A Hematopoietic stem cell transplantation for systemic erythematosus *Arthritis Res. Ther.* 2003, 5:207-209.

[5] Tsukamoto H, Nagafuji K, Horiuchi T, A phase I-II trial of autologous peripheral blood stem cell transplantation in the treatment of refractory autoimmune disease *Ann Rheum Dis* 2006; 65;508-514.

[6] Lisukov IA, Sizikova SA, Kulagin AD. High-dose Immunosuppression with Autologous Stem Cell Transplantation in Severe Refractory Systemic Lupus Erythematosus *Lupus* 2004; Vol 13: 89-94.

[7] Ikehara S. Bone marrow transplantation for autoimmune diseases. *Acta Haematol.* 1998; 99: 116-132.

[8] Van Bekkum D.W. Review: BMT in experimental autoimmune diseases. *Bone Marrow Transplant* 1993; 11: 183 –187.

[9] Knaan-Shanzer S., Houben P., Van Bekkum D.W. Remission induction of adjuvant arthritis in rats by total body irradiation and autologous bone marrow transplantation. *Bone Marrow Transplant* 1992; 8: 333-338.

[10] Van Bekkum D.W. Experimental basis for treating autoimmune diseases with bone marrow transplants. *Stem cells* 1996; 14: 463-465.

[11] Liu Yin J, Jowitt S. Resolution of immune-mediated diseases following allogeneic bone marrow transplantation for leukemia. *Bone Marrow Transplant* 1992; 9:31.

[12] Salzman P, Tami J, Jackson C, Clinical remission of myasthenia gravis after high dose chemotherapy and autologous transplantation with CD34+ stem cells. *Blood* 1994; 84 (abstract 206a).

[13] Tyndall A., Fassas A., Passweg J. et al. Autologous haematopoietic stem cell transplants for autoimmune diseases – feasibility and transplant-related mortality. *Bone Marrow Transplant* 1999; 24: 729–734.

[14] Tyndall A., Gratwohl A. Haematopoietic stem and progenitor cells in the treatment of severe autoimmune diseases. *Ann. Rheum. Dis.* 1996; 35: 149–151.

[15] Marmont A. Stem cell transplantation for severe autoimmune diseases: progress and problems. *Haematologica* 1998; 83: 733 – 743.

[16] Tyndall A, Gratwohl A. Blood and marrow stem cell transplants in autoimmune disease: a consensus report written on behalf of the European League Against Rheumatism (EULAR) and the European Group for Blood and Marrow Transplantation (EBMT). *British Journal of Rheumatology* 1997; 36: 390–392.

[17] Burt R, Slavin S, Burns W, Marmont A. Induction of tolerance in autoimmune diseases by hematopoietic stem cell transplantation: getting closer to a cure? *Blood* 2002; 99: 768-784.

[18] Jayne D, Passweg J, Marmont A et al. Autologous stem cell transplantation for systemic lupus erythematosus. *Lupus*; 2004;13 (3):168-76.

[19] Openshaw H, Nash R, McSweeney P. High-dose immunosupression and hematopoietic stem cell transplantation in autoimmune disease: clinical review. *Biol Blood Marrow Transplant* 2002; 8: 233-248.

[20] American College of Rheumatology, The American College of Rheumatology Response Criteria for Systemic Lupus Erythematosus Clinical Trials ARTHRITIS and RHEUMATISM 2004, Vol. 50, No. 11, pp 3418–3426.

[21] Bombardier C, Gladman D. Derivation of the SLEDAI. A disease activity index for lupus patients. The committee on prognosis studies in SLE. *Arthritis Rheum.* 1992; 35: 630-640.

[22] Isenberg D, Ramsey-Goldman R. Assessing patients with lupus: towards a drug responder index. *Rheumatology* 1999; 38: 1045-1049.

[23] Ketterer N, Salles G,. High CD34+ cell counts decrease hematologic toxicity of autologous peripheral blood progenitor cell transplantation. *Blood* 1998; 91: 3148–3155.

[24] Statkute1 L, Verda L Mobilization, harvesting and selection of peripheral blood stem cells in patients with autoimmune diseases undergoing autologous hematopoietic stem cell transplantation. *Bone Marrow Transplantation* 2007, 00, pp 1–13.

[25] Gottenberg JE, Roux S, Desmoulins F, ClercD, Mariette X. Granulocyte colony-stimulating factor therapy resulting in a flare of systemic lupus erythematosus: comment on the articleby Yang and Hamilton. *Arthr. Rheum.* 2001; 44: 2458–2460.

[26] Loberiza FR Jr, Zhang MJ, Lee SJ, et al. Association of transplant center and physician factors on mortality after hematopoietic stem cell transplantation in the United States. *Blood.* 2005;105:2979-2987.

[27] Burt R, Traynor A, Statkute L Nonmyeloablative Hematopoietic Stem Cell Transplantation for Systemic Lupus Erythematosus, *JAMA*, 2006, Vol 295, No. 5 527-535.

[28] Salzberger B, Bowden RA, Neutropenia in allogeneic marrow transplant recipients receiving ganciclovir for prevention of cytomegalovirus disease: risk factors and outcome. *Blood.* 1997;90:2502-2508.

[29] Kang I, Park SH. Infectious complications in SLE after immunosuppressive therapies. *Curr. Opin. Rheumatol.* 2003;15:528-534.

[30] Young N, Speck B. Antithymocyte and antilymphocyte globulins: clinical trials and mechanism of action. *Prog. Clin. Biol. Res.* 1984;148:221-226.

[31] Arzoo K, Sadeghi S, Liebman H. Treatment of refractory antibody mediated autoimmune disorders with an anti-CD20 monoclonal antibody (rituximab). *Ann. Rheum. Dis.* 2000; 61: 922-924.

[32] Looney R.J. Treating human autoimmune disease by depleting B cells. *Ann. Rheum Dis.* 2002; 61: 863-866.

[33] Eisenberg R. SLE: rituximab in lupus. *Arthritis. Res. Ther.* 2003;5:157-159.

[34] Anolik JH, Barnard J, Cappione A, et al. Rituximab improves peripheral B cell abnormalities in human systemic lupus erythematosus. *Arthritis. Rheum.* 2004;50:3580-3590.

[35] Willis F, Marsh JC, Bevan DH, et al. The effect of treatment with Campath-1H in patients with autoimmune cytopenias. *Br. J. Haematol.* 2001; 114:891-898.

[36] Cohen Y, Polliack A, Nagler A. Treatment of refractoryautoimmune diseases with ablative immunotherapy using monoclonal antibodies and/or high dose chemotherapy with hematopoietic stem cell support. *Curr. Pharm. Des.* 2003;9:279-288.

[37] Georgiou P.E., Politi E.N. et al. Outcome of lupus pregnancy: a controlled study *Rheumatology* 2000;39:1014-1019.

[38] Mok CC, Wong R W S Pregnancy in systemic lupus erythematosus *Postgrad Med. J.* 2001; Vol:77:157-165.

[39] Sannal G, Bertolaccini ML, Mathieu A Central nervous system lupus: a clinical approach to therapy. *Lupus* (2003) 12, 935–942.

[40] Schantz V, Oestergaard LL, Junker P. Shrinking spinal cord following transverse myelopathy in a patient with systemic lupus erythematosus and the phospholipid antibody syndrome. *J. Rheumatol.* 1998; 25: 1425–1428.

[41] Yazawa S, Kawasaki S, Ohi T *et al.* Development of severe longitudinal atrophy of thoracic spinal cord following lupus-related myelitis. *Intern. Med.* 2001; 40: 353–357.

[42] Dong Y, Zhang X, Tang F, Tian X, Zhao Y, Zhang F. Intrathecal injection with methotrexate plus dexamethasone in the treatment of central nervous system involvement in systemic lupus erythematosus. *Chin. Med. J. (Engl)* 2001; 114: 764–766.

[43] Hahn B.H. The potential role of autologous stem cell transplantation in patients with SLE. *J. Rheumatol.* 1997; 24 (Suppl 48): 89-93.

In: Progress in Systemic Lupus Erythematosus Research
Editor: Tomas I. Seward, pp. 193-210
ISBN 978-1-60021-861-3

Chapter 7

MR SPECTROSCOPY, DIFFUSION AND DIFFUSION TENSOR IMAGING IN SYSTEMIC LUPUS ERYTHEMATOSUS

Pia C. Sundgren[1], Patricia Cagnoli[2] and William McCune[2]
Departments of Radiology[1] and Rheumatology[2],
University of Michigan Health Systems,
Ann Arbor, MI 48109, USA

ABSTRACT

Although clinical assessment is the cornerstone of SLE and NPSLE diagnosis; it can be difficult to make and is frequently presumptive. MR findings play an important role in supporting a clinical diagnosis and findings include volume loss, focal white matter hyperintensity, diffusion abnormalities due to ischemic injuries, evidence of prior hemorrhage or infarct, and meningeal enhancement. Nevertheless, several previous studies have shown that conventional pre-and post-contrast enhanced brain MR appear normal in approximately one third of both symptomatic and asymptomatic NPSLE patients and even more frequently in SLE patients. It has been suggested that other modalities such as MR spectroscopy (MRS), diffusion weighted imaging (DWI) and diffusion tensor imaging (DTI) could be additional tools in the evaluation and monitoring of SLE and NPSLE patients. This chapter will describe these new MRI techniques, recent research results and trends, and discuss if these techniques may add any valuable information that may further elucidate the pathogenesis of NPSLE. These techniques may possibly aid in diagnosing and differentiating NPSLE from other diseases with similar acute clinical symptoms as well as in monitoring disease progression.

INTRODUCTION

Neuropsychiatric systemic lupus erythematosus (NPSLE) is a severe and life-threatening condition and has been reported to be a leading cause of morbidity and mortality in systemic lupus erythematosus (SLE) patients [1, 2]. The reported prevalence using the American College of Rheumatology (ACR) nomenclature from 1999 is 37-95 % [3-7].

Clinically, NPSLE can present in a variety of manners, with involvement of the central nervous system such as septic meningitis, cerebrovascular disease, demyelinating syndrome, headache, movement disorder, Guillain-Barré syndrome, myelopathy, seizure disorders, acute confusional state, anxiety disorder, cognitive dysfunction, mood disorder, and psychosis. NPSLE can also present with peripheral nervous system manifestations such as autonomic neuropathy, mononeuropathy, myasthenia gravis, cranial neuropathy, plexopathy and polyneuropathy [8].

Although clinical assessment is the cornerstone of the neuropsychiatric systemic lupus erythematosus (NPSLE) diagnosis, this diagnosis can be difficult to make and is frequently presumptive. Some of these clinical features are usually diagnosed promptly and reliably. However, the attribution of individual neuropsychiatric events to SLE remains a challenge and NPSLE may occur in the absence of serologic markers or CSF abnormalities. Although a wide range of neuroimaging tools have been used to evaluate CNS involvement in NPSLE no single technique has been proven to be definitive for most of the NPSLE syndromes and attribution is determined on the basis of exclusion using the best available clinical, laboratory, and imaging data [9].

Findings on magnetic resonance imaging (MRI) play an important role in supporting a clinical diagnosis of NPSLE. These findings include volume loss, white matter hyperintensity, diffusion abnormalities due to ischemic injuries, evidence of prior hemorrhage or infarct, and meningeal enhancement [10-12] (*Figure 1*). Nevertheless, studies have shown that conventional pre- and post-contrast enhanced brain MR appear normal in approximately one third of both symptomatic and asymptomatic NPSLE patients, leading to a delay in diagnosis and treatment of NPSLE [10-12]. In addition, conventional MRI, although the best available technique to study anatomical lesions in NPSLE, unfortunately has limited specificity and cannot reliably distinguish lupus-related lesions from those produced by other mechanisms. Previous studies have shown that MRI findings do not reliably predict clinical course or response to therapy [12]. Still, MRI provides superior clinical correlation to CT, with a high concordance of focal neurologic abnormalities on physical examination with localized abnormalities in the brain particularly in the periventricular and subcortical white matter, which can be in the territory of a major cerebral blood vessel [13-15] but also seen in small vessel disease. However, computed tomography (CT) remains a useful tool in the emergency setting for detecting large infarct cerebral hemorrhage, massive brain edema, and for excluding confusing disorders including brain abscess and mass lesions, or when MRI is unavailable, not tolerated (claustrophobia) or contraindicated.

The prevalence of MRI abnormalities in SLE patients without neuropsychiatric disease has been described [16] with ranges between 19% [13] to 70% [17]; and varies with age, severity of SLE or previous documented neurologic involvement [13, 16-19].

It has been suggested that other imaging modalities such as MR spectroscopy (MRS), single proton emission tomography (SPECT), positron emission tomography (PET), and magnetization transfer imaging (MTI) could be additional tools in the evaluation and monitoring of patients with NPSLE [10,11,20-34].

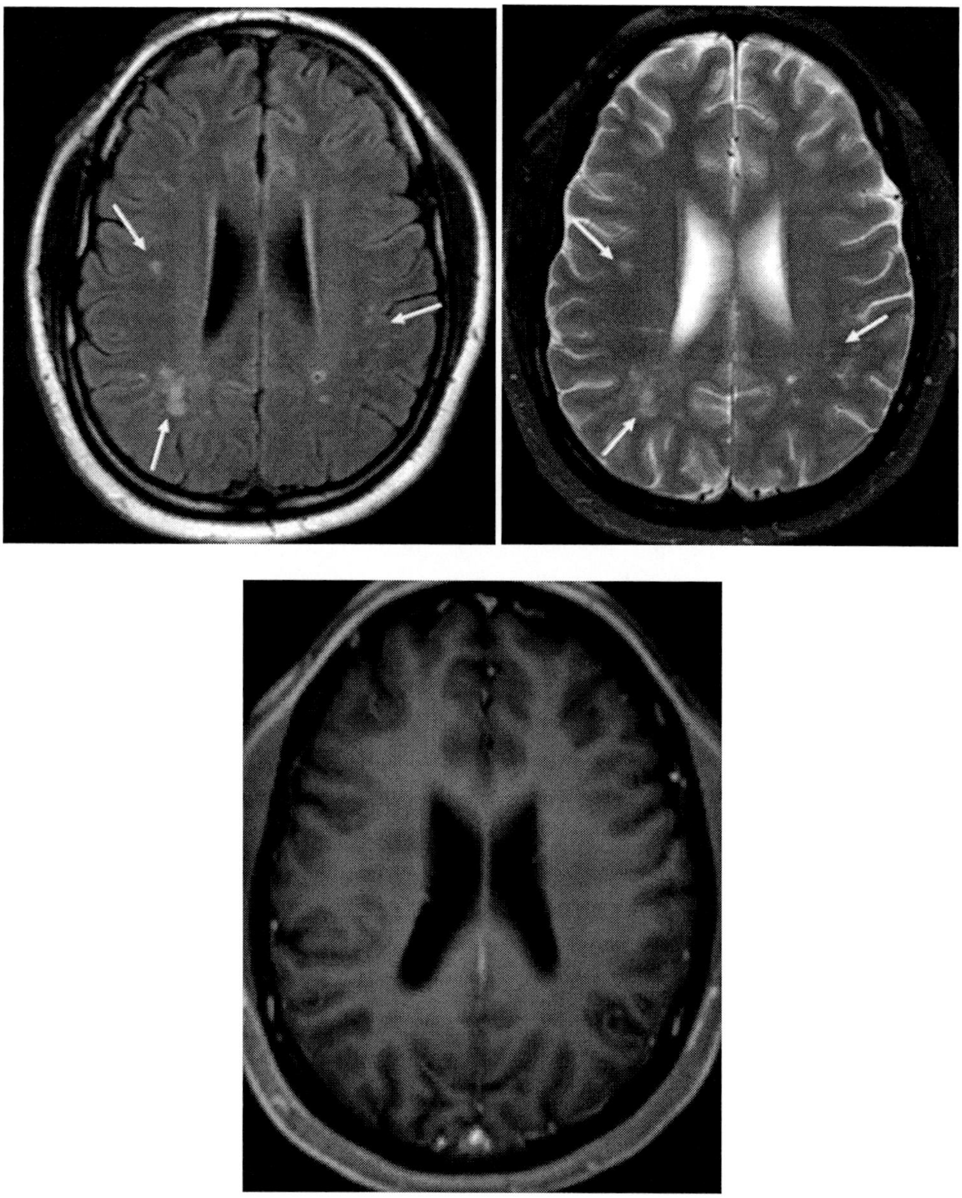

Figure 1 a-c. Axial fluid attenuated inversion recovery (FLAIR) (a), T2-weighted (b) and post contrast enhanced T1-weighted images (c) of the brain in a 42-year-old female with SLE. Focal non contrast enhancing areas of increased T2 hyperintensity in the deep and subcortical white matter (arrows) more in the right hemisphere than left present on axial FLAIR and T2 weighted images.

Of late, it has been suggested that other modalities such as diffusion imaging (DWI) [35,36,37] and even evaluation with more sophisticated techniques, such as diffusion tensor imaging (DTI), may further elucidate the pathogenesis of NPSLE and possibly play a role in diagnosing and differentiating NPSLE from other diseases having similar acute clinical symptoms and monitoring disease progression [38].

This chapter will focus on a few of these techniques namely MRS, DWI and DTI as possible imaging tools in the evaluation of SLE and NPSLE patients.

Magnetic Resonance Imaging Techniques

MR Spectroscopy

MR spectroscopy (MRS) is a non-invasive MRI technique that allows the biochemical metabolites in the brain tissue to be quantified. Most commonly used is ^{1}H (proton) MRS due to high natural abundance of protons and their high absolute sensitivity to magnetic manipulation, better spatial resolution, and relative simplicity of technique. Different biomolecules can be separated by their different chemical shift properties and can be quantified by the signal obtained at their specific frequencies and the information displayed as a spectrum. Metabolites in the CNS that are commonly evaluated with MRS in SLE and NPSLE patients include N-acetylaspartate, choline, creatine/phosphocreatine, myoinositol, the presence of lactate and lipids, and potentially glutamate/glutamine.

MRS can be performed using different techniques. Most commonly, in the clinical setting, spectra can be acquired using single voxel spectroscopy (SVS) with a spatial resolution in the order of one to eight cm^3 or the multiple voxel techniques also referred to as chemical shift imaging (CSI) or magnetic resonance spectroscopic imaging (MRSI), allowing the derivation of metabolite maps. Both techniques are commonly used in evaluation of SLE and NPSLE patients. Even if SVS allows evaluation of only small volumes of tissue, it is time-efficient and allows the acquisition of quantitative data. The CSI allows examination of a larger volume of tissue, which can then be evaluated using multiple smaller voxels within the investigated volume. These volumes can be as small as 1 cm^3. The two-dimensional CSI (2D-CSI or MRSI) technique still requires longer acquisition and post-processing time despite new improvements by the manufacturers. There are several limitations for MRS regardless of technique, and the spatial resolution of in vivo ^{1}H MRS is limited. MRS cannot be performed in or adjacent to tissue with high differences in magnetic susceptibility compared with brain tissue such as bone, air, large vessels, and hemorrhagic lesions. This is due to the artifacts arising from these structures and the resultant difficulty in obtaining a homogenous magnetic field, which is essential for good quality MRS study. In addition, susceptibility artifacts from metal and shunts may obscure the spectra.

The selection of appropriate MRS techniques, including measurement parameters such as echo time (TE), and repetition time (TR), depends on the clinical question. Long echo-time (TE) (135-270 msec) is sufficient for detection of the major metabolites such as N-Acetylaspartate (NAA), Choline (Cho) and creatine/phosphocreatine (Cr) and lactate/lipids (LL). N-Acetylaspartate (NAA) serves as a measure of normal healthy neuronal tissue.

Choline (Cho) has been implicated as a marker of cellularity and cell turnover, and therefore, may be used to infer a neoplastic process. Under most conditions, creatine/phosphocreatine (Cr), present in glial tissue and neurons, and is involved in phosphate transport, is a relatively stable metabolite used by most investigators as an internal control for quantifying other metabolites (i.e. metabolite ratios often include creatine as the denominator) [39]. Short echo times (TE=20-30 ms) evaluations are required when there is need for detection of metabolites with short relaxation times, such as glutamine, glutamate, myo-inositol and some amino-acids. Myoinositol is found in glial tissue and is thought to be involved as a second or third messenger for neurotransmitters and can be evaluated with MRS using a short TE [40]. Altered myoinositol have been shown to be associated with inflammatory injury [41, 42].

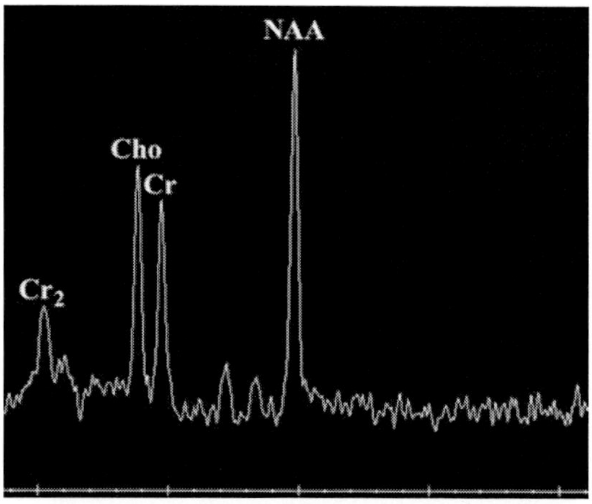

2a

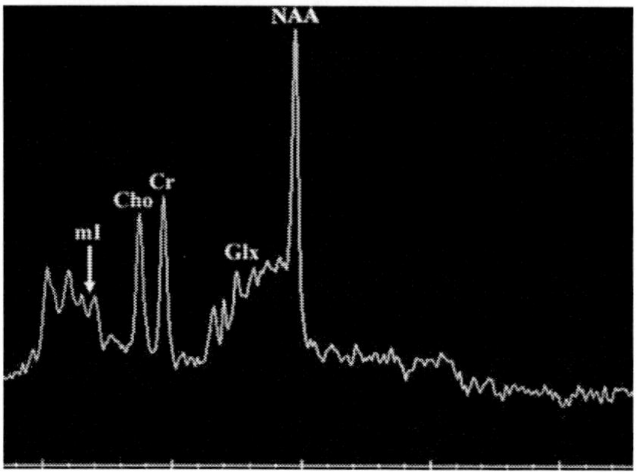

2b

Figure 2a-b. Normal magnetic resonance spectroscopy (MRS) spectrum using intermediate TE (144ms) showing the main metabolic peaks: N-Acetyl aspartate (NAA), choline (Cho), and creatine (Cr) (a). Normal magnetic resonance spectroscopy (MRS) spectrum using short TE (30ms) showing the main metabolic peaks of N-Acetyl aspartate (NAA), choline (Cho), creatine (Cr), glutamine/glutamate (Glx), and myoinositol (mI) peaks (b).

Lactate and macro-lipids are not present on a MRS spectrum performed in a normal brain. These metabolites are shown to increase in anaerobic metabolism. They have been demonstrated in cerebral necrosis and in some brain tumors but rarely in association with SLE and considered, by many, less relevant to the work-up for NPSLE. All the above metabolites have been reported in the SLE and NPSLE literature [10, 20-24, 29, 43-47]. Intermediate TE and short TE magnetic resonance spectroscopy with normal metabolic spectra are presented in Figure 2.

Diffusion Weighted Imaging - DWI

Diffusion weighted imaging (DWI) is a well established sequence used commonly in the detection of early signs of ischemia. It is well known that DWI measures the diffusivity of water molecules [48]. In routine DWI, water mobility is assessed in only three orthogonal directions. While this is sufficient to measure the scalar parameter, the apparent diffusion coefficient (ADC), routine DWI is unable to characterize the directionality of diffusion (*Figure 3*).

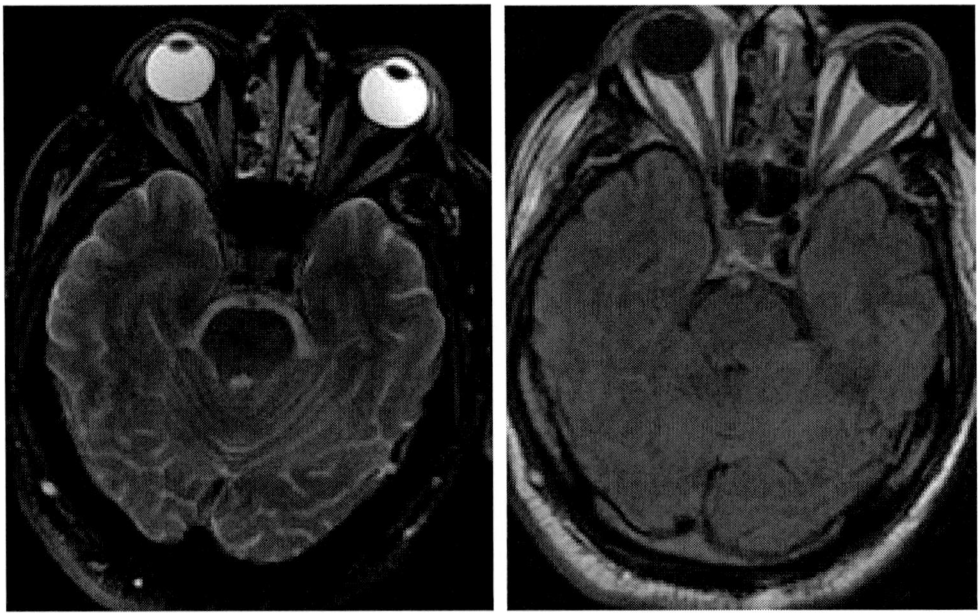

Figure 3 continued on next page.

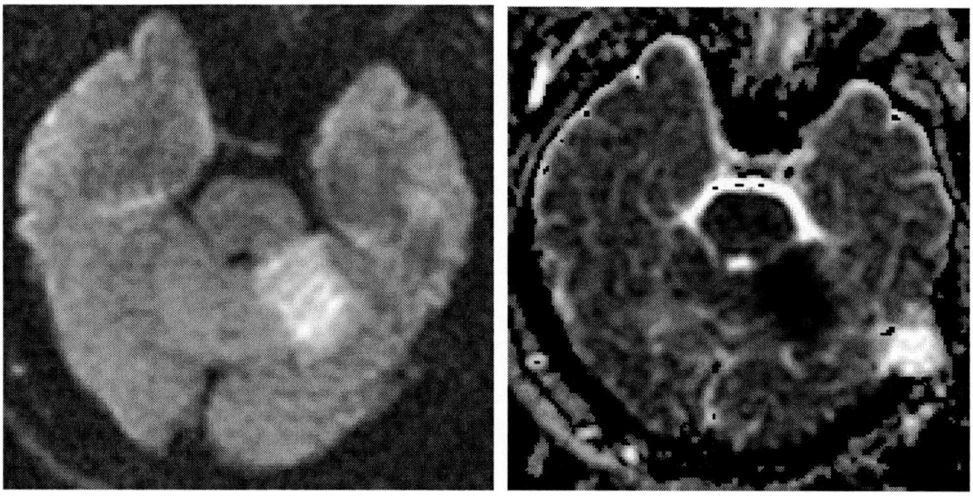

Figure 3 a-d. Axial fluid attenuated inversion recovery (FLAIR) (a), T2-weighted (b), diffusion weighted (DWI) (c) images, and apparent diffusion coefficient map of the brain in 62-year-old male demonstrating increased T2 hyperintensity in left cerebellum (a, b) and increased signal on the diffusion weighted images (trace) (c) and low signal on ADC map (d) consistent with acute stroke.

Diffusion Tensor Imaging

Diffusion tensor imaging DTI yields quantitative measures for tissue water mobility as a function of the direction of water motion. The diffusion of water molecules is characterized by Brownian motion. DTI of water is probed by application of diffusion-sensitization gradients in multiple directions [49]. Appropriate mathematical combination of the directional diffusion weighted images provides quantitative measures of water diffusion for each voxel via the apparent diffusion coefficient (ADC), as well as the degree of diffusion directionality, or anisotropy which can be measured by fractional anisotropy (FA) [50]. The diffusion is called isotropic when the motion is equal in all directions such as in simple fluids. FA has a value of 0 in isotropic tissues and approaches the value of 1 in highly anisotropic environments where water is constrained to move along a primary direction. The diffusivity as measured by ADC and the anisotropy as measured by FA represent just a part of the information available from the diffusion tensor. Examination of individual eigenvalues which reflect the diffusivity in longitudinal or transverse directions with respect to fiber tracts may add additional information and help in tissue characterization. By choosing the eigenvector associated with the largest eigenvalue, the principal diffusion direction of the brain structure to be examined can be encoded with color, resulting in color-coding maps or directionally encoded FA maps (DEC FA maps). In these color-encoded maps the fibers have been given different colors (red, green and blue) depending on their different diffusion directions [51]. The magnitude of the anisotropy in the tissue, such as FA, can be used as an illumination factor of the calculation of a directionally encoded color image [51] (*Figure 4*).

Imaging Findings in SLE and NPSLE Using MRS

Several studies utilizing MRS in the evaluation of SLE and NPSLE patients have been published over the last couple of years. However, there are large variations in the spectroscopy technique used i.e. single voxel spectroscopy (SVS) [10,21,22,24,52] or multivoxel chemical shift imaging (2D-CSI) [29,43,46], in patient selection, in the time of initial MR scanning, and in the inclusion of interval follow-up, making it difficult to compare the published data. For example, patient selection may vary from NPSLE patients with acute neurological symptoms [29] to reports that have focused mainly on NPSLE patients with major or minor symptoms regardless of when the MR study was performed with respect to initial symptoms, [21,22,46] or which have focused on SLE patients without any acute neuropsychiatric symptoms [10,20]. These differences may account for some of the discrepancies between the presented results.

Most reports demonstrate a decline in the NAA/Cr ratio and an increase in the Cho/Cr ratio in periventricular white matter and basal ganglia [21, 22, 29]. Other reports demonstrate more widespread significant decrease in the NAA/Cho ratio and a significant increase in the Cho/Cr ratio [10, 21, 22, 4, 29]. Such a decline in NAA has been suggested to be a sign of neuronal loss, whereas an increase in the choline compounds was assumed to be a sign of increased metabolic turnover/activity [22].

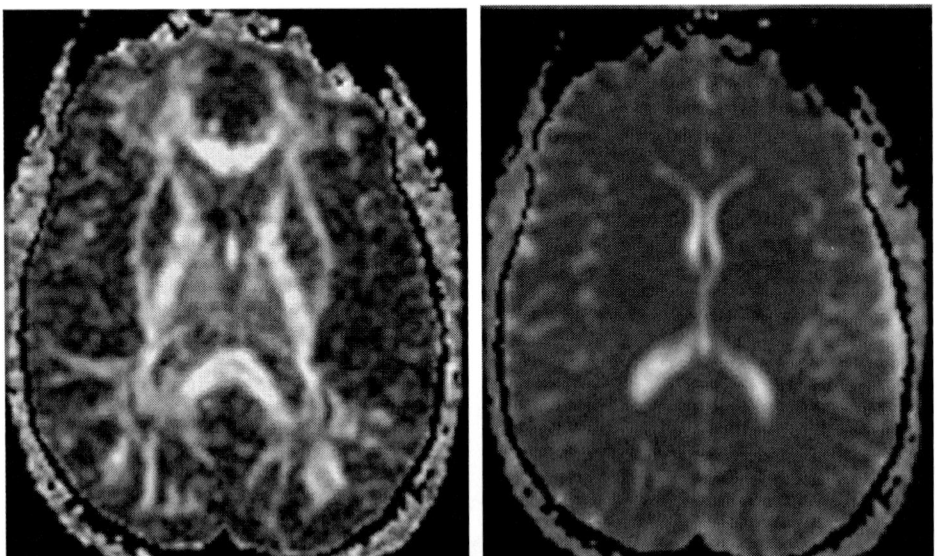

Figutr 4 continued on next page.

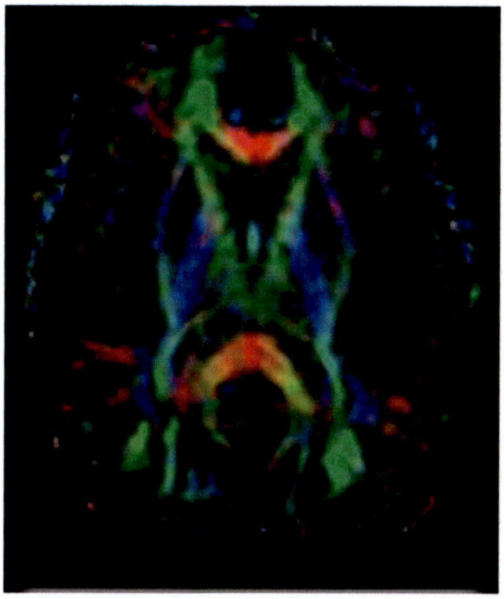

Figure 4 a-c. Apparent diffusion coefficient (ADC) map (a), fraction anisotropy (FA) map (b), and directionally encoded FA map (DEC FA maps) (c). In these color-encoded maps the fibers have been given different colors (red, green and blue) depending on their different diffusion directions.

Studies have demonstrated a reduction in NAA in injured areas of the brain in SLE patients as well as in normal appearing white and grey matter. Decreased NAA has been found in patients with active disease, cerebral atrophy, generalized seizures, psychosis, neurocognitive dysfunction or confusional states [10, 20, 21, 25, 26, 28, 43, 44, 53]. Decreased NAA/Cho ratios [47] and elevated Cho/Cr ratios [54] have been demonstrated in patients with cognitive impairment [54]. Both stroke, epilepsy and elevated IgG antiphospholipid antibodies (aPL) are more commonly seen in SLE patients with antiphospholipid antibody syndrome (aPLS) than those without (aPLS) [45] and the reduction of NAA/Cr was more closely related to the IgG-aPL than the presence of stroke or aPLS.[45].

Cho/Cr ratios have been found to be elevated in active NPSLE. Absolute choline levels have shown to be elevated in correlation with activity, stroke, inflammation and chronic white matter lesions but also in normal appearing white matter. [10, 20, 21, 24, 26, 46] and may, therefore, be regarded by some investigators as a poor quality indicator of prognosis [20, 21, 44, 47].

Few studies have followed patients over time [24, 27, 29]. Two of these studies [24,29] demonstrated a continued decrease in NAA over time, supporting the theory that diffuse permanent neuronal loss occurs in many or most NPSLE patients regardless of the clinically apparent severity of disease. In one study, 8 NPSLE patients with undergoing medical treatment for acute neurological symptoms where followed 3 and 6 months after initial examination [29]. Interval-significant decrease in the NAA/Cr ratios was demonstrated between the first and second examination and insignificant difference between the second and third examination. In contrast to a previous study demonstrating reversible changes with inactivity [27] the decline in NAA did not reverse over time [29]. In accordance with a few previous studies [22, 24] the mean Cho/Cr ratios were significantly increased in these 8

NPSLE patients and remained increased over the follow-up time compared to the normal controls at the time of presentation.

These findings may suggest that this decline will continue or remain permanent regardless of medical treatment and support the assumption that neuronal damage, seen as a decline in NAA, might be complete and irreversible even if the patient receives the appropriate treatment. Whether the decrease in NAA indicates cytotoxic injury, vasculitis, microinfarct due to microthrombosis, or the presence of additional processes resulting in brain injury has yet to be determined.

We have to keep in mind that reduced NAA changes and decreased NAA/Cr ratios can be seen in many other conditions and are not specific to NPSLE. Alterations in NAA and NAA/Cr ratios may become a measure of NPSLE severity and outcome rather than a measure of NPSLE activity. Larger longitudinal studies are needed to evaluate metabolite changes in response to treatment.

Interestingly, despite the suggestion that ischemia plays a role in the pathophysiology of NPSLE, obvious elevation of lactate levels (an indicator of anaerobic metabolism) has not been found in some earlier studies [20,21]. In a more recent study, alteration in LL/Cr ratio was present and the authors speculated as to whether it was due to an increase in lactate [29] or an increase in marco-lipids as suggested by others [20]. Most likely it is a combination of anaerobic/hypoxic injury at time of acute symptoms as well as indicating a host response to injury, such as an inflammatory reaction, membrane activation or demyelination [21]. The theory that demyelination is one component is supported by recent findings using diffusion weighted and diffusion tensor imaging.

An important role of imaging in NPSLE is deducing the etiology of acute focal (stroke-like) neurological deficits. The differential diagnoses vary and accurate assessment is of crucial importance, as the treatment for these alternative diagnoses differs. One of the parameters involved in the differential diagnostic process is the presence of antiphospholipid antibodies (APL-Ab) [55-57]. While there are correlations between MRI findings and the presence of APL-Ab there remains some controversy regarding the relationship between the presence of antiphospholipid antibodies and MRS findings in SLE patients. A few previous studies have demonstrated no significant differences in metabolic ratios between those with APLl-Ab and those without [29,46], while another study found significant differences in metabolic ratios between APL-Ab positive-and APL-ab negative patients [45].

Myoinositol (mI) has been found to be elevated early in the course of an active flare of NPSLE prior to changes on MRI. It can be speculated that determination of mI in combination with NAA levels can aid in determining the severity of NPSLE. Since increase mI with reduction of NAA is found in severe disease while elevated mI with normal NAA has been described with minor manifestations such as headaches and mild cognitive impairment [24].

There are potential benefits with the use of 2D-CSI in the work-up of NP-SLE patients. The CNS involvement in NP-SLE can be diffuse and maximum metabolic abnormalities may not necessarily be in areas that produce the dominant clinical symptoms or show the presence of abnormal MRI findings. The 2-D-CSI spectroscopy is able to cover larger areas of the brain and include both the areas of signal abnormalities or infarcts as well as areas that appear normal on conventional MR images. Individual voxels within the volume of interest

(VOI) can be placed in different regions of the brain including grey matter or white matter separately, and will facilitate comparisons between findings obtained from the small regions of interest (ROI) that can be used for measurements on ADC and FA maps. However, to investigate and measure a metabolite such as myoinositol short echo time (TE) on the order of 30ms are required and in those circumstances the SVS technique is still the method of choice. It will allow for quantification and the use of commercial fitting models such as LC model [58].

Imaging Findings in SLE and NPSLE Using DWI and DTI

It has previously been demonstrated that NPSLE patients have increased whole brain diffusivity compared to normal controls [35, 59-61]. This was true for both NPSLE patients with diffuse and chronic symptoms [35] and those with acute onset of neurological symptoms [60, 61]. The later study demonstrated differences separately in grey and white matter compared to normal controls [60] (*Figure 5*). These findings are suggestive of the presence of subtle and widespread damage in the brain parenchyma not confined to one tissue compartment only. Selective gray matter damage in normal appearing gray matter on conventional MRI in NPSLE patients has also been demonstrated with magnetization transfer imaging [33]. Reduced structural integrity in the brain, such as axonal loss and/or demyelination, is a possible etiology for the widespread damage [62, 63].

It is well-known that ADC values decrease and FA values increase when the motion of water molecules is directionally restricted, for example, by the boundaries of myelin sheets. Alternatively, loss of structural brain integrity would allow interstitial water molecules to move in a more unrestricted environment thus resulting in an increase in ADC and decrease in FA.

A few studies have measured the ADC and FA values both in lesions, and in normal appearing gray and white matter in SLE patients both with and without NPSLE [36-38, 64]. Signal hyperintensity in cerebral cortex associated with acute ischemic changes has been has been demonstrated with resolution after treatment [36, 37].

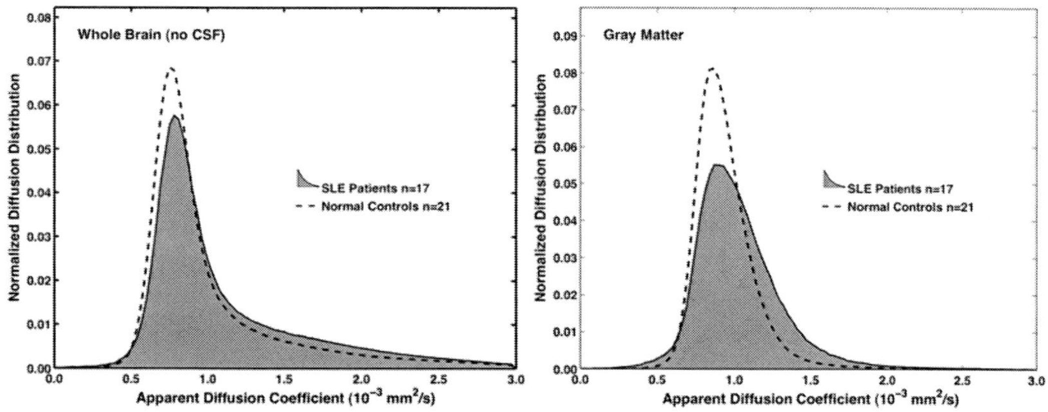

Figure 5 continued on next page.

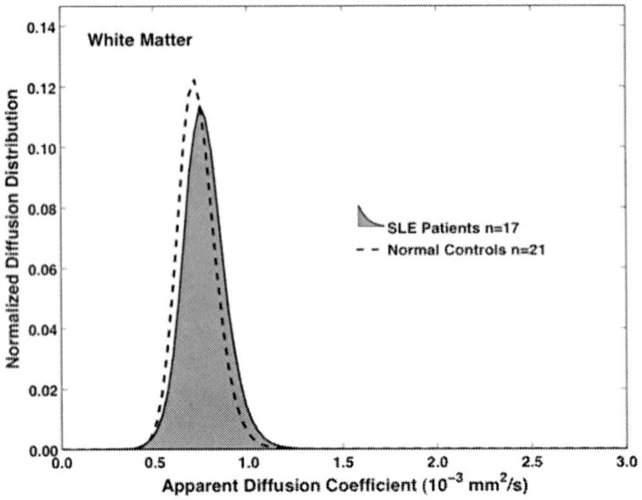

Figure 5 a-c Comparison of whole brain (excluding CSF) ADC histograms between NPSLE patients (shadow area) and normal controls (dashed lines) (a), Histograms of ADC in grey matter only (b) and of white matter only (c). The NPSLE patients demonstrate significantly increased mean ADC compared to normal controls and significant differences can also be seen between the groups in both grey and white matter.

Recent studies have demonstrated that diffusivity in different parts of the normal appearing brain can be higher in SLE and NPSLE patients compared to normal controls [38, 64]. Regional diffusion differences with increased diffusion in frontal lobe, splenium, anterior and posterior limbs of the internal capsule was found in a recent study [64]. They also found significantly decreased FA in the genu and splenium of corpus callosum compared to normal controls [64]. An increase in ADC and decrease in FA values in normal appearing white matter have also been demonstrated in a small group of NPSLE patients compared to normal controls [38]. Similar findings have also been demonstrated in a recent study of SLE patients compared to normal controls from the same research group [unpublished data]. We found significant increase in ADC values in normal appearing brain in SLE patients compared to normal controls [unpublished data]. Moreover, when we compared the ADC and FA values in a small group of NPSLE patients with those obtained in the same regions in a group of SLE patients, statistically significant differences ($p<0.05$) were found in both ADC and FA values in the internal capsule between the two groups. There were also significant increased FA values in the amygdala, insular cortex, orbitofrontal cortex, thalamus, and cingulate cortex in the SLE patients compared to NPSLE patients, and significant differences in ADC values in amygdala, insular cortex, and cingulate gyrus were also noted when comparing the two populations [65]. The NPSLE patients demonstrated significant increase in ADC in insular cortex compared to SLE ($p<0.05$) and decrease compared to normal controls. Significantly decreased ADC was present in the amygdala, internal capsule and cingulate gyrus between NPSLE compared to SLE patients and normal controls ($p<0.05$). These findings are, in part, in accordance with a previous report in which they demonstrated significant decrease in ADC in the amygdala in both SLE and NPSLE compared to normal controls, but without any significant differences between the two patient groups [66]. They also demonstrated that the decrease in ADC was more severe in patients with anti-NMDAR antibodies. These findings are similar to those found in mouse models [67]. These findings of possible effect on the limbic system in SLE patients that might result in altered emotions needs to be evaluated in larger studies in the future but is a indicator of limbic involvement that could in part explain some of the patients' emotional symptoms.

It seems that when following NPSLE patients over time with repeated MR imaging persistent and evolving alterations in their normal appearing brain parenchyma occur as demonstrated by recent unpublished data from our research group demonstrating statistically significant increase in FA values ($p<0.005$) in the internal capsule, orbitofrontal cortex, and insular cortex when comparing follow-up and initial examinations in a small number of NPSLE patients from the same cohort as mentioned above. There was also a general but non significant decrease in the ADC values in the same patients over time.

The pathogenesis of NPSLE is complex. The predominant pathologic process in NPSLE found at autopsy is small vessel disease in the absence of vasculitis or thrombosis, or a "bland vasculopathy". It is unclear whether these findings represent previous sites of inflammation or vaso-occlusion. Immune complex disease-mediated vasculitis, leukoagglutination, direct antibody mediated injury to vessels or neurons, antibody (aPL) - mediated thrombosis and direct injury endothelial injury by aPL antibodies or anti-endothelial may all play a role as well. In addition, some authors have suggested that superimposed demyelination may play a role in NPSLE [4, 11, 29, 38, 46]. This hypothesis that demyelination is a part of the pathogenesis is supported by histopathological studies that have described demyelination in brain parenchyma in patients with NPSLE [68]. This hypothesis can be supported by recent DTI study evaluating diffusivity parallel ($\lambda_{\parallel}$) to the long axis, a measure of axonal injury, and perpendicular ($\lambda_{\perp}$) to the long fiber axis, a measure of demyelination, in normal appearing white matter in 8 NPSLE patients compared to 10 normal controls [38]. The $\lambda_{\perp}$ was significantly higher in internal capsule, corpus callosum, thalamus, and in the parietal and frontal white matter bilaterally NPSLE patients compared to healthy and was suggested to be the result of demyelination. A breakdown of the myelin sheets as in demyelination would result in less restricted movement of the water molecules perpendicular to the fiber tracts.

Whole brain tractography performed in SLE patients and normal controls has shown generally less trackable fibers in the whole brain in SLE patients as compared to normal controls, which again points to global white matter damage in SLE [64].

CONCLUSION

Neuroimaging has made an important contribution to the understanding of NPSLE. Conventional MRI with gadolinium is considered the gold standard imaging technique at the moment, and the more sensitive tool to determine the anatomic location and extension of the lesions. The newer MRI functional approaches such as MRS, DWI and DTI that have been described above extend their scope beyond mere diagnostic tools of a structural abnormality with the potential to provide insight into the underlying disease mechanism and provide a reliable tool for objective clinical follow up in NPSLE.

Further research is still needed to gain knowledge of the limitations and advantages of each method and to determine the best combination to diagnose NPSLE.

References

[1] Gladman DD, Urowitz MB. In: *Klippel D*, editor. 1994.

[2] Sibley JT, Olszynski WP, Decoteau WE, Sundaram MB. The incidence and prognosis of central nervous system disease in systemic lupus erythematosus. *J. Rheumatol.* 1992;19(1):47-52.

[3] Brey RL, Neuropsychiatric syndromes in lupus: prevalence using standardized definitions. *Neurology* 2002;58:1214-1220.

[4] Hanly JG, McCurdy G, FougereL, Neuropsychiatric disease in systemic lupus erythematosus (SLE): attribution and clinical significance. *J. Rheumatol.* 2004;31:2156-2162.

[5] Sanna G, Neuropsychiatric manifestations in systemic lupus erythematosus: prevalence and association with antiphospholipid antibodies. *J. Rheumatol.* 2003;30:985-992.

[6] Sibbitt WL, Jr, The incidence and prevalence of neuropsychiatric syndromes in pediatric onset systemic lupus erythematosus. *J. Rheumatol.* 2002;29:1536-1542.

[7] Ainiala H, Validity of the new American College of Rheumatology criteria for neuropsychiatric lupus syndromes: a population-based evaluation. *Arthritis Rheum.* 2001 45:pp 419-423.

[8] The American College of Rheumatology nomenclature and case definitions for neuropsychiatric lupus syndromes. *Arthritis Rheum.* 1999; 42: 599-608.

[9] Hanly JG, Neuropsychiatric lupus. *Rheum. Dis. Clin. North Am.* 2005; 31(2): 273-98.

[10] Chinn RJS, Wilkinson ID, Hall-Crags MA et al., Magnetic resonance imaging of the brain and cerebral proton spectroscopy in patients with systemic lupus erythematosus, *Arthritis Rheum.* 1997;40:36–46.

[11] Hanly JG,Walsh NM, Sangalang V, Brain pathology in systemic lupus erythematosus. *J. Rheumatol.* 1992; 19: 732-741.

[12] Jennings JE, Sundgren PC, Atwood J, McCune J, Maly P. Value of MRI of the brain in patients with systemic lupus erythematosus and neurologic disturbances. *Neuroradiology* 2004; 46: 15-21.

[13] McCune WJ, MacGuire A, Aisen A, Gebarski S. Identification of brain lesions in neuropsychiatric systemic lupus erythematosus by magnetic resonance scanning. *Arthritis Rheum.* 1988; 31(2):159-166.

[14] West SG. Systemic lupus and the nervous system. In: Wallace DJ, Hanh BH, Dubois, editors. Lupus Erythematosus. 2002.

[15] Bell CL. Magnetic resonance imaging of central nervous system lesions in patients with lupus erythematosus. Correlation with clinical remission and antineurofilament and anticardiolipin antibody titers [see comments]. *Arthritis Rheum.* (1991; 34: 432-441.

[16] Kozora E, West SG, Kotzin BL et al. Magnetic resonance imaging abnormalities and cognitive deficits in systemic lupus erythematosus patients without overt central nervous system disease. *Arthritis Rheum.* 1998; 41: 41–47.

[17] M. Rovaris et al., Brain involvement in systemic immune mediated diseases: magnetic resonance and magnetisation transfer imaging study, *Journal of Neurology, Neurosurgery and Psychiatry* 68 (2000) (2), pp. 170–177.

[18] Jarek MJ,West SG, Baker MR, Rak KM. Magnetic resonance imaging in systemic lupus erythematosus patients without a history of neuropsychiatric lupus erythematosus. *Arthritis Rheum*. 1994; 37:1609–13.

[19] Nomura K, Yamano S, Ikeda Y et al. Asymptomatic cerebrovascular lesions detected by magnetic resonance imaging in patients with systemic lupus erythematosus lacking a history of neuropsychiatric events. *Internal. Med.* 1999;38:785–795.

[20] Brooks WM, Sabet A, Sibbitt WL Jr. et al., Neurochemistry of brain lesions determined by spectroscopic imaging in systemic lupus erythematosus, *J. Rheumatol.* 1997; 24: 2323–2329.

[21] Sibbitt WL, Haseler LJ, Griffey RR et al., Neurometabolism of active neuropsychiatric lupus determined with proton MR spectroscopy, *AJNR* 1997;18:1271–1277.

[22] Lim MK, Suh CH, H.J. Kim HJ et al., Systemic lupus erythematosus: brain MR imaging and single-voxel hydrogen 1 MR spectroscopy, *Radiology* 2000; 217:43–49.

[23] Peterson P, Howe FA. Clark CA et al., Quantitative magnetic resonance imaging in neuropsychiatric systemic lupus erythematosus, *Lupus* 2003;12: 1–6.

[24] Axford JS, Howe F.A, Heron C. Griffiths J.R. Sensitivity of quantitative ^{1}H magnetic resonance spectroscopy of the brain in detecting early neuronal damage in systemic lupus erythematosus, *Ann. Rheum. Dis.* 2001; 60: 106–111.

[25] Colamussi P, Trotta F, Ricci R et al. Brain perfusion SPET and proton magnetic resonance spectroscopy in the evaluation of two systemic lupus erythematosus patients with mild neuropsychiatric manifestations. *Nucl. Med. Commun.* 1997;18:269–73.

[26] Sibbitt WL Jr., Sibbitt RR. Magnetic resonance spectroscopy and positron emission tomography scanning in neuropsychiatric systemic lupus erythematosus. *Rheum. Dis. Clin. North Am.* 1993; 19: 851–68.

[27] Appenzeller S, Li LM, Costallat LT, Cendes F. Evidence of reversible axonal dysfunction in systemic lupus erythematosus: a proton MRS study. *Brain* 2005;128:2933–40.

[28] Handa R, Sahota P, Kumar M, Jagannathan NR, Bal CS, Gulati M, et al. In vivo proton magnetic resonance spectroscopy (MRS) and single photon emission computerized tomography (SPECT) in systemic lupus erythematosus (SLE). *Magn. Reson. Imaging* 2003;21:1033–1037.

[29] Sundgren PC, Jennings J, Attwood JT, Nan B, Gebarski S, McCune WJ, et al. MRI and 2D-CSI MR spectroscopy of the brain in the evaluation of patients with acute onset of neuropsychiatric systemic lupus erythematosus. *Neuroradiology* 2005;47:576–85.

[30] Bosma GP Th, Rood MJ, Zwinderman AH et al., Evidence of central nervous system damage in patients with neuropsychiatric systemic lupus erythematosus, demonstrated by magnetization transfer imaging, *Arthritis Rheum.* 43 (2000),pp. 48–54.

[31] Bosma GP, Rood MJ, T.W. Huizinga TW et al., Detection of cerebral involvement in patients with active neuropsychiatric systemic lupus erythematosus by the use of volumetric magnetization transfer imaging, *Arthritis Rheum.* 43 (2000) (11), pp. 2428–2436.

[32] Rovaris M, Viti B, Ciboddo G, et al., Brain involvement in systemic immune mediated diseases: magnetic resonance and magnetisation transfer imaging study, *J. Neurol. Neurosurg Psychiatry* 68 (2000) (2), pp. 170–177.

[33] Steens S.C.A, Admiraal-Behloul F, Bosma G.P et al. Selective gray damage in neuropsychiatric lupus. A magnetization transfer study. *Arthritis Rheum.* 2004;50(9):2877-2881.

[34] Emmer BJ, Steens SCA, Steup-Beekman GM, van der Grond J, Admiraal-Behloul F, Olofsen H, Bosma GP.Th, Ouwendijk WJN, Huizinga TWJ, van Buchem MA. Detection of change in CNS involvement in neuropsychiatric SLE. A magnetization transfer study. *J. Magn. Reson. Imag.* 2006;24(4):812-816.

[35] Bosma GP, Huizinga TW, Mooijaart SP, Van Buchem MA, Abnormal brain diffusivity in patients with neuropsychiatric systemic lupus Erythematosus. *Am. J. Neuroradiol.* 2003;24:850-854.

[36] Iguchi Y, Kimura K, Inoue T, Ueno Y, Sunada Y. Diffusion weighted magnetic resonance images in a patient with neuropsychiatric lupus. *Journal of clinical neuroscience* 2007;14:273-275.

[37] Moritani T, Shrier DA, Numaguchi Y et al. Diffusion weighted echoplanar MR imaging of CNS involvement in systemic lupus Erythematosus. *Acad. Radiol.* 2001;8:741-753.

[38] Hughes M, Sundgren PC, Fan X, Foerster B, Nan B, Welsh RC, Williamson JA, Attwood J, Maly PV, Chenevert TL, McCune W, Gebarski S. Diffusion tensor imaging in patients with acute onset of neuropsychiatric systemic lupus erythematosus: a prospective study of apparent diffusion coefficient, fractional anisotropy values, and eigenvalues in different regions of the brain. *Acta Radiol.* 2007;48(2):213-222.

[39] Burtscher IM, Holtas S. Proton MR Spectroscopy in Clinical Routine. *J. Magn. Reson. Imaging* 2001; 13:560-567.

[40] Peterson PL, Axford JS, Isenberg D. Imaging in CNS lupus Best Practice and Research *Clinical Rheumatol.* 2005;19(5):727-739.

[41] Haussinger D, Lubenberger J, Vom Dahl S et al. Proton magnetic resonance spectroscopy studies on human brain myo-inositol in hypoosmolarity and hepatic encephalopathy. *Gastroenterology* 1994;107:1475–1480.

[42] Videen JS, Michaelis T, Pinto P, Ross BD. Human cerebral osmolytes during chronic hyponatremia. A proton magnetic resonance study. *J. Clin. Invest* 1995;95:788–793.

[43] Sibbitt, WL, Haseler LJ, Griffey RH et al., Analysis of cerebral structural changes in systemic lupus erythematosus by proton MR spectroscopy, *AJNR* 1994;15:923–928.

[44] Davie CA, Feinstein A, Kartsounis LD et al., Proton magnetic resonance spectroscopy of systemic lupus erythematosus involving the central nervous system, *J. Neurol.* 1995;242:522–528.

[45] Sabet A, Sibbitt W Jr., Stidley CA et al., Neurometabolite markers of cerebral injury in the antiphospholipid syndrome of systemic lupus erythematosus, *Stroke* 1998;29 (11):2254–2260.

[46] Friedman SD, Stidley CA, Brooks WM et al., Brain injury and neurometabolic abnormalities in systemic lupus erythematosus, *Radiology* 1998;209 79–84.

[47] Brooks WM, Jung RE, Ford CC et al. Relationship between neurometabolite derangement and neurocognitive dysfunction in systemic lupus erythematosus, *J. Rheumatol.* 1999;26:81–85.

[48] Bammer R. Basic principles of diffusion-weighted imaging. *EJR* 2003;45:169-184.

[49] .Basser PJ, Pierpaoli C. Microstructural and physiological features of tissues elucidated by quantitative-diffusion-tensor MRI. *J. Magn. Reson* 1996; Series B 111:209 –219.

[50] Le Bihan, D, Mangin JF, Poupon C, Clark CA, Pappata S, Molko N. Diffusion Tensor Imaging: Concepts and Applications. *Magn. Reson. Imag.* 2001;13:534-546.

[51] Pajevic S, Pierpaoli C. Color schemes to represent the orientation of anisotropic tissues from diffusion tensor data; application to white matter fiber tract mapping in the human brain. *Magn. Reson. Med.*1999;42:526-540.

[52] Bosma GP Th, Steens SCA, Petropoulos H, Admiraal-Behloul F, van der Haak A, Doornbos J, Huizinga TWJ, Brooks WM, Harville A, Sibbitt WL Jr., van Buchem MA. Multisequence magnetic resonance imaging study of neuropsychiatric systemic lupus erythematosus. *Arthritis and Rheum.* 2004 pp 3195-3202.

[53] West SG, Emlen W, Wener MH, Kotzin BL. Neuropsychiatric lupus erythematosus: a 10-year prospective study on the value of diagnostic tests. *Am. J. Med.* 1995; 99: 153–63.

[54] Kozora E, Arciniegas DB, Filley CM, Ellison MC, West SG, Browns, MS et al. Cognition, MRS neurometabolites, and MRI volumetrics in non-neuropsychiatric systemic lupus Erythematosus: preliminary data. *Cog. Behav. Neurol.* 2005;18:159-162.

[55] Provenzale JM, Barboriak DP, Allen NB, Ortel TL. Patients with antiphospholipid antibodies: CT and MR findings of the brain. *AJR* 1996;167:1573-1578.

[56] Provenzale JM, Barboriak DP, Allen NB, Ortel TL. Antiphospholipid antibodies: findings at arteriography. *AJNR* 1998;19:611-616.

[57] Karassa FB, Ioannidis JP, Boki KA, et al Predictors of clinical outcome and radiologic progression in patients with neuropsychiatric manifestations of systemic lupus erythematosus. *Am. J. Med.* 2000;109:628-634.

[58] Provencher SW. Estimation of metabolite concentrations from localized in vivo proton NMR spectra. *Mag. Reson. Med.* 1993;30(6):672-679.

[59] Bosma GP, Van Buchem MA, Rood MJ, et al. Comparison of ADC histograms of patients with neuropsychiatric systemic lupus erythematosus and healthy volunteers. *Proc. Intl. SOC Mag. Res. Med.* 2000; 8: 1244.

[60] Welsh PC, Foerster B, Jennings J, Sundgren PC. Brain diffusivity in patients with neuropsychiatric Systemic Lupus Erythematosus and new acute neurological symptoms. *ASNR Proceedings Am. Soc. Neuroradiology* 2004; 395, SE 1.

[61] Welsh RC, Rahbar H, Foerster B, Thurnher M, Sundgren PC. Brain diffusivity in patients with neuropsychiatric systemic lupus erythematosus with new acute onset of neurological symptoms. *J. Magn. Reson.*. 2007 *in press*.

[62] Appenzeller S, Bonilha L, Rio[b] P , Li L, Lavras Costallat L, Cendes F. Longitudinal analysis of gray and white matter loss in patients with systemic lupus Erythematosus. *NeuroImage* 34 (2007) 694–701.

[63] Appenzeller S, Rondina JM, Li LM, et al. Cerebral and corpus callosum atrophy in systemic lupus erythematosus. *Arhtritis and Rheum*. 2005; 52: 2783.

[64] Zhang L, Harrison M, Heier LA, Zimmerman RD, Ravdin L, Lockshin M, Ylug AM. Diffusion changes in patients with systemic lupus erythematosus. *Magn. Reson. Imag.* 2007;;25:399-405.

[65] Williamson JA, Petrou M, Foerster B, Gebarski S, Cagnoli P, McCune W, Sundgren PC. Comparison of diffusion tensor imaging in systemic lupus erythematosus with and without neuropsychiatric symptoms: A prospective study of apparent diffusion coefficient and fractional anisotropy values in different regions of the brain. 2007; *Proceedings p 230, European Congress of Radiology*, Vienna Austria 2007.

[66] Emmer BJ, van der Grond J, Steup-Beekman GM, Huizinga TWJ, van Buchem M. Selective involvement of the amygdale in systemic lupus erythematosus. *PloSMedicine* 2006;4(12)2285-2289.

[67] Kowal C, DeGiorgio LA, Nakaoka T, Hertherington H, Huerta PT et al. Cognition and immunity: Antibody impairs memory. *Immunity* 2004;21:179-188.

[68] Johnson RT, Richardson EP. The neurological manifestation of systemic lupus erythematosus. A clinical-pathological study of 24 cases and review of the literature. *Medicine*1968;47:337-369.

In: Progress in Systemic Lupus Erythematosus Research ISBN 978-1-60021-861-3
Editor: Tomas I. Seward, pp. 211-226

Chapter 8

PERSONALIZED MEDICINE FOR SYSTEMIC LUPUS ERYTHEMATOSUS: A NEW CHALLENGE FOR THE NEAR FUTURE

Ana M. Bertoli and Luis M. Vilá*
From the Department of Medicine (Division of Rheumatology),
The University of Puerto Rico Medical Sciences Campus,
San Juan, Puerto Rico

ABSTRACT

Systemic lupus erythematosus (SLE) is a chronic disease with higher morbidity and mortality when compared to the general population. Disease outcome varies among patients, in part, because they do not respond the same to a given treatment modality. There is, therefore, a clear need for drug treatments to be selected according to the characteristics of an individual patient, in order to improve efficacy and reduce the number and severity of adverse drug reactions. Personalized medicine means the prescription of specific therapeutics best suited for an individual. This novel treatment approach should be regarded as an ongoing progression of healthcare which is advancing with genomic tools. Although still a translational challenge into the practice of rheumatologists, data for immunosuppressive drugs (mainly coming from transplant patients) is now available and waiting to be introduced in the field of autoimmune diseases such as SLE. Examples of that are genetic studies of drug metabolizing systems that can affect the efficacy, pharmacokinetic and tolerability profile of drugs such as azathioprine, cyclosporin A, mycophenolate mofetil, cyclophosphamide and glucocorticoids, among others. Although quite attractive, implementation of pharmacogenomics may not be so simple. Ideally the genetic trait should be accomplished with a well characterized patient from the socio-demographic, cultural and

* Address for correspondence: Luis M. Vilá, MD. Division of Rheumatology, Department of Medicine, University of Puerto Rico Medical Sciences Campus, PO Box 365067, San Juan, PR 00936-5067. Telephone: 787-758-2525, ext. 1825. Fax: 787-764-6839. E-mail: lvila@rcm.upr.edu

ethnic background as well as co-morbidities and drug exposure history, variables known as being modifier factors for drug efficacy and tolerability. Major efforts should also be made to systematically evaluate the patient; in this sense, validated outcome measures of disease activity, accumulated damage and health-related quality of life could be very valuable to quantify drug response. Worldwide integrated genomic information should also be an unequivocal subject for the future. Although quite attractive, personalized medicine is not without some drawbacks; cost, infrastructure and worldwide networking are not minor issues to overcome. Finally, personalized medicine must be strongly interpreted from the ethics perspective and regulated by the law.

Introduction

Systemic lupus erythematosus (SLE) is a disease characterized by multi-organ involvement and an unpredictable course that, sometimes, swings independently from the treatment. Moreover, as a chronic disease, SLE can impact patients' life; quality of life (QoL) is usually worse [1], while morbidity [2; 3] and mortality [4] are higher when compared to the general population.

Although a growing body of literature has focused in SLE, this disease still represents a clinical challenge. Remarkably, one of the most difficult and misunderstood aspects of SLE is its treatment. It is well recognized that the long-term outcome varies among patients from different ethnic populations [5-8] and that patients do not respond the same to a given treatment modality [9]. In this sense, many epidemiological studies have introduced the *nature versus nurture* argument highlighting the necessity to integrate existing genetic and environmental information available for this disease [10; 11].

While the biomedical research engine continues to fill the pipeline of drugs for the treatment of SLE, biomarkers for efficacy and tolerability remain, nevertheless, to be unraveled. There is a clear need for drug treatments to be selected according to the characteristics of an individual patient, improving, in this way, efficacy and reducing the number and severity of adverse drug reactions. Personalized medicine aims at this goal and it simply means the prescription of specific therapeutics best suited for an individual.

In this chapter, we will be addressing the following topics: 1) The Concept of Personalized Medicine, 2) Rationale for Personalized Medicine in SLE, 3) Implementing Personalized Medicine in SLE and 4) Future Directions.

The Concept of Personalized Medicine

Although pharmacokinetics is an useful tool to guide drug dosing and, eventually, predicting outcome, some studies have failed to fully explain the relationship between a given drug, the clinical response and adverse reactions merely based on the drug pharmacokinetic profile. This may indicate that pharmacotherapy should rely not only in the general approach of pharmacokinetics, but also in individual genetic variations. The latter can result in disparities in drug absorption, distribution, metabolism or pharmacological action. It is estimated that genetics can account for 20 to 95 percent of variability in drug kinetic and effect [12].

Personalized medicine is the use of detailed information about the patient's genotype and clinical data in order to select a medication, therapy or preventative measure that is particularly suited to that individual patient [13]. This novel treatment approach should be regarded as an ongoing progression of healthcare which is advancing with the use of nanobiotechnology (an area that applies the tools and processes of nano/microfabrication to build devices for studying biosystems).

Identifying particular alleles that contribute to variations in the effect and safety profile of a given drug treatment is the main challenge. Genomics, proteomics and metabolomics refer to the search of variations in genes that can cause disease, abnormal protein patterns and abnormal metabolite patterns, respectively [14]. These areas of expertise are the main source of technology development and knowledge advance in this field. The potential is enormous for pharmacogenetics (the study of individual genes) and pharmacogenomics (the study of the genome) to yield a powerful set of molecular diagnostic methods or markers that should become widely available to clinicians in order to select medications and dose for the individual patient [15]. As explained by Evans et al [16], "pathways" of genes may be more significant than individual "candidate" genes as the effect of several genes (and their polymorphisms) acting together are those responsible of a unique phenotype.

The main advantage of this new treatment approach is that a patient's genotype needs to be determined only once for any given gene, because, except for rare somatic mutations, it does not change. Other benefits of this approach are its accuracy, efficacy, safety and speed. Genotyping methods are improving so rapidly that it will be soon possible to analyze a panel of genotypes and test for those that are important determinants of drug disposition and effects [17]. However, medicine should not merely rely on these tests, but to take advantage of them, bringing all the genetic information together with a well clinically characterized patient.

Although the concept of pharmacogenomics applied to the individual patient sounds relatively simple and, at the same time, appealing there are many issues to accomplish before these "theragnostics" (the fusion of therapeutics and diagnostic medicine with the goal of providing individualized pharmacotherapy) [18] tests become widely available. First, the development of new automated technologies that allows rapid scoring of microsatellite alleles and single nucleotide polymorphisms are warranted. Indeed, recent expansions in this field show promise to achieve this goal [15; 19]. Second, healthcare infrastructure supporting the integration of genomic data and clinical records is necessary. The latter would involve physicians, hospitals, healthcare systems, pharmaceuticals and diagnostic-technology companies [20]. Third, financial outlays should be cost-effective. The implementation of these technologies may depend not only in the healthcare expenditures but also in the healthcare system prevailing in a given region; decision driven by the market may also impact this accomplishment. Although advances in molecular technology hold promise for reducing the cost and effort involved in genotyping individuals, these techniques remain expensive and specialized, hindering their widespread use [21]. Finally, personalized medicine must be strongly interpreted from the ethics standpoint and regulated by the law. Regulatory, ethical and privacy policies are still matters of concern and the perception of the public/consumers on personalized medicine remains yet to be elucidated.

The Personalized Medicine Coalition [20] has emerged as a necessity to accomplish the above mentioned issues. This is a non-profit organization composed by pharmaceutical, diagnostic, biotechnology and information technology companies as well as academic institutions and governmental agencies intended to provide consensus on public policy issues and to serve as a forum for debate and education.

Rationale for Personalized Medicine in SLE

Many reasons can be stated regarding the importance of implementing the personalized medicine approach to the care of lupus patients. First, SLE is one of the most common autoimmune diseases with a prevalence as high as 241 cases per 100,000 inhabitants [22]. It has also been recognized in all five continents; however, its distribution is not homogenous, e.g. patients from minority populations, mostly of African ancestry whether living in the US, the Caribbean Islands, the United Kingdom, or Continental Europe, tend to show a higher SLE incidence and prevalence rates compared to those living in Africa [23]. The latter could be possibly explained by the interplay genetic and environmental factors have in the occurrence of the disease. Second, these genetic (inherited) and non-genetic (acquired) factors are known not only to predispose to, but also to modulate the course and outcome of the disease. Ethnicity is perhaps the most representative feature implicated in the disease outcome [24-26]. For example, patients from minority populations in the U.S. and Europe, as a group, tend to have more abrupt disease onset, more severe disease manifestations and an overall higher degree of disease activity. They also tend to accrue more damage and show higher mortality rates when compared to Caucasians [27]. Although ethnicity is a broad defined construct, the genetic trait within certain ethnic group cannot be ignored. Lastly, although the management of SLE has improved in the past 50 years, there is still a 3–5-fold increased mortality compared to the general population [28], with major organ damage, infection and cardiovascular disease as the major challenges for the coming decade. These facts emphasize the need to better understand the factors predictive of poorer outcome in patients with lupus, treatment response and toxicity included.

Implementing Personalized Medicine in SLE

Medicine has always attempted to personalize patient-physician relationship and the patient healing approach has historical and cultural roots. Thanks to the genome project, we are now facing with renewed excitement the prospect of personalized medicine. Contrary to the "one size-fits all" model and the "blockbuster drug model" [29], pharmacogenetics and pharmacogenomics effort is focused in a new model to achieve health.

During the past decade we have witnessed impressive advances in the field of rheumatology [30] as many new drug treatments have dramatically changed patient's prognosis. While the biomedical research engine continues to fill the pipeline of drugs for the treatment of SLE, biomarkers for efficacy and tolerability are not, nevertheless, yet developed. In this enthusiasm of improving patients' outcome, rheumatologists should not forget the risks these new treatment modalities entail and assure that aggressive treatment is justified.

Balancing efficacy and the occurrence of adverse events of different drugs is not always easy to attain. This is particularly difficult for drugs with narrow therapeutic index, such as the immunosuppressants commonly used in SLE. For these drugs the difference in the concentrations exerting therapeutic benefit and those causing adverse events is small [31]. On the other hand, many other drugs show a wide interindividual variability regarding efficacy and safety; this is particularly remarkable for glucocorticoids, which are still one of the mainstay drug therapies in the treatment of SLE.

Pharmacogenomics would then, take place to better characterize not only individual patients' traits but also groups of patients who have been systematically treated and evaluated to make possible the assessment of the efficacy and adverse events profile of a certain drug. Although data built from drug studies in SLE are yet limited, advantage can be taken on important data from other fields of medicine, such as oncology and transplantation, in which immunosuppressive drugs are widely used.

More than 1.4 million single-nucleotide polymorphisms were identified in the initial sequencing of the human genome [32] with over 60,000 of them in the coding region of genes. Every gene contains some level of polymorphism, with single nucleotide polymorphisms (SNPs) occurring every 1000–3000 base pairs throughout the human genome. The current challenge is to elucidate which of these polymorphisms have relevance to the treatment of rheumatic diseases. Most drug effects are determined by the interplay of several gene products that influence the pharmacokinetics and pharmacodynamics of medications, including inherited differences in drug targets (i.e. receptors) and drug disposition (i.e. metabolizing enzymes and transporters). Genetic polymorphisms with indirect effects on drug response (neither direct targets of medications nor involved in their disposition) have also been shown to alter the response to treatment in certain situations [33].

Response to immunosuppressants can be related to several factors including age, sex, concomitant diseases, drug-drug interactions as well as inheritance. Another observation is that related to ethnic differences in dose requirements for immunosuppressants. However, ethnicity could be rather a crude marker for genotype [34; 35]. Although still a translational challenge in the practice of rheumatologists, data for immunosuppressive drugs are now available and awaiting to be introduced in the field of autoimmune diseases such as SLE.

Genetic studies of metabolizing systems that can affect the efficacy, pharmacokinetic and tolerability profile of drugs commonly used in SLE such as azathioprine, cyclosporin A, mycophenolate mofetil, cyclophosphamide and glucocorticoids, among others are already available [36] (Table 1). However, only few studies have exclusively addressed the relationship between a specific genotype and the treatment of lupus.

Table 1. Influence of different genotypes in the pharmacokinetics and pharmacodynamics of drugs commonly used in systemic lupus erythematosus (SLE)

Drug	Gene/allele	Affected enzyme/protein	Affected pathway	Consequence	Distribution
Azathioprine [37;69-74]	TPMT* coding (SNPs†)	TPMT	Metabolism (drug inactivation)	Less effectiveness More adverse events In SLE, only homozygous deficiency was associated with myelosuppression	90% of the population has normal activity
	HPRT‡ coding (SNPs)	HPRT	Metabolism (drug activation)	Less effectiveness	Less effectiveness
Mycophenolate mofetil [46-51]	UDP-GT¶ coding (SNPs)	UDP-GT	Metabolism (drug inactivation)	Bioavailability alteration Higher toxicity?	Variable depending on the SNP tested Usually low frequency
	MDR§2 (SNP)	Multi-drug resistance protein 2	Transporter (bioavailability)	C-24T SNP is associated with a lower oral clearance	
	IMPDH **coding (mutations)	IMPDH	Drug target	Less effectiveness	
Cyclosporine A [52-59]	MDR1 (SNP)	P-glycoprotein	Transporter (bioavailability)	From no changes to higher concentrations depending the SNP tested	45% to 80% in Caucasians
	CYP††3A4 coding (SNP)	CYP3A4	Metabolism (drug elimination)	From no changes to higher concentrations depending the SNP tested	SNPs found in 70% of Caucasians vs. 4% in African Americans
	CYP3A5 coding (SNP)	CYP3A5	Metabolism (drug elimination)	From no changes to higher concentrations depending the SNP tested	75% of Caucasians and 50% of African American show genetic inability of express functional CYP3A5

Drug	Gene/allele	Affected enzyme/protein	Affected pathway	Consequence	Distribution
Cyclophosphamide [38;39]	CYP2B6-coding (SNP)	CYP2B6	Metabolism (drug activation)	Higher likelihood of end-stage renal disease in SLE Lower likelihood of renal remission	12% in patients from a multiethnic SLE cohort
	CYP2C19-coding (SNP)	CYP2C19	Metabolism(drug activation) Higher likelihood of end-stage renal disease in SLE	Lower likelihood of renal remission Lower likelihood of ovarian failure	25% in patients form a multiethnic SLE cohort
	GST‡‡ coding (polymorphisms)	GST	Metabolism (drug inactivation)	GSTP1 codon 105 polymorphism increases the risks of myelosuppression and gastrointestinal toxicity in SLE patients	
Glucocorticoids [60-68]	Glucocorticoid-receptor coding (mutations)	Glucocorticoid receptor	Drug target	Mutations can be silent, associated with resistance or hypersensitivity, the latter displaying features of metabolic syndrome	Up to 60% in Caucasians
	GST coding (polymorphisms)	GST	Pharmacodynamics	Drug resistance	Up to 50% depending on the genotype; similar distribution in Caucasians and African Americans

*Thiopurine S –methyltransferase; †single nucleotide polymorphism; ‡hypoxanthine phosphoribosyltransferase; ¶uridine diphosphate glucuronosyltransferase; § multi-drug resistance-1 gene; ** inosine monophosphate dehydrogenase; ††member of the cytochrome P-450 family; ‡‡glutathione-S-transferase.

The relationship between single nucleotide polymorphisms of thiopurine S – methyltransferase (TPMT, an enzyme involved in drug inactivation), and azathioprine toxicity was examined by Naughton et al. [37]. In that study, they found that azathioprine was generally well tolerated in SLE patients and that only the TPMT homozygous deficiency was associated with myelosuppression. Owing that the homozygous deficiency was only found in one out of 120 patients, the authors concluded that TPMT genotyping would supplement, but not replace, regular blood monitoring in order to estimate the drug safety profile.

Another example would be that of cyclophosphamide, a drug extensively used in the treatment of severe clinical manifestations of SLE, such as lupus nephritis. Cyclophosphamide is a pro-drug that requires metabolic activation by cytochrome P450 (CYP) enzymes to 4-hydroxycyclophosphamide. Multiple CYPs have been involved in this activation and their polymorphisms implicated in the efficacy and the risk for adverse events. In the study by Takada et al [38], the authors found that SLE patients with renal involvement who were homozygous for *CYP2B6*5* or *CYP2C19*2* had a higher probability to evolve into end stage renal disease, while patients either heterozygous or homozygous for *CYP2C19*2* had a lower risk of developing premature ovarian failure. These findings are of outmost clinical importance since SLE mainly affects young women in their reproductive years of life, therefore, they could help making individualized treatment decisions. Cyclophosphamide metabolites are mainly detoxified by multiple glutathione S-transferases (GSTs). The relationship between GSTs mutations and the use of cyclophosphamide in SLE was studied by Zhong et al [39]. In that study the authors concluded that the GSTP1 codon 105 polymorphism increases the risks of cyclophosphamide toxicity in SLE patients.

Data for other immunosuppressant drugs such as mycophenolate mofetil and cyclosporine A are also available. Although these data come from non-lupus populations, they can, nevertheless, be very valuable in SLE patients. Similar to what it has been observed in the lupus population [40-42], African-American renal allograft recipients continue to exhibit poorer prognosis compared to Caucasian patients [43]. Thus, ethnic differences in the pharmacokinetics of immunosuppressants are a potential key factor in the differences observed. The latter are most likely mediated via several non-genetic as well as genetic factors, including known genetic variations that impair transporter/enzyme activity of genes such as CYP3A4, CYP3A5, multi-drug resistance 1 and 2 [44]. One of the most outstanding examples of such ethnic disparities is in the mycophenolate dose requirements in African-American compared to Caucasians; African-American patients require higher doses to attain equal response rates [45]. Many genetic variations of the enzymes responsible for mycophenolate inactivation as well as for the entero-hepatic recirculation have been described [46-51], however, up to date none of these gene polymorphisms can fully explain the response discrepancies between ethnic groups. Many gene polymorphisms mainly affecting the pharmacokinetics of Cyclosporine A, have also been described [52-59]. Although these genetic polymorphisms seem to be highly prevalent in the population, their impact in drug metabolism is very variable, with no evidence at this moment suggesting the necessity of any screening before treatment initiation.

Finally, recent findings in the glucocorticoid gene receptor mutations sound very valuable for their clinical application [60-68]. Although these mutations can be silent, they have also been associated with resistance or hypersensitivity, the latter displaying features of metabolic syndrome. Therefore, their implication in the daily clinical practice sound suitable if we are going to recognize *a priori* which patients are more likely to respond to glucocorticoids or, which is also very important in the lupus population, which of them are more prone to accrue, upon treatment, more cardiovascular risk factors.

Future Directions

Despite an increasing data on the variability of drug response phenotypes and their genetic basis, the challenge now is the translation into the practice of rheumatology. A first step toward achieving this goal should be minimizing spurious positive findings due to chance associations between genotypes and phenotypes. Therefore, logical strategies to identify candidate genetic polymorphisms and their application to the daily rheumatology practice are needed. These strategies should be directed to the following topics: 1) clinical areas where to translate and prove the applicability of pharmacogenomics, 2) conceding the value to the specialty care, 3) infrastructure development and 4) setting the role of public health and founding sources.

Ideally the genetic trait should be accomplished with a well characterized patient from the socio-demographic, cultural and ethnic background, co-morbidities and drug exposure history, as well as variables known as modifying factors for drug efficacy and tolerability. Major efforts should also be carried on to systematically evaluate the patient; in this sense, prospective cohort studies with nested designs focusing in drug treatment are an exceptional source of information regarding the interrelation between environment, socio-demographic, drug exposure history and the patient genetic trait. Another source of invaluable information is controlled clinical trials. The setting provided by this type of studies is ideal to better define the applicability of the genetic knowledge. During controlled clinical trials patients are well characterized, uniformly treated and systematically evaluated to objectively assess the drug response and safety profile.

As above mentioned, SLE represents a clinical challenge which requires the rheumatologist expertise, not only for treatment decisions but also for adequate patient follow-up. Outcome measures, which are increasingly being used in the routine clinical practice, can be merged with genomic and genetic data to provide new ways to choose therapy. The true value of any outcome measure is its ability to show the impact the disease has on the patient and to enable the clinician to follow the disease course, to evaluate the effect of therapeutic strategies and to better advise the patient. These outcome measures should assess at least four domains: disease activity, organ damage, health-related quality of life (HR-QoL) and survival [75; 76]. Among the different instruments used to evaluate these domains, rheumatologists should choose among those best suited for their clinical practice, both in terms of feasibility of its use and the relevance of the data obtained. Indexes to measure disease activity such as the British Isles Lupus Assessment Group (BILAG), European Consensus Lupus Activity Measurement (ECLAM), Systemic Lupus Erythematosus Disease Activity Index (SLEDAI), Systemic Lupus Activity Measure (SLAM) and Lupus Activity Index (LAI) have been validated prospectively and their reproducibility, validity and sensitivity to change compared [77]. Critical factors in the use of these indexes are the physician/investigator training and consensus among clinicians about how these indexes should be applied. Equally important is to understand the strengths and limitations each of these instruments have. Health status of lupus patients is not only related to disease activity but also to damage resulting from the disease itself, concomitant morbidities and treatment toxicity. The Systemic Lupus International Collaborating Clinics/American College of Rheumatology Damage Index has been validated to measure irreversible damage [78] and found to predict mortality [79]. A very valuable advantage of this index is that can reflect the positive and negative long-term effect of treatment. HRQoL instruments, such as the SF-36, are also available; the latter has been widely used to measure this domain although there are disease specific instruments under development [80].

Infrastructure development is also a first requirement if the gap between discovery and clinical development is to be bridged. Worldwide integrated genomic information should be an unequivocal subject for the future and multinational clinical trials could be a great opportunity to accomplish this. Networks supporting all the patient information and electronic medical records, among others, are important topics of concern for which founding sources are needed, especially for disadvantaged regions of the world. Lastly, the integration of public health with personalized medicine has yet to be accomplished [81; 82]. The next step is to set the role public health is going to play in this new treatment era.

Conclusion

Personalized Medicine should be sought as a new perspective to overcome the embarrassing dichotomy between the body of pharmacogenetic knowledge and its clinical application. The main objective of this novel "specialty" is to provide better margins of drug treatment efficacy and safety as new diagnostic tests become available. Although quite attractive, there are many important issues to be accomplished before this new treatment perspective can be widely used; infrastructure, financial outlays, a redirection of the public health and the public opinion as well as the ethics and law standpoints are matters of debate.

Lupus treatment armamentarium is not effective for all patients and, at the same time, encompasses a wide range of unpredictable adverse effects. Therefore, this disease is the perfect setting to apply all the knowledge gained through pharmacogenomics. If this is the future of medicine, scientists and physicians should collaborate all together in the difficult task of translating genetics and genomics into the clinical practice. There is a necessity, however, of being proficient enough to properly interpret these evolving concepts and discoveries in order to offer our patients the best results with the least cost in terms of adverse effects and financial outlays.

Reference List

[1] Jolly M. How does quality of life of patients with systemic lupus erythematosus compare with that of other common chronic illnesses?. *J. Rheumatol.* 2005; 32(9):1706-1708.

[2] de Leeuw K, Freire B, Smit AJ, Bootsma H, Kallenberg CG, Bijl M. Traditional and non-traditional risk factors contribute to the development of accelerated atherosclerosis in patients with systemic lupus erythematosus. *Lupus* 2006; 15(10):675-682.

[3] Bosch X, Guilabert A, Pallares L, Cerveral R, Ramos-Casals M, Bove A et al. Infections in systemic lupus erythematosus: a prospective and controlled study of 110 patients. *Lupus* 2006; 15(9):584-589.

[4] Bernatsky S, Boivin JF, Joseph L, Manzi S, Ginzler E, Gladman DD et al. Mortality in systemic lupus erythematosus. *Arthritis. Rheum.* 2006; 54(8):2550-2557.

[5] Lau CS, Yin G, Mok MY. Ethnic and geographical differences in systemic lupus erythematosus: an overview. *Lupus* 2006; 15(11):715-719.

[6] Toloza SM, Roseman JM, Alarcon GS, McGwin G, Jr., Uribe AG, Fessler BJ et al. Systemic lupus erythematosus in a multiethnic US cohort (LUMINA): XXII. Predictors of time to the occurrence of initial damage. *Arthritis Rheum.* 2004; 50(10):3177-3186.

[7] Borchers AT, Keen CL, Shoenfeld Y, Gershwin ME. Surviving the butterfly and the wolf: mortality trends in systemic lupus erythematosus. *Autoimmun. Rev.* 2004; 3(6):423-453.

[8] Petri M. The effect of race on incidence and clinical course in systemic lupus erythematosus: The Hopkins Lupus Cohort. *J. Am. Med. Womens Assoc.* 1998; 53(1):9-12.

[9] Adler M, Chambers S, Edwards C, Neild G, Isenberg D. An assessment of renal failure in an SLE cohort with special reference to ethnicity, over a 25-year period. *Rheumatology* (Oxford) 2006; 45(9):1144-1147.

[10] Alarcon GS, Friedman AW, Straaton KV, Moulds JM, Lisse J, Bastian HM et al. Systemic lupus erythematosus in three ethnic groups: III. A comparison of characteristics early in the natural history of the LUMINA cohort. LUpus in MInority populations: NAture vs. Nurture. *Lupus* 1999; 8(3):197-209.

[11] Reveille JD, Moulds JM, Ahn C, Friedman AW, Baethge B, Roseman J et al. Systemic lupus erythematosus in three ethnic groups: I. The effects of HLA class II, C4, and CR1 alleles, socioeconomic factors, and ethnicity at disease onset. LUMINA Study Group. Lupus in minority populations, nature versus nurture. *Arthritis Rheum.* 1998; 41(7):1161-1172.

[12] Kalow W, Tang BK, Endrenyi L. Hypothesis: comparisons of inter- and intra-individual variations can substitute for twin studies in drug research. Pharmacogenetics 1998; 8(4):283-289.

[13] Personalized medicine. Accessed at http://en.wikipedia.org/wiki/personalizedmedicine. Last accessed on 02/10/2007.

[14] Linda Bren. Metabolomics: Working Toward Personalized Medicine. Accessed at http://www.fda.gov/fdac/features/2005/605_metabolomics.html. Last accessed on 02/10/2007.

[15] Brennan MD. High throughput genotyping technologies for pharmacogenomics. *Am. J. Pharmacogenomics* 2001; 1(4):295-302.

[16] Evans WE, Relling MV. Moving towards individualized medicine with pharmacogenomics. *Nature* 2004; 429(6990):464-468.

[17] Evans WE, McLeod HL. Pharmacogenomics--drug disposition, drug targets, and side effects. *N. Engl. J. Med.* 2003; 348(6):538-549.

[18] Ozdemir V, Williams-Jones B, Cooper DM, Someya T, Godard B. Mapping translational research in personalized therapeutics: from molecular markers to health policy. *Pharmacogenomics* 2007; 8(2):177-185.

[19] Jannetto PJ, Laleli-Sahin E, Wong SH. Pharmacogenomic genotyping methodologies. *Clin. Chem. Lab. Med.* 2004; 42(11):1256-1264.

[20] Munroe JB. A coalition to drive personalized medicine forward Personalized Medicine. *Personalized Medicine* 2007; 1(1):9-13.

[21] Relling MV, Dervieux T. Pharmacogenetics and cancer therapy. *Nat. Rev. Cancer* 2001; 1(2):99-108.

[22] Ward MM. Prevalence of physician-diagnosed systemic lupus erythematosus in the United States: results from the third national health and nutrition examination survey. *J. Womens Health (Larchm)* 2004; 13(6):713-718.

[23] Bae SC, Fraser P, Liang MH. The epidemiology of systemic lupus erythematosus in populations of African ancestry: a critical review of the "prevalence gradient hypothesis". *Arthritis Rheum.* 1998; 41(12):2091-2099.

[24] Alarcon GS, McGwin G, Jr., Bartolucci AA, Roseman J, Lisse J, Fessler BJ et al. Systemic lupus erythematosus in three ethnic groups. IX. Differences in damage accrual. *Arthritis Rheum.* 2001; 44(12):2797-2806.

[25] Serdula MK, Rhoads GG. Frequency of systemic lupus erythematosus in different ethnic groups in Hawaii. *Arthritis Rheum.* 1979; 22(4):328-333.

[26] Ward MM, Pyun E, Studenski S. Long-term survival in systemic lupus erythematosus. Patient characteristics associated with poorer outcomes. *Arthritis Rheum.* 1995; 38(2):274-283.

[27] Bertoli AM, Alarcon G. Epidemiology of Systemic Lupus Erythematosus. Tsokos GC, Gordon C and Smolen JS. *Systemic Lupus Erythematosus. A companion to rheumatology.* Mosby E, editor. Pages 1-18, 2007.

[28] Urowitz MB, Gladman DD, Abu-Shakra M, Farewell VT. Mortality studies in systemic lupus erythematosus. Results from a single center. III. Improved survival over 24 years. *J. Rheumatol.* 1997; 24(6):1061-1065.

[29] Drug Researcher.Com. *Market Reports: Pharmaceutical and Science.* Accessed at http://www.drugresearcher.com/marketreport. Last accessed on 02/10/2007.

[30] Pisetsky DS. Rheumatology in 2. *Bull. Hosp. Jt. Dis.* 2006; 64(1-2):9-11.

[31] Benet LZ. Relevance of pharmacokinetics in narrow therapeutic index drugs. *Transplant Proc.* 1999; 31(3):1642-1644.

[32] Sachidanandam R, Weissman D, Schmidt SC, Kakol JM, Stein LD, Marth G et al. A map of human genome sequence variation containing 1.42 million single nucleotide polymorphisms. *Nature* 2001; 409(6822):928-933.

[33] MacPhee IA, Fredericks S, Holt DW. Does pharmacogenetics have the potential to allow the individualisation of immunosuppressive drug dosing in organ transplantation? *Expert Opin. Pharmacother* 2005; 6(15):2593-2605.

[34] Fredericks S, Holt DW, MacPhee IA. The pharmacogenetics of immunosuppression for organ transplantation: a route to individualization of drug administration. Am. J. *Pharmacogenomics* 2003; 3(5):291-301.

[35] Fredericks S, Holt DW. Pharmacogenomics of immunosuppressive drug metabolism. *Curr. Opin. Nephrol. Hypertens* 2003; 12(6):607-613.

[36] Cattaneo D, Perico N, Remuzzi G. From pharmacokinetics to pharmacogenomics: a new approach to tailor immunosuppressive therapy. *Am. J. Transplant* 2004; 4(3):299-310.

[37] Naughton MA, Battaglia E, O'Brien S, Walport MJ, Botto M. Identification of thiopurine methyltransferase (TPMT) polymorphisms cannot predict myelosuppression in systemic lupus erythematosus patients taking azathioprine. *Rheumatology* (Oxford) 1999; 38(7):640-644.

[38] Takada K, Arefayene M, Desta Z, Yarboro CH, Boumpas DT, Balow JE et al. Cytochrome P450 pharmacogenetics as a predictor of toxicity and clinical response to pulse cyclophosphamide in lupus nephritis. *Arthritis Rheum.* 2004; 50(7):2202-2210.

[39] Zhong S, Huang M, Yang X, Liang L, Wang Y, Romkes M et al. Relationship of glutathione S-transferase genotypes with side-effects of pulsed cyclophosphamide therapy in patients with systemic lupus erythematosus. *Br. J. Clin. Pharmacol.* 2006; 62(4):457-472.

[40] Korbet SM, Schwartz MM, Evans J, Lewis EJ. Severe lupus nephritis: racial differences in presentation and outcome. *J. Am. Soc. Nephrol.* 2007; 18(1):244-254.

[41] Alarcon GS, McGwin G, Jr., Petri M, Ramsey-Goldman R, Fessler BJ, Vila LM et al. Time to renal disease and end-stage renal disease in PROFILE: a multiethnic lupus cohort. *PLoS Med.* 2006; 3(10):e396.

[42] Johnson SR, Urowitz MB, Ibanez D, Gladman DD. Ethnic variation in disease patterns and health outcomes in systemic lupus erythematosus. *J. Rheumatol.* 2006; 33(10):1990-1995.

[43] Foster CE, III, Philosophe B, Schweitzer EJ, Colonna JO, Farney AC, Jarrell B et al. A decade of experience with renal transplantation in African-Americans. *Ann. Surg.* 2002; 236(6):794-804.

[44] Dirks NL, Huth B, Yates CR, Meibohm B. Pharmacokinetics of immunosuppressants: a perspective on ethnic differences. *Int. J. Clin. Pharmacol. Ther.* 2004; 42(12):701-718.

[45] Neylan JF. Immunosuppressive therapy in high-risk transplant patients: dose-dependent efficacy of mycophenolate mofetil in African-American renal allograft recipients. U.S. Renal Transplant Mycophenolate Mofetil Study Group. *Transplantation* 1997; 64(9):1277-1282.

[46] Huang YH, Galijatovic A, Nguyen N, Geske D, Beaton D, Green J et al. Identification and functional characterization of UDP-glucuronosyltransferases UGT1A8*1, UGT1A8*2 and UGT1A8*3. *Pharmacogenetics* 2002; 12(4):287-297.

[47] Mackenzie PI, Miners JO, McKinnon RA. Polymorphisms in UDP glucuronosyltransferase genes: functional consequences and clinical relevance. *Clin. Chem. Lab. Med.* 2000; 38(9):889-892.

[48] Bowne SJ, Sullivan LS, Blanton SH, Cepko CL, Blackshaw S, Birch DG et al. Mutations in the inosine monophosphate dehydrogenase 1 gene (IMPDH1) cause the RP10 form of autosomal dominant retinitis pigmentosa. *Hum. Mol. Genet.* 2002; 11(5):559-568.

[49] Bernard O, Tojcic J, Journault K, Perusse L, Guillemette C. Influence of nonsynonymous polymorphisms of UGT1A8 and UGT2B7 metabolizing enzymes on the formation of phenolic and acyl glucuronides of mycophenolic acid. *Drug Metab. Dispos.* 2006; 34(9):1539-1545.

[50] Kuypers DR, Naesens M, Vermeire S, Vanrenterghem Y. The impact of uridine diphosphate-glucuronosyltransferase 1A9 (UGT1A9) gene promoter region single-nucleotide polymorphisms T-275A and C-2152T on early mycophenolic acid dose-interval exposure in de novo renal allograft recipients. *Clin. Pharmacol. Ther.* 2005; 78(4):351-361.

[51] Naesens M, Kuypers DR, Verbeke K, Vanrenterghem Y. Multidrug resistance protein 2 genetic polymorphisms influence mycophenolic acid exposure in renal allograft recipients. *Transplantation* 2006; 82(8):1074-1084.

[52] Rivory LP, Qin H, Clarke SJ, Eris J, Duggin G, Ray E et al. Frequency of cytochrome P450 3A4 variant genotype in transplant population and lack of association with cyclosporin clearance. *Eur. J. Clin. Pharmacol.* 2000; 56(5):395-398.

[53] von Ahsen N, Richter M, Grupp C, Ringe B, Oellerich M, Armstrong VW. No influence of the MDR-1 C3435T polymorphism or a CYP3A4 promoter polymorphism (CYP3A4-V allele) on dose-adjusted cyclosporin A trough concentrations or rejection incidence in stable renal transplant recipients. *Clin. Chem.* 2001; 47(6):1048-1052.

[54] Kuehl P, Zhang J, Lin Y, Lamba J, Assem M, Schuetz J et al. Sequence diversity in CYP3A promoters and characterization of the genetic basis of polymorphic CYP3A5 expression. *Nat. Genet.* 2001; 27(4):383-391.

[55] Kim RB, Leake BF, Choo EF, Dresser GK, Kubba SV, Schwarz UI et al. Identification of functionally variant MDR1 alleles among European Americans and African Americans. *Clin. Pharmacol. Ther.* 2001; 70(2):189-199.

[56] Hoffmeyer S, Burk O, von Richter O, Arnold HP, Brockmoller J, Johne A et al. Functional polymorphisms of the human multidrug-resistance gene: multiple sequence variations and correlation of one allele with P-glycoprotein expression and activity in vivo. *Proc. Natl. Acad. Sci. USA* 2000; 97(7):3473-3478.

[57] Min DI, Ellingrod VL. C3435T mutation in exon 26 of the human MDR1 gene and cyclosporine pharmacokinetics in healthy subjects. *Ther. Drug. Monit.* 2002; 24(3):400-404.

[58] Min DI, Ellingrod VL, Marsh S, McLeod H. CYP3A5 polymorphism and the ethnic differences in cyclosporine pharmacokinetics in healthy subjects. *Ther. Drug. Monit.* 2004; 26(5):524-528.

[59] Foote CJ, Greer W, Kiberd BA, Fraser A, Lawen J, Nashan B et al. MDR1 C3435T polymorphisms correlate with cyclosporine levels in de novo renal recipients. *Transplant Proc.* 2006; 38(9):2847-2849.

[60] van Rossum EF, Roks PH, de Jong FH, Brinkmann AO, Pols HA, Koper JW et al. Characterization of a promoter polymorphism in the glucocorticoid receptor gene and its relationship to three other polymorphisms. *Clin. Endocrinol.* (Oxf) 2004; 61(5):573-581.

[61] van Rossum EF, Lamberts SW. Glucocorticoid resistance syndrome: A diagnostic and therapeutic approach. *Best Pract. Res. Clin. Endocrinol. Metab.* 2006; 20(4):611-626.

[62] Russcher H, Smit P, van den Akker EL, van Rossum EF, Brinkmann AO, de Jong FH et al. Two polymorphisms in the glucocorticoid receptor gene directly affect glucocorticoid-regulated gene expression. *J. Clin. Endocrinol. Metab.* 2005; 90(10):5804-5810.

[63] van Rossum EF, Lamberts SW. Polymorphisms in the glucocorticoid receptor gene and their associations with metabolic parameters and body composition. *Recent Prog. Horm. Res.* 2004; 59:333-357.

[64] van Rossum EF, Koper JW, van den Beld AW, Uitterlinden AG, Arp P, Ester W et al. Identification of the BclI polymorphism in the glucocorticoid receptor gene: association with sensitivity to glucocorticoids in vivo and body mass index. *Clin. Endocrinol.* (Oxf) 2003; 59(5):585-592.

[65] Di Blasio AM, van Rossum EF, Maestrini S, Berselli ME, Tagliaferri M, Podesta F et al. The relation between two polymorphisms in the glucocorticoid receptor gene and body mass index, blood pressure and cholesterol in obese patients. *Clin. Endocrinol.* (Oxf) 2003; 59(1):68-74.

[66] van Rossum EF, Koper JW, Huizenga NA, Uitterlinden AG, Janssen JA, Brinkmann AO et al. A polymorphism in the glucocorticoid receptor gene, which decreases sensitivity to glucocorticoids in vivo, is associated with low insulin and cholesterol levels. *Diabetes* 2002; 51(10):3128-3134.

[67] Davies SM, Bhatia S, Ross JA, Kiffmeyer WR, Gaynon PS, Radloff GA et al. Glutathione S-transferase genotypes, genetic susceptibility, and outcome of therapy in childhood acute lymphoblastic leukemia. *Blood* 2002; 100(1):67-71.

[68] Anderer G, Schrappe M, Brechlin AM, Lauten M, Muti P, Welte K et al. Polymorphisms within glutathione S-transferase genes and initial response to glucocorticoids in childhood acute lymphoblastic leukaemia. *Pharmacogenetics* 2000; 10(8):715-726.

[69] Clunie GP, Lennard L. Relevance of thiopurine methyltransferase status in rheumatology patients receiving azathioprine. *Rheumatology* (Oxford) 2004; 43(1):13-18.

[70] Baker DE. Pharmacogenomics of azathioprine and 6-mercaptopurine in gastroenterologic therapy. *Rev. Gastroenterol. Disord* 2003; 3(3):150-157.

[71] McLeod HL, Siva C. The thiopurine S-methyltransferase gene locus -- implications for clinical pharmacogenomics. *Pharmacogenomics* 2002; 3(1):89-98.

[72] Ansari AA, Mayne A, Sundstrom JB, Gravanis MB, Kanter K, Sell KW et al. Frequency of hypoxanthine guanine phosphoribosyltransferase (HPRT-) T cells in the peripheral blood of cardiac transplant recipients. A noninvasive technique for the diagnosis of allograft rejection. *Circulation* 1995; 92(4):862-874.

[73] Chocair PR, Duley JA, Simmonds HA, Cameron JS. The importance of thiopurine methyltransferase activity for the use of azathioprine in transplant recipients. *Transplantation* 1992; 53(5):1051-1056.

[74] Jun JB, Cho DY, Kang C, Bae SC. Thiopurine S-methyltransferase polymorphisms and the relationship between the mutant alleles and the adverse effects in systemic lupus erythematosus patients taking azathioprine. *Clin. Exp. Rheumatol.* 2005; 23(6):873-876.

[75] Strand V. Clinical trial design in systemic lupus erythematosus: lessons learned and future directions. *Lupus* 2004; 13(5):406-411.

[76] Strand V, Gladman D, Isenberg D, Petri M, Smolen J, Tugwell P. Endpoints: consensus recommendations from OMERACT IV. Outcome Measures in Rheumatology. *Lupus* 2000; 9(5):322-327.

[77] Liang MH, Socher SA, Larson MG, Schur PH. Reliability and validity of six systems for the clinical assessment of disease activity in systemic lupus erythematosus. *Arthritis Rheum.* 1989; 32(9):1107-1118.

[78] Gladman DD. The Systemic Lupus International Collaborating Clinics/American College of Rheumatology (SLICC/ACR) Damage Index for Systemic Lupus Erythematosus International Comparison. *J. Rheumatol.* 2000;373-6.

[79] Nived O, Jonsen A, Bengtsson AA, Bengtsson C, Sturfelt G. High predictive value of the Systemic Lupus International Collaborating Clinics/American College of Rheumatology damage index for survival in systemic lupus erythematosus. *J. Rheumatol.* 2002; 29(7):1398-1400.

[80] Panopalis P, Clarke AE. Quality of life in systemic lupus erythematosus. *Clin. Dev. Immunol.* 2006; 13(2-4):321-324.

[81] Holford TR, Windemuth A, Ruano G. Designing physiogenomic studies. *Pharmacogenomics* 2006; 7(2):157-158.

[82] Ruano G. Quo vadis personalized medicine? *Personalized Medicine* 2004; 1: 1-7.

In: Progress in Systemic Lupus Erythematosus Research
Editor: Tomas I. Seward, pp. 227-243
ISBN 978-1-60021-861-3

Chapter 9

THERAPEUTIC POTENTIAL OF HMG-COA REDUCTASE INHIBITORS (STATINS) IN SYSTEMIC LUPUS ERYTHEMATOSUS

Przemyslaw J. Kotyla and Bogna Sliwinska-Kotyla
Department of Internal Medicine and Rheumatology
Medical University of Silesia, Katowice, Poland

ABSTRACT

Systemic lupus erythematosus is a connective tissue disorder of unknown origin and a relatively bad prognosis. In the last fifty years the big progress in the treatment of the condition has been made, resulting in the improvement of prognosis and prolongation of the life span. Nowadays we are prepare enough to manage the acute form of the disease, treat acute vasculitis lupus nephritis, decrease inflammation. As the result of extension of the life span the lupus face has been changed. Today a premature atherosclerosis is considered the main risk factor for increased mortality among lupus patients. The premature development of atherosclerosis is a well known clinical phenomena since the work of Urowitz and colleagues who described the term bimodal peak of mortality and attributed the second peak of mortality to premature development of atherosclerosis and its fatal complications. For almost two decades the mechanism of the atherosclerosis in lupus had not been explained satisfactory. In the early nineties of the last century Ross suggested that atherosclerotic process is an inflammation in its nature. Now atherosclerosis is considered a chronic inflammatory condition of the vessel wall. In the recent years many immunological mechanisms in the development and progression of the atherosclerotic lesions have been recognized. Since the atherosclerosis and atherosclerosis in lupus patients share the same pattern of inflammation it would be reasonable to treat the patients with a drug that cools the inflammation on one side and halts progression of atherosclerosis on the other.

Statins, inhibitors of HMG-CoA reductase, a key enzyme in the pathway of cholesterol synthesis have been commonly used in the therapy of ischemic coronary events and the control of hypercholesterolemia. In last years evidence was accumulated suggesting that action of statins go far beyond lipid lowering properties and may affect function of immune system cells. An array of anti-inflammatory effects has now been identified, including reduced production of pro-inflammatory cytokines, chemokines and adhesion molecules; reduced expression of inducible major histocompatibility complex (MHC) class II molecules by antigen presenting cells (APC); lowering of C-reactive protein levels and reduced production of reactive oxygen species. The effect that is separated from lipid lowering properties is sometimes called pleiotropic action of statins. The beneficial effect is often seen before the normalization of lipid profile suggesting that action of statins comprises at least two mechanism – cholesterol synthesis inhibition and direct effect on arterial wall and endothelium.

Such pleiotropic effect may benefit patients with autoimmune rheumatic diseases, including lupus.

The repertoire of drugs used in the treatment of systemic autoimmune disorders is characterized by unfavorable influence on lipid profile in patients treated, thus may perpetuate the development of atherosclerosis evoked by the inflammatory process itself.

In this regard statins may act on two main fields; being a concomitant therapy for autoimmune disorders and normalize the lipid profile abnormalities in patients with connective tissue disorders.

This overview assesses the evidence for using statins in patients with systemic lupus erythematosus.

Introduction

Systemic lupus erythematosus is an autoimmune disorder of unknown background that serves as a prototype for the other autoimmune disease. It affects mainly young people, especially women, a population that is not at risk of atherosclerosis development. In the former time acute course of lupus with lupus nephropathy, hematological complication and infection had been attracted the attention of physicians. However, with an improvement of the lupus management we are now able to control well acute phase of disease that contributes significantly to the improvement of the prognosis and prolongation of the life span. Many years after the onset of lupus survivals from acute lupus phase face the problem of unexpected premature cardiovascular incidents.

Epidemiology

The problem of premature atherosclerosis in young lupus patients was described for the first time by Urowitz and colleagues [1]. They coined the term "bimodal mortality" and explained that the first peak of mortality is caused by acute phase of disease, but the last one was attributed to the fatal complication of atherosclerosis. These observations were confirmed by Bulkey and Roberts, who in series of autopsies of young lupus female patients found significant atherosclerotic lesions at least in one coronary artery in majority of cases [2]. These findings were substantiated by subsequent studies that additionally showed incidence of myocardial infarction being 5 times as high in lupus patients as in general population. Moreover, the specific target population for the disease was a group of young women where a age- specific incidence increased by a factor as much as 50 has been observed [3, 4].

The epidemiological studies showed prevalence of cardiovascular events in SLE at the level 6-26% [5,6]. With the use of novel non-invasive techniques the ratio of subclinical atherosclerosis was substantially higher and was established as high as 17-40% [7, 8].

Atherosclerosis and Inflammation

The pathogenesis of accelerated atherosclerosis in SLE is not completely understood. It is believed that atherosclerosis in SLE is the result of combination of traditional risk factors, treatment, and inflammation [9, 10]. However, the traditional risk factors are failed to fully explain the process of accelerated atherosclerosis that suggests the main role of inflammatory process in beginning and progression of atherosclerotic lesions among the patients with SLE. Moreover, the role of corticosteroid therapy and subsequent development of atherosclerosis in SLE is still subject of controversies and the results obtained from the studies gave contradictory results [4, 11]. Since the traditional risk factors, corticosteroid use are enable to fully explain the burden of accelerated atherosclerosis, SLE alone (but also the other connective tissue disorders) should be recognized as novel independent risk factor.

The phenomena of atherosclerosis in patients with autoimmune disease was not explained well. In nineties of the last century Ross [12] explained that atherosclerosis is equal to inflammation. In recent years this new understanding of the pathogenesis of atherosclerosis has included insights in the role of inflammatory mediators in cardiovascular disease, and characterization of immunologic phenomena that is present in coronary vascular disease but also may be found in classic autoimmune diseases [13-15]. This contributes to recognition of atherosclerosis in systemic lupus erythematosus as a chronic inflammatory disease characterized by circulating autoantibodies, activated T lymphocytes, immune complexes and proinflammatory cytokines. The level of inflammation in the course of SLE is high enough to start and progress the atherosclerosis in the patients.

The Role of Endothelium

The anatomic substrate for development of atherosclerosis is endothelium. Besides the cytokine and immunocompetent cells, the endothelium is the third major player in atherosclerosis. Expression of functionally important endothelial cell surface is influenced by circulating cytokines and other stimuli [16]. On the other side the endothelium is the source of anti–inflammatory and anti-thrombotic compounds that posse the ability to neutralize strong atherogenic stimuli. This protective role of endothelium is only observed with endothelium untouched. Under the stimulation of many diverse agents which include cytokines, autoantibodies, antiphospholipid antibodies, and modified LDL the endothelium can express a series of changes that allow it to participate in inflammation and immune response [17]. To characterize better these changes the endothelium activation term was introduced by Willms-Kretschmer [18] and than reintroduced by Pober, who showed the role of cytokines in the activation of endothelium [19, 20]. Endothelium activation consists of five main changes- loss of vascular integrity, expression of leukocyte adhesion molecules, change in phenotype from anti-thrombotic to pro-thrombotic, cytokine production and up-regulation of HLA molecules [21-25].

Loss of endothelial integrity promotes the influx the fluid from intravascular space into subendothelium. Up-regulation of leukocyte adhesion molecules, such as E-selectin, ICAM-1 and VCAM-1 allows leukocyte to interact with endothelial surface and than to penetrate into the tissue [26]. This transmigration is driven by several factors with monocyte chemoattractant protein-1 (MCP-1) being the most prominent compound that is synthesized by endothelial and smooth cells layers [27].

Endothelium activation and subsequent dysfunction has been implicated in acute inflammatory response and it has been correlated with elevated level of C-reactive protein [28, 29]. It also occurs in patients with SLE suggesting the involvement of the same mechanism in spite of disease origin [30]. Moreover the patients with SLE are characterized by higher nitric oxide production and larger baseline diameter of peripheral artery. The extent of nitric oxide production, expression of nitric oxide synthase in endothelium and baseline of brachial artery diameter correlates well with lupus activity but also with the progression of atherosclerosis [31].

Endothelium is also the site where expression of MHC class II molecules takes place. Being not a classical antigen presenting cells (APC) the endothelial cells may also express MHC molecules, that occurs in particular after endothelial stimulation with activated T cells, interferon gamma (IF- γ) and lymphokine [32-34]. The role of MHC molecules in atherosclerotic processes has been intensively debated. The main area of interest is premature atherosclerosis in transplanted organs [35, 36]. Accelerated atherosclerosis in this particular clinical states correlates well with increased expression of MHC molecules in graft organs, being at least partially responsible for subsequent graft rejection [37].

COX/Metalloproteinases Role

In last few years the role of metalloproteinases MMP-2 and MMP-9 has been intensively discussed. Both enzymes are highly expressed in human atherosclerotic plaques and represents the principal mechanism of collagen breakdown that leads directly to plaque instability and subsequent thrombus formation [38, 39]. Macrophages are the main source of MMP-2 and MMP-9, which synthesis is regulated via PGE2 / dependent pathway cAMP [40]. Several inflammatory stimuli including IL-1, TNF alpha and CD40L induce PGE 2 synthase that in turn activates COX-2 leading to increased biosynthesis of PGE 2 leading eventually to activation of MMPs [41, 42]. Taking into account expression of COX-2 it is speculated that cyclooxygenenase-2 might play a role in lipid accumulation in lesional smooth muscle cells (SMC) and macrophages and favoring formation of foam cells within atheroma. [43].

Cytokine Involvement

Systemic lupus erythematosus is a disease that is characterized by production of autoantibodies that is supported by Th2 response. The T helper cells can differentiate into two TH1 and Th2 subgroups [44]. Thl response promotes cell mediated immunity and inflammation via T cell expansion and monocyte activation while Th2 response is characterized by humor activity with antibody production. In SLE it is believed that imbalance between TH1 and TH2 response exists favouring Th2 activity and B cell-dependent autoantibody production [45]. B cell function is orchestrated by a family of Th2 dependent cytokines ((IL-4, Il-5, Il-6 and Il-10) that work together with released from monocytes and macrophages IL-1,IL-6 and TNF alpha [46,47]. The latest contributed significantly to the development of atherosclerosis being present in atherosclerotic plaques, affecting smooth cells proliferation and inducing the local inflammation in vessel wall and activation of macrophages [48].

The role of TNF alpha in SLE is controversial. Some studies show a positive correlation between disease activity and TNF alpha especially with increased triglycerides and low HDL [49]. However others have found a higher level in inactive disease postulating a protective role [50]. The others have found no difference in basal levels of TNF alpha in healthy controls versus SLE [51] Other papers postulate serum TNF-alpha and IL-6 as sensitive markers of SLE disease activity. They may play a role as independent markers for prediction of SLE disease activity and to differentiate normal subjects from those having SLE [52]. Being a marker of disease activity TNF alpha may also contribute to the development of atherosclerosis and play a role in atherosclerotic plaque breakdown via activating MMPs. It also influences lipid profile disturbances by elevation of triglyceride level [41, 42, 53].

Antiatherosclerotic Properties of Statins

Statins a 3- hydroxymethyl-3-methylglutaryl coenzyme A (HMG-CoA) reductase inhibitors belong to a class of drugs that characterize by inhibition a key enzyme in the pathway of cholesterol synthesis [54, 55]. Strong correlation between total and LDL cholesterol levels and atherosclerotic disease gave the background for use the statins in primary and secondary prevention of coronary artery disease [55]. Data from angiographic studies, however showed only minimal changes of atherosclerotic lesions in patients treated with statins as compared to the control. On the other hand despite of weak influence upon vessel wall morphology subjects on statins therapy dramatically benefit from the treatment. This gave the strong suspicion that statins as a class of drug may work at least on two fields; suppress cholesterol biosynthesis on one side and directly influence the atherosclerotic process via cholesterol independent way [56].

Statins therapy causes regression of atherosclerotic plaque that may contribute significantly to the clinical benefits observed in patients on statins therapy [54]. Moreover therapy with statins decreases the accumulation of cholesterol in arterial wall that is believed to be a marker of atherosclerosis [57]. The Scandinavian Simvastatin Survival Study (4S) was the first that showed that cholesterol lowering treatment decreases significantly all-cause mortality in patients with coronary heart disease and myocardial infarction [58]. The promising results form this study gave background for subsequent studies. West of Scotland Coronary Prevention study was the first primary prevention study that showed significantly reduction of MI and cardiac death [59].

Statins not only reduced morbidity and mortality from coronary heart disease but also prolonged life span in patient with hyper and normocholesterolemia. The latest suggest that action of statins is at least partially independent from lipid lowering properties of HMG-CoA reductase inhibitors [55].

The role of cholesterol in the pathogenesis of atherosclerosis is well established. Some doubts exist regarding relation between cholesterol level and development of cerebrovascular disease. Several studies addressed this question and some data obtained from these studies indicate that similarly to the cases of coronary heart disease therapeutic potential of statins can be seen in central nervous system vessels [60-63].

Atherogenesis and plaque formation begin with accumulation of low-density lipoproteins cholesterol in the endothelial compartment of blood vessel followed by its oxidation. Oxidated lipoproteins accumulated within endothelial space are the main target for monocytes and macrophages. Enzymes release from monocytes/macrophaes break down fibrous cap at the top of the plaque and lead to the rupture [64, 65]. Statins posse ability to stabilize atherosclerotic plaques. Several clinical studies showed potential of statins to decrease evolution rate of atherosclerotic lesion towards rupture. The one of the possible mechanism involved into this process is suppression of COX-2 and microsomal prostaglandin synthase-1 (mPGES-1) by statins. As the result of this process plaque stabilization is occurred, that prevents its rupture and subsequent thrombus formation that is the main mechanism leading toward acute myocardial infarction [43, 66].

Platelets activation and aggregation is a key step in thrombus formation. Since they are already activated they release potent factors involved into amplification platelets aggregation and recruitment, and thrombosis [67, 68]. Platelets can be activated by different stimuli including thrombin, adenosine diphosphatate and proinflammatory cytokines (including Il-1 and interferon gamma) [69]. Platelets are also important source of thromboxan A_2 (TXA_2), one of the most potent vasoconstrictor in the body. Statins may minimize platelet aggregation and thromboxan release through partial inhibition of ADP and ATP release from activated platelets and exerting antioxidant effects [70].

Fibrinogen, an important factor in coagulation exerts its proatherosclerotic action by stimulation of proliferation, and migration of the smooth cells. These processes are realized via affecting permeability of vascular endothelium and function of platelets, monocyte/macrophages as well as exerting proinflammatory and pro-coagulatory effects [71,72]. The results obtained from the studies indicate that effect of statin on the level of fibrinogen is relatively mild [73, 74]. However in patients suffering from connective tissue diseases fibrinogen level may reflect the level of inflammation. This is why fibrinogen is well known acute phase marker with its level raised significantly in the course of inflammation [75]. Statins may act on this field by cooling the inflammation following decreasing fibrinogen level.

Another potent coagulation factor that is found in atherosclerotic plaques is tissue factor (TF) [76].It is synthesized by damaged or stimulated monocytes, macrophages smooth and endothelial cells. After binding to activated factor VII, TF promotes coagulation [77]. Statins reduce level and activity of TF in human monocytes cultures activated but also non-activated by inflammatory stimuli [78, 79]. This effect is not only restricted to the mononuclear cells but also can be seen in smooth muscle cells of artery wall as well as endothelial cells [80, 81].

The several studies have addressed the influence of statin upon thrombin formation. The special emphasis was put on some thrombin generation parameters including such as thrombin fragment (F1+2), fibrinopeptide A (FPA), and thrombin-antihrombin III (TAT) complexes [75]. According to data obtained from the studies simvastatin inhibits conversion of prothrombin to thrombin [82]. Additionally in ex vivo studies simvastatin decreased thrombin generation and the total activity of the enzyme in patients with significantly high cholesterol level [83]. Statin are also shown to inhibit platelet-dependent formation of thrombin. The mechanism of this activity that is supposed to be involved is improvement of impaired interaction between platelets and coagulation factors, since platelets activity and aggregability do not change during the treatment [84].

Pleiotropic Properties of Statins

Statin were designed as potent cholesterol lowering drugs. Within many years passed they proven their efficacy in normalization lipid profile disturbances in secondary and primary prevention of cardiovascular events [58, 59, 85]. Large trials have demonstrated that one of the mechanism involved is lowering serum lipid levels, specifically low density lipoproteins, that is one of the most important risk factors for coronary artery disease [86]. The primary pharmacological function of statins is to suppress HMG-CoA reductase in the hepatic cells that decreases significantly de novo cholesterol synthesis in the liver. As the result of this inhibition overexpression of low density lipoprotein receptors on the hepatocytes surface occurs [87]. By upregulating LDL receptor expression hepatocytes increase cholesterol clearance. Increased cholesterol utilization and decreased LDL production contribute enormously to the decreased cardiovascular morbidity and mortality [88]. Decreasing cholesterol level is really of great patophysiological importance and exerts clinical benefits to the patients treated. However most studies suggest that non-cholesterol lowering properties of statin may be of the special biological importance [89-92].

These diverse properties which are apart from lipid lowering potential are sometimes called pleiotropic effect (Gk. Pleio – meaning many, tropos meaning manner). The term is a little controversial, since in vivo it is difficult to differentiate what effects are really independent from lowering cholesterol, as the decrease cholesterol level itself may exert many biological consequences. Statins block cholesterol synthesis at the level of mevalonate formation. Mevalonic acid is not only a substrate for subsequent cholesterol synthesis but also provides substrate for farnesylpyrophosphate and geranylgeranylpyrophosphate. These compounds are important for isoprenylation of cellular small molecular weight G-proteins of the Ras superfamily (Ras Rac Rho).G-proteins are involved in regulation of growth, cell-to-cell interaction and apoptosis [91, 93,]. Isoprenylation of small G proteins is essential for those proteins to achieve new regulatory functions [94]. Equilibrium between activity of these proteins provides strong positive stimuli upon endothelium and promotes to exert vasorelaxation [95]. Influence of cardiovascular risk factors on the cascade of small G proteins results with activation of small RhoA protein, and Rho kinase (ROCK) leading to destabilization of nRNA for eNOS synthase [96]. In the same moment strong positive regulatory effect on prepro ET-1 synthesis could be observed. It provides imbalance between NO synthesis and overproduction of ET-1. As the result vasoconstriction of vessel is observed. Endothelial and muscle smooth cells also express another small G protein Rac1 that is the major component of NAD(P)H oxidase that serves in many pathological states as the source of free radical species. Free radical species can interact with NO and decrease its bioavailability leading to endothelial dysfunction [95]. Another biological function of RhoA and ROCK proteins is regulation of endothelial barrier dysfunction by increasing phosphorylation of myosin light chain. Rho A plays also the role in signal transduction to muscle and non-muscle myosin II [97]. All those events eventually lead to the blood vessel contraction and promote development of atherosclerotic plaque. Statins may interfere with isoprenylation of small G protein and block their patophysiological function. It is suggested that this is one of the main mechanism that explains well pleiotropic properties of HMG-CoA reductase inhibitors [89].

Lessons derived from experimental models suggest that statins upregulate eNOS expression and inhibit smooth muscle proliferation via inhibition Rho-ROCK pathway. The effect is enhanced by cotemporary inhibition of Ras. Animal models showed that Ras plays the significant role in formation of atherosclerotic plaques, which was shown in apolipoprotein knock-out mice [98].

Many studies have proven that statins may posse immunomodulatory properties that might be of the special benefit in the treatment of autoimmune disorders. Statin may inhibit nuclear factor κB (NFκB) resulting with inhibition of endothelial activation [99, 100]. Statins regulate Class II Transactivator that reduce induced by interferon gamma (IFγ) expression of MHC class II molecules on antigen – presenting cells (APS). MHC molecule expression on the surface of APC is required for antigen presentation, thus antigen is recognized by T cells in the context of MHC II antigens. Decreased expression is resulting in antigen tolerance and down regulation of T cell response [101, 102]. Interaction with the process of MHC II presentation contributes to the shift of T cell from Th1 response to the protective Th2 response [103, 104]. Statins may also interfere with second signal transmission, since they are able to decrease expression of CD80/86 molecule on APC (mainly on B cells). Co-stimulation is essential to evoke full activation of T cells; in the absence of strong Co-stimulation signal T cell may develop immune tolerance and subsequent lack of activity. In this model treatment with atorvastatin stopped the progression of lupus in lupus-prone New Zeland F_1 mice [105]. This model may also explain good therapeutic response to statin therapy observed by Abud-Mendoza in patients with refractory SLE and lupus nephropathy [106]. In another study four weeks treatment with simvastatin in patients with SLE resulted with marked suppression of TNF alpha level and decreased lupus activity in SLEDAI scale [107].

The therapeutic and immunomodulatory effects of statins could also be observed in collagen-induced arthritis that represents an animal model of rheumatoid arthritis. In this study simvastatin suppresses significantly articular inflammation and decreases pro-inflammatory cytokine synthesis, IFNγ, tumor necrosis factor α (TNFα) and interleukin-12 (IL-12) [103]. This phenomenon could be also observed in patients with refractory rheumatoid arthritis, where administration of HMG-CoA reductase inhibitor - simvastatin resulted in suppression of inflammation [106]. This effect was confirmed in a larger double blind, randomized, placebo-controlled trail with atorvastatin. According to the data obtained from the study atorvastatin has a significant effect on disease activity and reduces the markers of inflammation [108]. In another study Yokota et al reported inhibition of production of IL-6, IL-8 and TNFα in fibroblast like synoviocytes from patients with RA [109].

Systemic lupus erythematosus is often complicated by antiphospholipid antibody syndrome that is believed to at least partially responsible for thrombotic episodes observed among the patients with SLE. Endothelium plays an essential role in the beginning and progression of thrombotic changes in the SLE patients. Under influence of stress factors such as pro-inflammatory cytokines, anti-phospholipid antibodies the phenotype of endothelium is changed from anti-adhesive toward pro-inflammatory and pro-adhesive. Statins showed their potential as a anti-inflammatory drugs in antiphospholipid antibody syndrome where they can inhibit activation of endothelium [110]. In animal model statins are shown to minimize prothombotic and pro-inflammatory influence of the antiphospholipid antibodies [111]. In another study monocytes from patients with APS treated with fluvastatin, showed markedly suppression of tissue factor. Moreover the effect was seen to six month after the end of the treatment [112].

In the beginning of 21st century we recognize SLE as a complex systemic disease with late complication from cardiovascular system. Since statins proven their efficacy in treatment of atherosclerosis in population not affected by connective tissue diseases and showed non-cholesterol lowering properties it is reasonable to use this group of compounds in primary and secondary prevention of cardiovascular diseases among the patients with SLE. This problem was recently addressed by Wajed and colleagues who proposed very tight control of lipid and cholesterol levels in patients with SLE [113]. It comes form understanding the SLE as coronary heart disease equivalent, that explains why total and in more extent LDL cholesterol levels should be as low as in patients with coronary heart disease. The ideal control of lipid risk factors is to maintain the LDL-cholesterol at the level of 2,6 mmol/l. This can be easily achieved by the use of statins. The usage of latest may also provide some additional benefits effects that are driven from immunomodulatory activity of HMG-CoA reductase inhibitors [114].

REFERENCES

[1] Urowitz MB, Bookman AA, Koehler BE, Gordon DA, Smythe HA, Ogryzlo MA. The bimodal mortality pattern of systemic lupus erythematosus. *Am. J. Med.* 1976; 60:221-225.

[2] Bulkley BH, Roberts WC. The heart in systemic lupus erythematosus and the changes induced in it by the corticosteroid therapy. A study of 36 necropsy patients. *Am. J. Med.* 1975; 58: 243-264.

[3] Johnsson H, Nived O, Sturfelt G. Outcome in systemic lupus erythematosus: a prospective study of patients from a defined population. *Medicine* (Baltimore) 1989; 68:141-150.

[4] Manzi S, Meilan EN, Rairie JE, et al. Age specific incidence rates of myocardial infarction and angina in women with systemic lupus erythematosus: comparison with the Framingham Study. *Am. J. Epidemiol.* 1997; 145: 408-415.

[5] Toloza SMA, Uribe AG, McGwin G et al. Systemic lupus erythematosus in a multiethnic US cohort (LUMINA) *Arthritis Rheum.* 2004; 50: 3947-3957.

[6] Morelli S, Bernardo M, Viganego F, et al. Left sided heart valve abnormalities and risk of ischemic cerebrovascular accidents in patients with systemic lupus erythematosus. *Lupus* 2003;12:805-812.

[7] Doria A, Shoenfeld Y, Wu R, et al. Risk factors for subclinical atherosclerosis in a prospective cohort of patients with systemic lupus erythematosus. *Ann. Rheum Dis.* 2003; 62:1071-1077.

[8] Bruce IN, Burns RJ, Gladmann DD, et al. Single photon emission computed tomography dual isotope myocardial imaging in women with systemic lupus erythematosus. I. Prevalence and distribution of abnormalities. *J. Rheumatol.* 2000; 27:2372-2377.

[9] Petri M, Detection of coronary artery disease and the role of traditional risk factors in the Hopkins lupus cohort. *Lupus* 2000; 9:170-5.

[10] Esdaile JM, Abrahamowicz M, Grodzicky T, et al. Traditional Framingham risk factors fail to fully account for accelerated atherosclerosis in systemic lupus erythematosus. *Arthritis Rheum.* 2001:44: 2331-2337.

[11] Roman MJ, Salmon JE, Sober R et al. Prevalance and relation to risk factors of carotid atherosclerosis and left ventricular hypertrophy in systemic lupus erythematosus and antiphospholipid antibody syndrome. *Am. J. Cardiol.* 2001, 87: 663-666.

[12] Ross R. Atherosclerosis an inflammatory disease. *N. Eng. J. Med.* 1999; 340: 115-126.

[13] Cristea A, Rus H, Niculescu F, Bedeleanu D, Vlaicu R. Characterization of circulating immune complexes in heart disease. *Immunol. Lett.* 1986; 13: 45-49.

[14] Liuzzo G, Kopecky SL, Frye RL, et al. Perturbation of the T-cell repertoire in patients with unstable angina. *Circulation* 1999; 100: 2135-2139.

[15] Mustafa A, Nityanand S, Berglund L, Lithell H, Lefvert AK. Circulating immune complexes in 50-year-old men as a strong and independent risk factor for myocardial infarction. *Circulation* 2000; 102: 2576-2581.

[16] Mantovani A, Garlanda C, Introna M, Vecchi A. Regulation of endothelial cell function by pro- and anti-inflammatory cytokines. *Transplant. Proc.* 1998; 30: 4239-4243.

[17] Hunt BJ. The endothelium in atherogenesis. *Lupus* 2000; 9: 189-193.

[18] Willms-Kretschmer K, Flax HM, Cotran RS. The fine structure of the vascular response in hapten-specific delayed hypersensitivity and contact dermatitis. *Lab. Invest.* 1967:17: 334-349.

[19] Pober JS. Cytokine-mediated activation of vascular endothelium. *Am. J. Pathol.* 1988; 133: 426-433.

[20] Pober JS. Immunobiology of human vascular endothelium. *Immunol. Res.* 1999; 19: 225-232.

[21] Adams DH, Shaw S. Leukocyte-endothelial interactions and regulation of leukocyte migration. *Lancet* 1994;343:831-836.

[22] Hwang SJ, Ballantyne CM, Sharrett AR, et al. Circulating adhesion molecules VCAM-1 ICAM-1 and E-selectin in carotid atherosclerosis and incident coronary heart diseases cases: the Atherosclerosis Risk in Communities (ARIC) Study. *Circulation* 1997; 96: 4219-4225.

[23] Ridker PM, Hennekens CH, Roitman-Johnson et al. Plasma concentration of soluble intercellular adhesion molecule 1 and risks of future myocardial infarction in apparently healthy men. *Lancet* 1998; 351: 88-92.

[24] Belmont HM, Abramson SB, Lie JT. Pathology and pathogenesis of vascular injury in systemic lupus erythematosus. *Arthritis Rheum.* 1996; 39: 9-22.

[25] Steihoff G, Wonigeit K, Pichlmayr R. Analysis of sequential changes in major histocompability complex expression in human livergrafts after transplantation. *Transplantation* 1988; 45:394-401.

[26] Hansson GK. Immune mechanisms in atherosclerosis. *Arterioscler. Thromb. Vasc. Biol.* 2001; 21: 1876-1890.

[27] Wang JM, Sica A, Peri G et al. Expression of monocyte chemotactic protein-1 and interleukin-8, by cytokine-activated human vascular smooth cells. *Arterioscler Thromb.* 1991;11:1166-1174.

[28] Hingorani AD, Cross J, Kharbanda RK, et al. Acute systemic inflammation impairs endothelium dependent- vasodilatation in humans. *Circulation* 2000; 102: 994-999.

[29] Fichtlscherer S, Zeiher AM. Endothelial dysfunction in acute coronary syndromes: association with elevated C-reactive protein levels. *Ann. Med.* 2000; 32: 515-518.

[30] Lima DSN, Sato EI, Lima VC, Miranda F, Hatta FH. Brachial Endothelial Function is impaired in patients with systemic lupus erythematosus. J Rheumatol 2002, 29: 292-7

[31] Belmont HM, Levartovsky D, Goel A, et al. Increased nitric oxide production accompanied by up regulation of inducible nitric oxide synthase in vascular endothelium from patients with systemic lupus erythematosus. *Arthritis. Rheum.* 1997; 40: 1810-1816.

[32] Pober JS, Gimbrone MA, Cotran RS, et al. Ia expression by vascular endothelium is inducible by activated T cells and by human gamma interferon. *J. Exp. Med.* 1983; 157:1339-1353.

[33] Groenewegen G, Buurman WA, van de Linden CJ. Lymphokine dependence of in vivo expression of MHC class II antigens by endothelium. *Nature* 1985; 316; 361-363.

[34] Collins T, Korman AJ, Wake CT, et al. Immune interferon activates multiple class II major histocompatibility complex genes and the associated invariant chain gene in human endothelial cells and dermal fibroblasts. *Proc. Natl. Acad. Sci. USA* 1984; 81: 4917-4921.

[35] Labarrere CA, Nelson DR, Faulk WP. Endothelial activation and development of coronary artery disease in transplanted human hearts. *JAMA* 1997; 278: 1169-1175.

[36] Kuffova L, Holan V, Lumsden L Forrester JV, Filipec M. Cell subpopulation in failed human corneal grafts. *Br. J. Ophtalmol.* 1999; 83: 1364-1369.

[37] Pober JS, Orosz CG, Rose ML, Savage CO. Can graft endothelial cells initiate a host anti-graft immune response? *Transplantation* 1996; 61: 343-349.

[38] Loftus IM, Naylor R, Goodall S, et al. Increased matrix-metalloproteinase-9 activity in unstable carotid plaques: a potential role in acute plaque disruption. *Stroke* 2000;31: 40-47.

[39] Galis ZS, Sukhova GK, Lark MW, Libby P. Increased expression of matrix metalloproteinases and matrix degrading activity in vulnerable regions of human atherosclerotic plaques. *J. Clin. Invest* 1994; 94:2493-2503.

[40] Cipollone F, Prontera C, Pini B, et al. Overexpression of functionally coupled cyclooxygenase-2 and prostaglandin E synthase in symptomatic atherosclerotic plaques as a basis of prostaglandin E(2)-dependent plaque instability. *Circulation* 2001; 104;921-927.

[41] Arias-Negrete S, Kelley K, Chadee K. Proinflammatory cytokines regulate cyclooxygenase-2 expression in human macrophages. *Biochem. Biophys. Res. Commun.* 1995; 208: 582-589.

[42] Mitchell J, Belvisi M, Akarasereenont P, et al. Induction of cyclooxygenase-2 by cytokines in human pulmonary epithelial cells; regulation by dexamethasone *Br. J. Pharmacol.* 1994; 113: 1008-1014.

[43] Mezzetti A. Pharmacological modulation of plaque instability. *Lupus* 2005;14: 769-772.

[44] Mosmann TR, Cherwinski H, Bond MW, et al. Two types of murine helper T cell clone. Definition according to profiles of activities and secreted proteins. *J. Immunol.* 1986;136: 2348-2357.

[45] Kirou KA, Crow MK,. New pieces to SLE cytokine puzzle. *Clin. Immuniol.* 1999; 91:1-5.

[46] Handwerger BS, Rus V, da Siva L, Via CS. The role of cytokines in the immunopathogenesis of lupus. *Semin. Imunopathol.* 1994; 16:153-180.

[47] Horowitz DA, Jacob CO, The cytokine network in the pathogenesis of systemic lupus eythematosus and possible therapeutic implications. *Semin. Immunopathol.* 1994; 16; 181-200.

[48] Mc Mahon M, Grossman J. Pathogenesis of atherosclerosis in lupus In: Wallace DJ, Hahn BH. *Dubois'Lupus Erythematosus Philadelpha Lippincott Williams and Wilkins* 2007; 356-369.

[49] Svenungsson E, Gunnarsson I, Fei GZ, Lundberg IE, Klareskog L, Frostegard J. Elevated triglycerides and low levels of high-density lipoprotein as markers of disease activity in association with up-regulation of the tumor necrosis factor/tumor necrosis factor receptor system in systemic lupus erythematosus. *Arthritis. Rheum.* 2003;48:2533-40.

[50] Gomez D, Correa PA, Gomez LM, Cadena J, Molina JF, Anaya JM.Th1/Th2 cytokines in patients with systemic lupus erythematosus: is tumor necrosis factor alpha protective? *Semin. Arthritis. Rheum.* 2004; 33: 404-441.

[51] Scuderi F, Convertino R, Molino N, Provenzano C, Marino M, Zoli A, Bartoccioni E. Effect of Pro-inflammatory/Anti-inflammatory Agents on Cytokine Secretion by Peripheral Blood Mononuclear Cells in Rheumatoid Arthritis and Systemic Lupus Erythematosus. *Autoimmunity* 2003;36: 71-77.

[52] Sabry A, Sheashaa H, El-Husseini A, et al. Proinflammatory cytokines (TNF-alpha and IL-6) in Egyptian patients with SLE: its correlation with disease activity. *Cytokine.* 2006;35: 148-153.

[53] Svenungsson E, Fei GZ, Jensen-Urstad K, de Faire U, Hamsten A, Frostegard J. TNF-α: a link between hypertriglyceridaemia and inflammation in SLE patients with cardiovascular disease. *Lupus* 2003;12:454-461.

[54] Corsini A, Pazzucconi F Arnaboldi I, et al. Direct effects of statins on the vascular wall. *J. Cardiovasc. Pharmacol.* 1998; 31:773-778.

[55] Vaughan CJ, Gotto AM, Basson CT. The evolving role of statins in the management of atherosclerosis. *J. Am. Coll. Cardiol.* 2000;35:1-10.

[56] Pierre-Paul D, Gahtan V. Noncholesterol-lowering effects of statins. *Vasc. Endovasc. Surg.* 2003; 37:301-313.

[57] Sparrow CP, Burton CA, Hernandez M, et al. Simvastatin has anti-inflammatory and antiatherosclerotic activities independent of plasma cholesterol lowering. *Arterioscl. Thromb. Vasc. Biol.* 2001; 21:115-121.

[58] Scandinavian Simvastatin Survival Study Group: Randomised trial of cholesterol lowering in 4,444 patients with coronary heart disease: The Scandinavian Simvastatin Survival Study (4S). *Lancet* 1994; 344:1383-1389.

[59] Shepherd J, Cobbe SM, Ford I, et al. for the West of Scotland Coronary Prevention Study group: Prevention of coronary heart disease with pravastatin in men with hypercholesterolemia. *N. Engl. J. Med.* 1995; 333: 1301-1307.

[60] Lewis SJ, Sacks FM, Mitchell JS, et al for the CARE investigators: Effect of pravastatin on cardiovascular events in women after myocardial infarction: The Cholesterol and Reccurent Events (CARE) trial. *J. Am. Coll. Cardiol.* 1998; 32: 40-46.

[61] Sacks FM, Pfeffer MA, Moye LA, et al for the Cholesterol and Reccurent Events Trial Investigators: The effect of pravastatin on coronary events after myocardial infarction in patients with average cholesterol levels. *N. Engl. J. Med.* 1996; 335: 1001-1009.

[62] Blauw GJ, Lagaay AM, Smelt AHM, et al. Stroke, statins and cholesterol: A meta-analysis of randomized, placebo controlled, double-blinded trials with HMG-CoA reductase inhibitors.*Stroke* 1997; 28: 946-950.

[63] Crouse JR III, Byington RP, Hoen HM, et al. Reductase inhibitor monotherapy and stroke prevention. *Arch. Intern. Med.* 1997; 157: 1305-1310.
[64] Navab M, Berliner JA,Watson AD, et al. The yin and yang of oxidation in the development of fatty streak: A review based on 1994 George Lymann Duff Memorial Lecture. *Atheroscler. Thromb. Vasc. Boil.* 1996; 16: 831-842.
[65] Henney AM, Wakeley PR, Davies MJ, et al. Location of stromyelysin gene in atherosclerotic plaques using in situ hybridization. *Proc. Natl. Sci. USA* 1991; 88: 8154- 8158.
[66] Cipollone F, Fazia M, Iezzi A et al. Suppression of the functionally coupled cyclooxygenase-2/prostaglandin E synthesis as a basis of simvastatin dependent plaque stabilization in humans. *Circulation* 2003; 107: 1479-1485.
[67] Fuster V, Badimon I, Badimon JJ, et al. The pathogenesis of coronary artery disease and acute coronary syndromes. *N. Engl. J. Med.* 1992; 326: 310-318.
[68] Daniel JL, Dangelmaier C, Jin J, et al. Role of intracellular signaling events in ADP-induced platelet aggregation. *Thromb. Haemost.* 1999; 82: 1322-1326.
[69] Schror K. Antiplatelet drugs. A comparative review. *Drugs* 1995; 50: 7-28.
[70] Kaneider NA, Egger P, Dunzendorfer S, et al. Rho-GTPase-dependent platelet-neutrophil interaction affected by HMG-CoA reductse inhibition with altered adenosisne nucleotide release and function. *Arterioscler. Thromb. Vasc. Biol.* 2002; 22: 1029-1035.
[71] Warkentin TE. Hemostasis and atherosclerosis. *Can. J. Cardiol.* 1995;11 suppl C: 29-34.
[72] Heinrich J Assmann G. Fibrinogen and cardiovascular risk. *J. Cardiovascular. Risk* 1995; 2: 197-205.
[73] Song JC White CM. Do HMG-CoA reductase inhibitors affect fibrinogen. *Ann. Pharmacother* 2001; 35: 236-241.
[74] Rosenson RS, Tangney CC, Schaefer EJ. Comparative study of HMG-CoA reductse inhibitors on fibrinogen. *Atherosclerosis* 2001; 155: 463-466.
[75] Krysiak R, Okopień B, Herman ZS. Effects of HMG-CoA reductase inhibitors on coagulation and fibrinolysis processes. *Drugs* 2003; 63: 1821-1854.
[76] Rosenson RS, Tangney CC. Antiatherothrobotic properties of statins: implications for cardiovascular event reduction. *JAMA* 1998;279:1643-1650.
[77] Dahlback B. Blood coagulation. *Lancet* 2000; 355: 1627-1632.
[78] Ferro D, Basili S, Alessandri C, et al. Inhibition of tissue-factor-mediated thrombin generation by simvastatin. *Atherosclerosis* 2000; 149: 111-116.
[79] Colli S, Eligini S, Lalli M, et al. Vastatin inhibit tissue factor in cultured human macrophages: a novel mechanism of protection against atherothrombosis. *Arterioscler. Thromb. Vasc. Biol.* 1997; 17: 265-272.
[80] Eto M, Kozai T, Cosentino F et al. Statins prevents tissue factor expression in human endothelial cells: role of Rho/Rho-kinase and Akt pathways. *Circulation* 2002; 87: 748-755.
[81] Camera M, Toschi V, Comparato C, et al. Cholesterol-induced thrombogenicity of the vessel wall: inhibitory effect of fluvastatin. *Thromb. Haemost.* 2002; 87: 748-755.

[82] Musial J, Undas A, Undas R, et al. Treatment with simvastatin and low-dose aspirin depresses thrombin generation in patients with coronary heart disease and borderline-high cholesterol levels. *Thromb. Haemost.* 2001; 85:221-225.

[83] Szczeklik A, Musial J, Undas A, et al. Inhibition of thrombin generation by simvastatin and lack of additive effects of aspirin in patients with marked hypercholesterolemia. *J. Am. Coll. Cardiol.* 1999; 33:1286-1293.

[84] Aoki I, Aoki N, Kawano K et al. Platelet-dependent trombin generation in patients with hyperlipidemia. *J. Am. Coll. Cardiol.* 1997; 30: 91-96.

[85] Downs JR, Clearfield M, Weis S et al. Primary prevention of acute coronary events with lovastatin in men and women with average cholesterol levels: results of AFCAPS/TecCAPS. Air Force/Texas Coronary Atherosclerosis prevention Study. *JAMA* 1998; 279:1615-1622.

[86] Jury EC, Ehrenstein MR. Statins: immunomodulators for autoimmune rheumatic disease? *Lupus* 2005; 14: 192-196.

[87] Brown MS, Goldstein JL. A receptor-mediated pathway for cholesterol homeostasis. *Science* 1986; 232:34-37.

[88] Sacks FM, Tonkin AM, Shephard J, et al. Effect of pravastatin on coronary disease events in subgroups defined by coronary risk factors: the Prospective Pravastatin pooling Project. *Circulation* 2000; 102: 1893-1900.

[89] Takemoto M, Liao JK. Pleiotropic effects of 3-hydroxy-3-methylglutaryl coenzyme A reductase inhibitors. *Arterioscler. Thromb. Vasc. Biol.* 2001; 11:328-343.

[90] Gotto AM Jr, Farmer JA. Pleiotropic effects of statins: do they matter? *Curr. Opin. Lipidol.* 2001; 12: 391-394.

[91] Comparato C, Altana C, Bellosta S et al. Clinically relevant pleiotropic effects of statins: drug properties or effects of profound cholesterol reduction? *Nutr. Metab. Cardiovasc. Dis.* 2001:11:328-343.

[92] LaRosa JC. Pleiotropic effects of statins and their clinical significance. *Am. J. Coll. Cardiol.* 2001; 88:291-293

[93] Glomset JA, Farnsworth CC. Role of protein modification reactions in programming interactions between ras-related GTPases and cell membranes. *Ann. Rev. Cell. Biol.* 1994;10:181-205.

[94] Corsini A, Mazzotti M, Raiteri M, et al. Relationship between mevalonate pathway and arterial myocyte proliferation: In vitro studies with inhibitors of HMG-CoA reductase. *Atherosclerosis* 1993; 1001: 117-125.

[95] Barandier C, Ming XF, Yang Z. Small G proteins as an novel therapeutic targets in cardiovascular medicine. *New Physiol. Sci.* 2003;18:18-22.

[96] Eto M, Barandier C, Ratheb L et al. Thrombin suppresses endothelial nitric oxide synthase and upregulates endothelin converting enzyme-1 expression by distinct pathways: role of Rho/ROCK and mitogen activated protein kinase. *Circ. Res.* 2001; 89: 583-590.

[97] Somlyo AP, Somlyo AV. Signal transduction by G-proteins, Rho-kinase and protein phosphatase to smooth muscle and non-muscle myosin II. *J. Physiol.* 2000; 522:177-185.

[98] George J, Afek A, Keren P et al. Functional inhibition of Ras by s-trans, trans-farnesyl thiosalicylic acid attenuates atherosclerosis in apolipoprotein knockout mice. *Circulation* 2002; 105:2416-2422.

[99] Vaughan CJ, Gotto AM. Update on statins:2003. *Circulation* 2004;110:886-892.

[100] Meroni PL, Tremoli E. Modulation of adhesion molecule expression on endothelial cells: to be or not to be? *J. Thromb. Haemost.* 2003;1: 2280-2282.

[101] Kwak B, Mulhaupt F, Myit S, Mach F. Statins as newly recognized type of immunomodulator. *Nature Medicine* 2000;6: 1399-1402.

[102] Sadeghi MM, Tiglio A, Sadigh K et al. Inhibition of interferon-gamma-mediated microvascular endothelial cell major histocompatibility complex class II gene activation by HMG-CoA reductase inhibitors. *Transplantation* 2001; 71:1262-1268.

[103] Leung BP, Sattar N, Crilly A et al. A novel anti-inflammatory role for simvastatin in inflammatory arthritis. *J. Immunol.* 2003; 170: 1524-1530.

[104] Aktas O, Waiczies S, Smorodchenko A, et al. Treatment of relapsing paralysis in experimental encephalomyelitis by targeting Th1 cells through atorvastatin. *J. Exp. Med.* 2003;197:725-733.

[105] Lawman S, Mauri C, Jury EC Cook HT, Ehrenstein MR. Atorvastatin inhibits autoreactive B cell activation and delays lupus development in New Zeland Black/White F_1 mice. *J. Immunol.* 2004; 173: 7641-7646.

[106] Abud-Mendoza C, de la Fuente H, Cuevas-Orta E, Baranda L, Cruz-Rizo J, Gonzalez-Amaro R. Therapy with statins in patients with refractory rheumatic diseases: a preliminary study. *Lupus* 2003;12(8):607-11.

[107] Kotyla P.J. Sliwinska-Kotyla B. Kucharz E.J.TNF alpha as a potential target in the treatment of SLE: A Role for the HMG-CoA reductase inhibitor simvastatin. *J. Rheumatol.* 2006; 33:2361

[108] Mc Carey DW, McInnes IB, Madhok R et al. Trail of atorvastatin in rheumatoid arthritis (TARA): double blind, randomized placebo controlled trial. *Lancet* 2004; 363: 2015-2021.

[109] Yokota K, Miyazaki T, Hirano M, Akiyama Y, Mimura T. Simvaststin inhibits production of interleukin 6 (IL-6) and IL-8 and cell proliferation induced by tumor necrosing factor -α in fibroblast-like synoviocytes from patients with rheumatoid arthritis.

[110] Meroni PL, RaschiE, Testoni C et al. Statins prevent endothelial cell activation induced by anti-phospholipid (anti-beta $_2$glycoprotein I) antibodies: effect on the pro-adhesive and proinflammatory phenotype. *Arthritis. Rheum.* 2001; 44: 2870-2878.

[111] Ferrara DE, Liu X, Espinola RG et al. Inhibition of thrombogenic and inflammatory properties of antiphospholipid antibodies by fluvastatin in an in-vivo animal model. *Arthritis Rheum.* 2003; 48: 3272-3279.

[112] Cuadrado MJ, Buendia P, Aguirre A, et al. Effect of fluvastatin on monocyte tissue expression in primary antiphospholipid syndrome: preliminary results of an in vivo study. *Arthritis Rheum.* 2005; 52: 253.

[113] Wajed J, Ahmad P, Durrington N, Bruce IN. prevention of cardiovascular disease in systemic lupus erythematosus- proposed guidelines for risk factor management *Rheumatology* 2004; 43: 7-12.

[114] McInnes IB, McCarey DW, Sattar N. Do statins offer therapeutic potential in inflammatory arthritis. *Ann. Rheum. Dis*. 2004; 63: 1535-1537.

INDEX

A

abortion, 186
accidents, 72, 107, 164, 236
accuracy, 54, 66, 213
acetylcholine, 136
achievement, xi, 178
acid, 12, 111, 142, 163, 224, 233, 242
activation, viii, ix, 30, 40, 56, 63, 78, 81, 90, 91, 105, 106, 107, 123, 129, 132, 133, 134, 136, 138, 149, 150, 151, 202, 216, 217, 218, 229, 230, 231, 232, 234, 235, 237, 238, 242
acute confusional state, 156, 194
acute coronary syndrome, 68, 96, 237, 240
acute lymphoblastic leukemia, 225
acute renal failure, 184
adaptive immune system, 137
ADC, 198, 199, 201, 203, 204, 205, 209
adenosine, 232
adhesion, xii, 40, 41, 80, 95, 165, 166, 228, 230, 237, 242
adipose, 41
adipose tissue, 41
adjustment, 41, 80
ADP, 232, 240
adsorption, 3, 7
adults, 43, 61, 64, 65, 70, 101
adventitia, 52
adverse event, 125, 215, 216, 218
aerobic exercise, 24
aetiology, 85, 92
Africa, 214
African American(s), 106, 216, 217, 224
age, ix, 2, 4, 9, 19, 41, 43, 45, 59, 79, 83, 85, 87, 106, 108, 112, 114, 115, 117, 119, 120, 121, 128, 141, 143, 187, 194, 215, 229
ageing, 158
agent, 2, 42, 109, 161
aggregation, 40, 232
aging, 143
agonist, 13, 136, 148
albumin, 1, 3, 4, 164
alcohol, 85, 109
alcohol use, 85
algorithm, 142
allele, 90, 216, 217, 224
allergic reaction, 3, 145
ALT, 185
altered peptide ligand, 136, 147, 148
alternative, 133, 137, 202
alters, 127
Alzheimer's disease, 163, 173
amino acid, x, 131, 137, 142, 143, 149, 151
amygdala, 204
anaemia, 33, 64
ANC, x, 178, 182, 183, 184, 186
androgens, 86
anemia, 10, 11, 189
angina, 43, 46, 47, 93, 236
angiogenesis, 52
angiography, 43, 44
angioplasty, 47
animal models, 41, 48, 133, 137, 139, 142
animals, 12, 108, 134
anisotropy, 199, 201, 208, 210
ankylosing spondylitis, 61
Annexin V, 82
antagonism, 147
anthrax, 125

antibiotic, 64, 187
antibody, ix, 3, 4, 6, 7, 15, 33, 65, 80, 91, 103, 105, 110, 111, 116, 118, 122, 126, 133, 138, 139, 144, 146, 153, 157, 158, 159, 160, 161, 164, 167, 168, 169, 170, 171, 183, 192, 201, 205, 206, 231, 235, 236
anticardiolipin, 6, 33, 41, 59, 60, 63, 68, 75, 80, 95, 97, 168, 174, 175, 183, 184, 206
anticoagulant, 33, 43, 80, 94, 101
anticoagulation, 64, 87
anticytoststic drugs, xi
antigen, xii, 122, 123, 126, 133, 134, 135, 136, 137, 139, 141, 144, 145, 148, 150, 157, 228, 230, 234
antigen-specific cells, 135
anti-inflammatory, xii, 5, 31, 49, 83, 84, 107, 122, 228, 235, 237, 239, 242
anti-inflammatory drugs, 5, 31, 49, 235
antimalarial agents, 71
antimalarials, 13, 40, 84, 89
antinuclear antibodies, 48, 183
antioxidant, 82, 232
antiphospholipid antibodies, viii, 7, 15, 30, 37, 39, 41, 43, 50, 53, 61, 62, 63, 64, 68, 73, 80, 82, 94, 97, 173, 174, 201, 202, 206, 209, 229, 235, 242
antiphospholipid syndrome, 9, 59, 60, 61, 62, 69, 74, 75, 96, 138, 150, 174, 209, 242
antipsychotic, 186
anxiety, x, 155, 194
anxiety disorder, 194
aorta, 81, 95
aortic valve, 63
APC, xii, 133, 136, 140, 145, 228, 230, 234
APL, 11, 136, 202
apoptosis, 44, 52, 57, 62, 132, 144, 152, 158, 161, 162, 163, 165, 234
apoptotic cells, 62, 102, 107, 122, 123, 128, 129, 163, 173
Argentina, 9
arginine, 82, 97
argument, 212
arterial hypertension, 50, 72, 73, 74
arteriography, 209
arteritis, 53
artery(ies), 19, 30, 41, 42, 43, 44, 45, 46, 50, 51, 53, 54, 62, 63, 70, 74, 79, 80, 94, 95, 97, 228, 230, 233
arthritis, 5, 10, 184, 185, 186, 190, 235
aseptic, 102
aspartate, 160, 169, 197
aspirin, 5, 11, 12, 15, 48, 50, 71, 72, 241
assessment, 25, 27, 35, 43, 45, 46, 50, 51, 53, 65, 71, 79, 88, 91, 157, 164, 174, 188, 202, 215, 221
astrocytes, 164
asymptomatic, vii, viii, xi, 30, 31, 43, 45, 47, 50, 51, 58, 64, 70, 78, 193, 194
ataxia, 186
atherogenesis, 38, 40, 69, 80, 237
atherosclerosis, vii, viii, xii, 29, 30, 37, 38, 39, 40, 41, 42, 43, 45, 46, 47, 49, 50, 62, 63, 65, 66, 67, 68, 69, 70, 71, 72, 77, 79, 80, 81, 82, 83, 84, 92, 93, 94, 95, 96, 97, 221, 227, 228, 229, 230, 231, 232, 235, 236, 237, 238, 239, 240, 242
atherosclerotic plaque, 37, 38, 40, 41, 42, 44, 45, 48, 70, 79, 80, 82, 230, 231, 232, 233, 234, 238, 240
ATP, 232
atrium, 53
atrophy, 192, 201, 210
attacks, 25, 163
attribution, 194, 206
auscultation, 33
Austria, 210
autoantibodies, ix, x, 1, 34, 37, 38, 41, 53, 60, 61, 62, 65, 75, 95, 106, 107, 116, 121, 123, 127, 131, 133, 135, 137, 138, 141, 142, 144, 146, 151, 155, 157, 158, 159, 160, 162, 163, 165, 167, 168, 169, 170, 172, 174, 229, 231
autoantigens, 62, 134, 136, 139, 141, 151, 159, 162, 163, 170
autoimmune disease, vii, ix, x, xi, 1, 2, 6, 9, 18, 24, 25, 26, 60, 71, 75, 105, 106, 107, 114, 116, 118, 121, 122, 123, 129, 131, 132, 133, 134, 136, 137, 138, 146, 147, 148, 150, 158, 159, 162, 177, 178, 187, 190, 191, 192, 211, 214, 215, 228, 229
autoimmune diseases, ix, xi, 1, 2, 6, 18, 24, 25, 60, 71, 75, 123, 131, 132, 133, 134, 138, 146, 147, 148, 150, 158, 159, 162, 178, 187, 190, 191, 211, 214, 215, 229
autoimmune disorders, ix, xii, 67, 105, 107, 178, 192, 228, 234
autoimmune hepatitis, 61
autoimmunity, ix, 67, 69, 70, 106, 114, 119, 120, 125, 129, 132, 133, 137, 138, 139, 146, 147, 148, 150, 152, 173
autologous bone marrow transplant, 186, 190
autonomic neuropathy, 194
autopsy, 31, 33, 79, 205
autoreactive T cells, 137, 138, 145, 146, 148
autosomal dominant, 224
availability, 39
avoidance, 86

azathioprine, x, xi, 2, 9, 89, 177, 179, 180, 184, 186, 211, 215, 218, 223, 225, 226
Azathioprine, 5, 13, 216
azotemia, 48

B

B cells, ix, 90, 101, 131, 132, 133, 134, 138, 141, 143, 144, 147, 149, 150, 188, 192, 234
BAC, 96
bacteria, vii, 89, 90
bacterial infection, 160
banking, 13
barriers, 48
basal ganglia, 200
base pair, 215
basement membrane, 117, 121
BBB, 158, 159, 160, 161, 164, 165
BD, 70, 101, 172, 208
behavior, 39, 170
behavioral disorders, 161
beneficial effect, xii, 5, 18, 71, 84, 87, 88, 98, 145, 146, 228
bias, 137
bilirubin, 185
binding, 3, 60, 62, 75, 80, 82, 90, 96, 101, 102, 103, 133, 136, 138, 141, 142, 148, 149, 151, 157, 160, 161, 162, 166, 170, 174, 233
bioavailability, 216, 234
biological activity, 90
biological consequences, 233
biological markers, 84
biomarkers, 68, 145, 212, 214
biomolecules, 196
biopsy, 8, 34, 35, 67
biosynthesis, 230, 231
biotechnology, 214
birth, 10, 11
birth rate(s), 11
birth weight, 11
births, 10, 11
bladder, 186
bleeding, 184
blocks, 65, 111, 133
blood, vii, 3, 4, 5, 13, 17, 18, 20, 25, 26, 32, 33, 38, 39, 40, 41, 46, 50, 58, 83, 84, 108, 158, 166, 175, 181, 182, 194, 218, 225, 232, 234
blood flow, 18, 25, 46
blood pressure, 13, 17, 18, 20, 25, 26, 32, 39, 50, 83, 84, 225
blood vessels, 5, 25, 33, 40
blood-brain barrier, 166, 175
bloodstream, 3, 6
body composition, 225
body fat, 39, 83
body mass index, 82, 225
body weight, 4, 88, 181, 187
bone marrow, x, 132, 177, 181, 183, 185, 187, 190
bone marrow transplant, 190
bone mass, 87, 99, 100
bone mineral content, 101
bone resorption, 86
bowel, 186
bradycardia, 11, 65
brain, xi, 57, 157, 158, 160, 161, 164, 165, 167, 172, 174, 193, 194, 195, 196, 198, 199, 201, 202, 203, 204, 205, 206, 207, 208, 209, 210
brain abscess, 194
brain damage, 160
brain structure, 199
brain tumor, 198
branching, 136
breakdown, 123, 161, 205, 230, 231
breast feeding, 13
breast milk, 12
breastfeeding, 12, 13, 14
Brownian motion, 199
buffer, 110, 112
bundle branch block, 64
burn, ix, 105, 107, 108, 109, 111, 112, 113, 114, 115, 116, 117, 118, 119, 120, 122, 123

C

calcification, 42, 43, 45, 63, 70, 75, 82, 94
calcium, 44, 55, 56, 59, 88, 97, 98
calcium channel blocker, 55, 56
California, 131, 146
Canada, 84
cancer, 187, 188, 222
candidates, 6, 147
capillary, 117, 118, 119
capsule, 204, 205
cardiac catheterization, 51, 54
cardiac involvement, vii, 29, 30, 65
cardiac myocytes, 34
cardiac output, 31
cardiac tamponade, 31, 32

cardiovascular disease, vii, viii, ix, 29, 30, 37, 41, 51, 60, 64, 65, 67, 68, 69, 70, 71, 75, 77, 78, 79, 93, 94, 95, 98, 214, 229, 235, 239, 242
cardiovascular morbidity, 233
cardiovascular risk, vii, 30, 39, 45, 81, 83, 93, 96, 97, 219, 234, 240
cardiovascular system, 235
Caribbean, 85, 93, 214
Caribbean Islands, 214
catabolism, 38, 107
catheter, 50
Caucasians, 214, 216, 217, 218
CD34, x, 178, 181, 183, 185, 187, 191
CD34+, x, 178, 181, 183, 185, 187, 191
CD44, 145, 152
CD8+, 107, 137, 138, 143, 144, 152, 186
cDNA, 119, 173
CE, 50, 223
cell, ix, x, 35, 37, 40, 41, 48, 52, 53, 56, 57, 62, 63, 69, 73, 80, 81, 82, 90, 95, 105, 107, 113, 117, 121, 122, 123, 125, 126, 128, 129, 131, 132, 133, 134, 137, 138, 141, 142, 143, 144, 145, 146, 147, 148, 149, 150, 151, 152, 155, 158, 159, 163, 166, 167, 168, 172, 178, 181, 182, 183, 185, 187, 188, 190, 191, 192, 197, 229, 231, 233, 234, 237, 241, 242
cell adhesion, 40, 145
cell death, 52, 132, 163
cell growth, 69
cell line, 158
cell membranes, 241
cell surface, 56, 125, 163, 167, 229
cell transplantation, 178, 190, 191, 192
cellular adhesion, 40
cellular immunity, 90
cellulose, 3, 4, 7
central nervous system, x, 157, 159, 166, 167, 168, 169, 171, 174, 177, 181, 189, 190, 192, 194, 206, 207, 208, 209, 232
cerebellum, 199
cerebral blood flow, 161
cerebral cortex, 203
cerebral hemorrhage, 194
cerebrospinal fluid, 157, 159, 168, 171, 172, 174
cerebrovascular disease, viii, 37, 38, 77, 79, 93, 163, 194, 232
channel blocker, 59
chemokines, xii, 107, 119, 166, 228
chemotherapy, 188, 191, 192
chicken, 140
childbearing, 9
childhood, 225
children, 11, 13, 43, 64, 65, 158, 164, 168, 189
China, 31
Chinese, 99, 100, 102, 173
chloroquine, 47, 71, 98
cholesterol, xii, 41, 43, 47, 70, 71, 81, 84, 98, 225, 227, 231, 232, 233, 235, 239, 241
chorea, 164
choroid, 158
chronic active hepatitis, 60
chronic autoimmune hepatitis, 60
chronic fatigue syndrome, 60, 75
chronic illness, 221
circulation, 17, 18, 19, 25, 26, 41, 46, 65, 160, 163
classes, 41
classification, 27, 30, 86, 156
claustrophobia, 194
clinical assessment, xi, 193, 194, 226
clinical diagnosis, xi, 193, 194
clinical symptoms, xi, 91, 193, 196, 202
clinical trials, 48, 139, 145, 192, 219, 220
clone, 123, 238
closure, 128
clustering, 83
CNS, 159, 160, 162, 164, 167, 170, 172, 174, 179, 180, 181, 183, 185, 189, 194, 196, 202, 208
CO2, 109, 111
coagulation, 4, 38, 232, 233, 240
coagulation factor(s), 233
coding, 199, 215, 216, 217
codon, 90, 217, 218
coenzyme, 48, 231, 241
cognition, 170
cognitive deficit(s), 156, 207
cognitive dysfunction, 160, 164, 170, 194
cognitive function, 167, 174
cognitive impairment, 156, 160, 164, 170, 201
cognitive performance, 157
cohort, vii, 30, 39, 41, 42, 43, 50, 51, 63, 67, 68, 69, 71, 73, 83, 93, 94, 95, 97, 99, 101, 102, 103, 108, 114, 124, 158, 159, 161, 163, 168, 169, 171, 205, 217, 219, 221, 223, 236
collagen, 36, 39, 40, 230, 235
coma, 189
combination therapy, 55, 58
communication, 159
community, 89
complement, ix, 3, 33, 40, 78, 81, 90, 91, 96, 102, 144, 158, 183, 189

complement components, 183
complement inhibitors, 91
complement system, 40, 90, 91, 158
complementarity, 144, 151, 152
complexity, 2
compliance, 124
complications, viii, ix, x, xii, 1, 2, 5, 10, 12, 31, 35, 37, 43, 45, 47, 49, 55, 64, 65, 77, 78, 79, 84, 85, 88, 92, 98, 101, 105, 106, 107, 121, 138, 155, 178, 183, 184, 187, 188, 192, 227
components, 40, 60, 90, 91, 106, 123, 132, 157, 165
compounds, 200, 229, 233, 235
comprehension, 125
computed tomography, vii, 30, 42, 43, 45, 46, 47, 174, 194, 236
concentration, 5, 13, 93, 96, 103, 110, 117, 152, 158, 237
conception, 9, 11, 14
concordance, 194
conditioning, x, 26, 177, 178, 181, 184, 185, 187, 188
conduction, 13, 30, 62, 64, 65
confusion, 189
congestive heart failure, 59
Congress, iv, 210
connective tissue, xii, 25, 37, 57, 62, 65, 227, 228, 229, 232, 235
consciousness, 164
consensus, 12, 74, 142, 149, 151, 152, 160, 161, 189, 191, 214, 220, 226
consent, 4
constrictive pericarditis, 31
consumers, 49, 213
consumption, 90
contact dermatitis, 237
control, ix, xii, 6, 10, 12, 13, 17, 18, 19, 21, 22, 23, 24, 25, 26, 61, 65, 68, 82, 84, 90, 102, 103, 105, 108, 112, 113, 114, 115, 117, 120, 121, 122, 125, 131, 132, 133, 137, 139, 142, 144, 146, 148, 149, 157, 187, 189, 197, 227, 228, 231, 235
control group, 10, 17, 18, 19, 21, 22, 23, 24, 25, 26, 61, 108
controlled studies, 3, 5, 12, 49, 50, 57
controlled trials, viii, 6, 30, 36, 48, 50, 57, 58, 59, 65
conversion, 233
cooling, 232
coronary angioplasty, 47, 50
coronary arteries, 43, 45, 62
coronary artery disease, viii, 37, 40, 42, 43, 47, 69, 71, 77, 93, 98, 231, 233, 236, 238, 240
coronary heart disease, 45, 46, 49, 50, 68, 69, 72, 79, 81, 93, 94, 97, 232, 235, 237, 239, 241
corpus callosum, 204, 205, 210
correlation(s), ix, 27, 45, 54, 65, 81, 106, 107, 122, 152, 158, 159, 160, 161, 162, 164, 169, 170, 187, 194, 201, 202, 224, 231, 239
cortex, 204, 205
corticosteroid therapy, 67, 84, 87, 185, 229, 236
corticosteroids, ix, x, 2, 5, 12, 13, 31, 36, 37, 39, 40, 48, 49, 63, 64, 78, 83, 84, 87, 88, 89, 92, 100, 101, 138, 178, 179, 180, 184, 186, 189, 190
cortisol, 12
coverage, 134
CPC, 158
cranial nerve, 189
C-reactive protein, xii, 37, 38, 40, 42, 43, 48, 68, 71, 81, 91, 95, 103, 228, 230, 237
creatine, 33, 196, 197
creatinine, 4, 5, 81, 183, 186
cross-sectional study, 61, 85
CRP, 37, 38, 40, 71, 81
CSF, x, 157, 158, 159, 160, 161, 164, 177, 181, 182, 185, 187, 194, 204
CT scan, 186
cues, 107
culture, 162
curing, 137
CVD, 64, 79, 80, 81, 82, 83, 84, 85, 92
cyanosis, 18
cycles, 112, 190
cyclooxygenase, 238, 240
cyclooxygenase-2, 238, 240
cyclophosphamide, xi, 2, 5, 8, 9, 36, 57, 72, 84, 89, 101, 138, 146, 159, 182, 211, 215, 218, 223
cyclosporin, xi, 180, 186, 211, 215, 224
cyclosporine, 9, 186, 218, 224, 225
cystitis, 182
cytochrome, 217, 218, 224
cytokines, ix, xii, 36, 37, 40, 44, 48, 53, 82, 83, 86, 93, 105, 107, 119, 122, 123, 125, 126, 128, 129, 133, 135, 136, 137, 143, 144, 145, 146, 150, 152, 162, 166, 228, 229, 231, 232, 235, 237, 238, 239
cytokinesis, 163, 173
cytomegalovirus, 192
cytoplasm, 119, 162
cytoskeleton, 157
cytotoxicity, 42, 69, 158

D

danger, 122, 123, 147
data analysis, 98
database, 49, 178
death(s) ix, 5, 11, 37, 41, 43, 47, 48, 49, 78, 79, 89, 92, 107, 109, 114, 132, 184, 232
decision making, 48
decisions, 218, 219
defects, 18, 64, 89, 90, 91, 122, 129, 163
deficiency, 86, 90, 91, 216, 218
definition, 10, 83, 159
deformation, 25
degenerate, 149
degradation, 52
dehydroepiandrosterone sulphate, 87, 98
delivery, 10, 12, 13, 135, 137, 139
dementia, 158
demyelinating disease, 147
demyelination, 202, 203, 205
dendritic cell, 133, 136, 148
density, viii, 38, 41, 67, 78, 81, 85, 94, 95, 96, 97, 98, 99, 100, 233, 239
Department of Defense, 124
depolarization, 165
deposition, 62, 63, 81, 91, 106, 111, 117, 118, 119, 121, 123, 144, 169
deposits, 33, 35, 44, 118, 119, 127
depression, 18, 25, 158, 161, 162, 164, 186, 189
depressive symptoms, x, 155
dermatitis, 113, 186
dermatomyositis, 25
dermis, 113, 120
desensitization, 137
destruction, 132
detection, 35, 43, 51, 61, 65, 70, 94, 103, 111, 158, 159, 185, 196, 198
deviation, 150
diabetes, 12, 18, 46, 47, 49, 50, 72, 80, 83, 84, 138, 150
diabetes mellitus, 12, 46, 47, 49, 50, 80, 83
diagnostic criteria, 162
dialysis, 184
diastole, 58
diastolic blood pressure, 19
diastolic dysfunction, viii, 30, 58, 59, 74
diastolic pressure, 19, 58
diet, 88, 182
differentiation, 122, 149
diffusion, xi, 164, 193, 194, 196, 198, 199, 201, 202, 204, 208, 209, 210
diffusion-weighted imaging, 209
diffusivity, 198, 199, 203, 204, 205, 208, 210
digestion, 44
dilated cardiomyopathy, 35, 67
dilation, 18, 25
diluent, 111
dimethylarginine, viii, 77, 82, 96, 97
directionality, 198, 199
discordance, 65
discrimination, 61
disease activity, x, xi, 3, 4, 25, 31, 36, 38, 49, 59, 67, 78, 81, 82, 84, 86, 89, 95, 97, 100, 102, 126, 160, 162, 177, 178, 183, 184, 185, 187, 189, 191, 212, 214, 219, 226, 231, 235, 239
disease progression, x, xi, 117, 122, 123, 177, 178, 193, 196
disease-free survival, 185
disinfection, 109
dislocation, 108, 109, 111
disorder, vii, xii, 1, 4, 30, 78, 136, 162, 185, 194, 227, 228
dispersion, 65, 75
disposition, 213, 215, 222
dissociation, 84
distribution, 44, 83, 127, 148, 212, 214, 217, 236
diversity, 139, 224
DNA, x, 2, 3, 4, 5, 6, 7, 11, 91, 97, 106, 107, 110, 116, 118, 128, 138, 139, 141, 142, 143, 144, 145, 149, 151, 152, 153, 155, 160, 161, 169, 182, 183, 185, 189
donors, 121
Doppler, vii, 30, 34, 46, 51, 54, 57, 58, 59, 71, 73, 75, 186
dosage, 49, 135
dosing, 212, 223
down-regulation, 126, 144, 152
drainage, 32
drug interaction, 215
drug metabolism, 218, 223
drug reactions, xi, 211, 212
drug resistance, 216, 217, 218
drug safety, 218
drug targets, 215, 222
drug therapy, 89
drug treatment, xi, 1, 211, 212, 213, 214, 219, 220
drugs, x, xi, xii, 2, 5, 12, 13, 36, 40, 47, 48, 49, 50, 56, 57, 64, 66, 71, 72, 84, 87, 89, 98, 102, 106,

138, 155, 178, 183, 184, 187, 211, 212, 214, 215, 216, 218, 222, 228, 231, 233, 240
dry ice, 111
ductus arteriosus, 12
duration, 6, 37, 45, 59, 65, 70, 78, 81, 86, 89, 99, 133, 135, 152, 186, 190
duties, 124
DWI, xi, 193, 196, 198, 199, 203, 205
dyslipidemia, 38, 67, 96
dyspnea, 31, 33, 51, 58, 186
dysthymic disorder, 162

E

EAE, 137
ears, 108, 109
echocardiogram, 12, 55
edema, 11, 35, 194
education, 178, 214
Education, 83
effusion, 31
eigenvalue, 199
eigenvector, 199
electrocautery, 109
electrolyte, 64, 189
electron, vii, 30, 42, 43, 45, 47
ELISA, 110, 116, 117, 118, 159, 164, 168, 171, 182, 183
ELISA method, 164
embolism, 64
emission, 45, 174, 195, 236
emotion(s) 25, 170, 205
emotional disorder, 161
employees, 124
encephalomyelitis, 135, 242
encephalopathy, 164
encoding, 91, 138, 149
endocarditis, 63, 64, 75
endocardium, 30
endothelial cells, 41, 52, 62, 63, 73, 80, 81, 82, 95, 96, 117, 162, 172, 230, 233, 238, 240, 242
endothelial dysfunction, 40, 79, 82, 93, 96, 162, 234
endothelin receptor antagonists., viii, 30
endothelium, xii, 39, 41, 42, 52, 63, 80, 165, 166, 172, 228, 229, 230, 232, 234, 235, 237, 238
end-stage renal disease, 96, 217, 223
energy, 100, 158
engagement, 132, 144
England, 168
enlargement, 53
enterocolitis, 185
enthusiasm, 214
environment, 136, 203, 219
environmental factors, 52, 91, 106, 132, 214
enzyme(s), xii, 36, 38, 49, 59, 61, 72, 82, 182, 183, 215, 216, 217, 218, 224, 227, 230, 231, 233, 241
enzyme inhibitors, 36, 49
enzyme-linked immunoassay, 61
eosinophilia, 35
epidemiology, 124, 222
epidermal ulcers, ix, 106
epidermis, 113, 120
epilepsy, 201
epinephrine, 161
epithelial cells, 238
Epstein-Barr virus, 139
equilibrium, 132
equipment, 55
erythrocyte sedimentation rate, 83, 183
erythrocytes, 167
Escherichia coli, 69
ESR, 182, 183
estradiol, 86
estrogen, 87
ethanol, 113
ethanolamine, 163, 165
ethics, xii, 184, 212, 213, 220
ethnic background, xi, 85, 212, 219
ethnic groups, 171, 218, 221, 222
ethnicity, 214, 215, 221
etiology, ix, 59, 105, 107, 121, 202, 203
EU, 1
Europe, 87, 214
euthanasia, 108, 109, 115
evolution, 3, 55, 137, 232
examinations, 205
exclusion, x, 35, 86, 155, 157, 194
exercise, 17, 18, 19, 20, 21, 22, 23, 24, 25, 26, 27, 50, 51, 57
expenditures, 213
experimental allergic encephalomyelitis, 149
experimental autoimmune encephalomyelitis, 137, 147, 148
expertise, 213, 219
exposure, xi, 83, 86, 87, 106, 123, 125, 161, 212, 219, 224
extracellular matrix, 37

F

fabric, 123
failure, viii, 3, 9, 30, 35, 49, 54, 55, 58, 59, 74, 86, 87, 123, 126, 184, 185, 217, 218
family, 85, 125, 144, 163, 217, 231
family history, 85, 125
fasting, 71
fat, 113
fatigue, 2, 18, 24, 26, 51, 60, 64, 167
feet, 19
females, viii, 4, 78, 106, 181
fertility, 13, 189
fetal abnormalities, 88
fetus, 12
fever, 33, 35, 64, 182, 184, 185, 186, 187
fibers, 34, 36, 163, 199, 201, 205
fibrin, 38, 63, 107
fibrinogen, 35, 95, 232, 240
fibrinolysis, 240
fibroblasts, 73, 238
fibromyalgia, 106
fibrosis, 33, 35, 36, 53, 59
fibrous cap, 37, 232
fibrous tissue, 63
filtration, 182
fitness, 25
fluctuations, 159
fluid, 3, 31, 34, 167, 195, 199, 230
focal seizure, 164
focusing, 219
folic acid, 39, 84
follicle, 12
Ford, 209, 239
fractures, viii, 78, 79, 85, 87, 88, 92, 98, 99, 101
fragility, 99
frontal lobe, 204
functional approach, 205
fungal infection, 91
fusion, 171, 213

G

gadolinium, 205
gallium, 33, 34
gamma globulin, 5
gastrointestinal bleeding, 184
gene(s), 60, 75, 91, 102, 103, 106, 108, 112, 119, 120, 123, 126, 127, 134, 137, 149, 168, 172, 213, 215, 217, 218, 224, 225, 226, 238, 240, 242
gene expression, 112, 120, 126, 127, 225
gene promoter, 224
gene therapy, 137
generalized seizures, 201
generation, 38, 136, 141, 233, 240, 241
genetic factors, 218
genetic information, 213
genetics, 102, 103, 213, 220
genital herpes, 186
genome, 213, 214, 215
genomics, 220
genotype, 103, 213, 215, 217, 224
gestation, 11, 12, 186
glass, 111
glatiramer acetate, 137
glomerulonephritis, ix, 6, 8, 106, 107, 117, 118, 119, 122, 123, 128, 135, 141, 142, 146, 181, 184
glucocorticoid receptor, 225
glucocorticoids, xi, 211, 215, 219, 225
glucose, 39, 71, 83, 84
glucose metabolism, 83
glutamate, 160, 169, 196, 197
glutamic acid, 138, 150
glutathione, 217, 218, 223, 225
glycerol, 163
glycine, 82, 97
glycolysis, 158
glycoprotein, 37, 41, 62, 69, 80, 94, 96, 150, 159, 216, 224
gold, 34, 35, 43, 53, 55, 205
grants, 146
grey matter, 201, 202, 203, 204
groups, 17, 19, 21, 22, 23, 24, 25, 26, 37, 57, 60, 63, 84, 113, 136, 162, 204, 215
growth, 72, 107, 119, 125, 233
growth factor, 72, 107, 119, 125
growth factors, 107, 119, 125
guanine, 226
guidelines, 67, 242

H

haemoglobin, 185
hair follicle, 113
hair loss, 10
half-life, 84, 135
hallucinations, 164

hands, 19
harm, 84, 132
harvesting, 191
Hawaii, 222
HDL, 38, 46, 47, 81, 82, 231
headache, 156, 163, 164, 186, 194
healing, 107, 123, 125, 214
health, ix, xi, 18, 19, 26, 48, 78, 98, 105, 106, 124, 125, 137, 212, 214, 219, 220, 222, 223
health care, 19, 125
health problems, ix, 105, 106
health status, 48
heart block, 11, 35, 65
heart disease, 49, 50, 235, 236
heart failure, 35, 50, 51, 58, 59, 74, 75, 79
heart rate, 58
heart,, vii, 181
heat, 37, 69, 70, 138, 150
heat shock protein, 37, 69
height, 87
hematopoiesis, xi, 178, 183, 184, 185, 187
hematopoietic stem cells, x, 177, 181
hematuria, 11, 146
hemoglobin, 182
hemorrhage, xi, 5, 184, 193, 194
hemostasis, 173
hepatic encephalopathy, 208
hepatitis, 161
hepatocytes, 233
hepatomegaly, 51
herpes, 102, 125
herpes zoster, 102, 125
high blood pressure, 38
hip, 86, 88
hippocampus, 160
histogram, 204, 209
histone, 106, 135, 140, 141, 145
histopathology, 44
HLA, 134, 141, 147, 159, 168, 172, 221, 230
homeostasis, 107, 132, 137, 241
homocysteine, viii, 37, 39, 45, 50, 64, 68, 77, 83, 84, 97
Hong Kong, 102
hormone, 13, 26
hospitalization, 49
hospitals, 61, 213
host, 90, 107, 132, 134, 202, 238
HSCT, 187
human brain, 208, 209
human genome, 215, 223
humidity, 108
hybrid, 128
hydrocortisone, 13, 36
hydrogen, 110, 207
hydrogen peroxide, 110
hyperactivity, 127
hypercholesterolemia, viii, xii, 46, 47, 68, 71, 77, 80, 84, 96, 98, 227, 239, 241
hypergammaglobulinemia, ix, 106, 107, 121
hyperhomocysteinemia, 39
hyperlipidemia, 39, 241
hyperparathyroidism, 86
hyperplasia, 31
hyperprolactinemia, 87
hyperreactivity, 136
hypersensitivity, 217, 219, 237
hypertension, vii, viii, 10, 11, 12, 18, 30, 38, 49, 52, 54, 55, 57, 63, 71, 72, 73, 77, 80, 83, 84, 98, 189
hypertrophy, 50, 53, 59, 236
hyperuricemia, 11
hyponatremia, 208
hypothesis, 42, 53, 61, 69, 81, 82, 123, 157, 205, 222

I

iatrogenic, x, 155
ibuprofen, 5, 12
ICAM, 230, 237
identification, 84, 134, 138
idiopathic, 53, 57, 73, 74
IFN, 40, 122, 126, 133, 141, 145, 235
IFNγ, 107
IL-6, ix, 53, 81, 86, 97, 106, 107, 120, 122, 231, 235, 239, 242
IL-8, 97, 122, 235, 242
illumination, 199
images, 66, 195, 199, 202, 208
imaging, xi, 33, 34, 35, 46, 55, 66, 73, 157, 183, 193, 194, 195, 196, 198, 199, 200, 202, 205, 206, 207, 208, 210, 236
imaging modalities, 195
imaging techniques, 33
imbalances, 122
immune complex deposition, ix
immune disorders, 4
immune function, 89, 122
immune reaction, 69
immune regulation, 69, 138, 149
immune response, 48, 106, 107, 122, 126, 129, 132, 136, 139, 146, 149, 151, 229, 238

immune system, vii, xii, 2, 5, 89, 103, 132, 134, 146, 163, 178, 228
immunity, 3, 68, 107, 123, 126, 146, 147, 169, 210, 231
immunization, 103, 139
immunocompetent cells, 26, 229
immunocompromised, 107
immunogenicity, 135, 163
immunoglobulin, 35, 41, 48, 90, 128, 149, 185
immunoglobulins, 3, 6
immunomodulation, 150, 152
immunomodulator, 242
immunomodulatory, 48, 103, 234, 235
immunopathogenesis, 238
immunosuppression, 127, 178, 185, 186, 188, 223
immunosuppressive agent, ix, 1, 78, 89, 91
immunosuppressive drugs, xi, 2, 3, 6, 15, 32, 36, 55, 57, 64, 89, 91, 211, 215
immunosuppressive therapies, 53, 192
immunotherapy, 106, 133, 135, 139, 142, 145, 146, 147, 148, 150, 192
implementation, xi, 8, 211, 213
in situ, 53, 160, 240
in situ hybridization, 240
in vitro, 8, 40, 65, 82, 126, 129, 139, 141, 142, 144, 152, 158, 160, 172, 187
in vivo, 62, 91, 103, 128, 143, 144, 147, 149, 186, 196, 209, 224, 225, 233, 238, 242
incidence, 6, 7, 9, 37, 43, 45, 55, 59, 87, 89, 93, 97, 107, 113, 114, 115, 122, 138, 158, 160, 206, 214, 221, 224, 228, 236
inclusion, 48, 181, 200
India, 102
indication, 189
indicators, 189
indices, x, 58, 177
indirect effect, 215
indium, 33, 34
individualization, 223
indomethacin, 12
inducer, 146
induction, 69, 87, 106, 107, 122, 128, 134, 135, 138, 141, 147, 163, 165, 190
infants, 12
infarction, 35, 41, 43, 44, 47, 48, 79
infection, ix, 42, 69, 70, 78, 89, 90, 91, 101, 102, 103, 105, 107, 109, 126, 138, 161, 186, 187, 188, 214, 228
infertility, 12
inflammation, vii, xii, 2, 5, 33, 34, 35, 36, 37, 38, 39, 40, 42, 44, 49, 63, 68, 69, 71, 81, 83, 86, 87, 95, 107, 117, 119, 126, 132, 137, 201, 205, 227, 229, 231, 232, 235, 237, 239
inflammatory arthritis, 242, 243
inflammatory cells, 33, 40, 44, 53, 63, 107
inflammatory disease, 83, 229, 236
inflammatory mediators, 229
inflammatory response, 81, 91, 107, 119, 230
inflammatory responses, 107
information technology, 214
informed consent, 181
infrastructure, xi, 212, 213, 219, 220
inguinal, 109, 115
inheritance, 215
inhibition, xii, 38, 74, 81, 82, 84, 152, 165, 169, 228, 231, 232, 233, 234, 235, 240, 242
inhibitor, viii, 40, 72, 77, 82, 112, 235, 240, 242
inhibitory effect, 164, 240
initiation, 40, 107, 125, 162, 218
injections, 136, 138, 144, 148
injuries, xi, 193, 194
inositol, 163, 197, 208
insight, 80, 205
instability, 38, 40, 68, 230, 238
institutions, 19, 214
instruction, 148
instruments, 219
insulin, viii, 41, 77, 83, 84, 97, 98, 225
insulin resistance, viii, 77, 83, 84, 97
insulin sensitivity, 41, 84
integration, 213, 220
integrity, 46, 112, 120, 157, 160, 161, 165, 203, 230
intellect, 186
intensity, 6, 18, 25, 26, 35, 70
interaction(s), ix, 37, 94, 97, 131, 132, 134, 141, 145, 151,159, 233, 234, 237, 240, 241
intercellular adhesion molecule, 38, 237
interference, 144
interferon, 5, 53, 127, 133, 138, 147, 230, 232, 234, 237, 238, 242
interferon (IFN), 133, 138
interferon gamma, 53, 230, 232, 234
Interleukin-1, 127, 128
interleukin-8, 237
interleukin-beta, ix, 106
interstitial lung disease, 27
interval, 4, 65, 113, 200, 224
intervention, 3, 85, 92, 138, 139
intervention strategies, 85, 92

intima, 46, 80, 82
intrauterine growth retardation, 10, 11
intravenously, 160, 181, 182
inversion, 195, 199
inversion recovery, 195, 199
iodine, 109
irradiation, 190
ischemia, 198, 202
isotope, 236
Italy, 1, 155

J

Japan, 3, 4, 17, 18, 19
joint pain, 5
joints, vii, 2

K

keratinocytes, 107
kidney(s), vii, 86, 108, 111, 117, 118, 119, 123, 127, 144, 147, 160, 189
kinetics, 122

L

labeling, 62
lack of control, 32, 39, 48
lactate level, 202
lactation, 13
LCA, 159
LDL, 37, 40, 41, 43, 47, 48, 69, 80, 81, 82, 94, 229, 231, 233, 235
leakage, 123, 158, 164
learning, 160, 169
left ventricle, 58
lesions, vii, ix, xii, 30, 37, 42, 52, 53, 63, 80, 105, 107, 108, 109, 113, 114, 115, 120, 121, 128, 194, 196, 201, 203, 205, 206, 207, 227, 228, 229, 231
lethargy, 189
leukemia, 190
leukocytes, 81, 107, 185
leukocytosis, 91
LFA, 145, 152
life span, xii, 189, 227, 228, 232
lifestyle, 18, 80, 84, 92
lifetime, 98
ligand(s), 123, 128, 133, 146, 149, 159
likelihood, 217
limbic system, 205
limitation, 45, 56
lipase, 38, 40, 67, 81, 82, 95, 96
lipid metabolism, 48
lipids, 37, 44, 48, 50, 68, 71, 97, 98, 196, 198, 202
lipoproteins, 41, 94, 232, 233
lipoxygenase, 52
listening, 17, 18
liver, 11, 40, 60, 185, 189, 233
liver disease, 60
liver enzymes, 11
location, 35, 142, 205
locus, 226
longitudinal study, 103, 172
Los Angeles, 131
lovastatin, 241
low-density lipoprotein, 8, 37, 69, 71, 80, 94, 232
LPS, 122, 160
lumbar spine, 86, 100
lumen, 44, 46, 52
lung, x, 25, 53, 73, 177, 181, 183, 186, 189
lung function, 25
lungs, vii, 52
lupus, iv, vii, viii, ix, x, xi, xii, 2, 5, 6, 7, 8, 9, 10, 11, 14, 15, 17, 18, 26, 27, 30, 31, 33, 35, 38, 41, 42, 45, 48, 51, 60, 61, 62, 63, 64, 65, 66, 67, 68, 69, 70, 71, 73, 75, 77, 78, 80, 81, 82, 83, 85, 86, 88, 89, 90, 91, 93, 94, 95, 97, 98, 102, 105, 106, 107, 108, 113, 114, 115, 116, 117, 118, 119, 121, 122, 123, 124, 125, 127, 128, 129, 131, 135, 136, 138, 139, 140, 141, 142, 143, 144, 145, 146, 147, 148, 149, 150, 151, 152, 153, 161, 163, 164, 167, 168, 169, 170, 171, 172, 173, 174, 177, 181, 183, 184, 185, 186, 187, 188, 189, 190, 191, 192, 194, 206, 207, 208, 209, 210, 211, 212, 214, 215, 216, 218, 219, 220, 221, 222, 223, 227, 228, 230, 231, 234, 235, 236, 238, 242
lupus anticoagulant, 41, 60, 61, 62, 63, 64, 69, 75, 80, 94, 174, 183
lupus erythematosus, iv, ix, xi, xii, 7, 9, 14, 27, 68, 78, 93, 95, 102, 105, 124, 125, 167, 168, 170, 171, 174, 194, 206, 207, 209, 211, 212, 216, 221, 222, 227, 228, 231, 235, 236
lymph, ix, 106, 107, 109, 113, 115, 116, 127, 135, 136, 140
lymph node, 109, 115, 116, 127, 135, 136, 140
lymphadenopathy, ix, 106, 107, 113
lymphocytes, 33, 37, 40, 53, 106, 122, 132, 144, 152, 159, 167, 186, 187
lymphoma, 188

lymphoproliferative mutation., ix
lysine, 136
lysis, 137

M

macrophages, 37, 40, 41, 44, 80, 94, 107, 122, 128, 129, 230, 231, 232, 233, 238, 240
magnetic field, 196
magnetic resonance, 33, 35, 57, 66, 161, 168, 194, 196, 197, 198, 206, 207, 208, 209
magnetic resonance imaging, 33, 57, 66, 161, 168, 194, 207, 209
magnetic resonance scanning, 206
magnetic resonance spectroscopy, 197, 198, 207, 208, 209
magnetization, 195, 203, 208
magnetization transfer imaging, 195, 203, 208
major depressive disorder, 162
major histocompatibility complex, xii, 132, 149, 228, 238, 242
males, 106
mammalian cells, 163
management, ix, 2, 3, 6, 7, 25, 47, 56, 67, 131, 137, 214, 228, 239, 242
mania, 189
manipulation, 196
manners, 194
manufacturer, 182, 183
mapping, 209
market, 213
marrow, 122, 128, 181, 184, 190, 191, 192
Maryland, 27, 169
mass spectrometry, 141
mast cells, 107
matrix, 40, 111, 117, 238
matrix metalloproteinase, 40, 238
MBP, 135, 137
MCP, 40, 81, 230
MCP-1, 40, 81, 230
measurement, 25, 26, 46, 51, 54, 55, 88, 91, 103, 196
measures, viii, xi, 30, 36, 43, 47, 49, 54, 57, 86, 91, 198, 199, 212, 219
mechanical ventilation, 32
media, 46, 80, 82
median, xi, 114, 178, 183, 185
medication, 48, 80, 84, 86, 87, 88, 109, 185, 188, 213
medicine, xi, 211, 212, 213, 214, 215, 220, 221, 222, 226, 241
membranes, 2, 117, 157
membranoproliferative glomerulonephritis, 127
membranous nephropathy, 127
memory, 160, 169, 185, 186, 188, 210
men, 13, 18, 41, 48, 49, 69, 85, 94, 95, 96, 99, 100, 107, 236, 237, 239, 241
meningitis, 194
menopause, 81
mental status change, 189
mental status changes, 189
messenger RNA, 173
meta-analysis, 90, 103, 239
metabolic changes, 84
metabolic syndrome, viii, 77, 81, 83, 96, 97, 217, 219
metabolism, 39, 82, 99, 100, 101, 198, 202, 212
metabolites, 196, 198, 218
metabolizing, xi, 211, 215, 224
metalloproteinase, 238
methionine, 39
methylation, 82, 97
methylprednisolone, viii, 31, 36, 78, 83, 180, 184, 185
Mexico, 29, 31, 33, 34, 36, 52, 66
MHC, xii, 132, 134, 136, 137, 138, 139, 140, 143, 148, 150, 228, 230, 234, 238
MHC class II molecules, 140, 230, 234
mice, ix, 65, 105, 107, 108, 109, 112, 113, 114, 115, 116, 117, 118, 119, 120, 121, 122, 123, 127, 128, 129, 134, 135, 136, 137, 138, 139, 140, 141, 142, 143, 144, 145, 147, 148, 150, 151, 152, 153, 160, 161, 164, 234, 242
microfabrication, 213
micrograms, 135
microorganism(s), 42, 90
microscope, 109
microscopy, 62, 111
Microsoft, 112
microtubules, 157, 173
migraine, 158
migration, 38, 41, 232, 237
mild cognitive impairment, 202
military, 107, 123, 124
milligrams, 135
minority, 214, 221
miscarriage, 10, 15
mitogen, 241
mitral regurgitation, viii, 30, 63
mitral valve, viii, 30, 63
MMP, 230

MMP-2, 230
MMP-9, 230
MMPs, 230, 231
mobility, 85, 198, 199
models, ix, x, 42, 48, 105, 126, 131, 135, 139, 142, 144, 151, 164, 203, 234
molecular mechanisms, vii, 30, 68, 72, 149
molecular mimicry, 125
molecular structure, 143
molecular weight, 11, 233
molecules, xii, 40, 41, 53, 80, 90, 125, 133, 136, 137, 143, 144, 145, 148, 152, 163, 165, 166, 198, 199, 203, 205, 228, 230, 237
monoclonal antibody, 34, 128, 142, 147, 152, 160, 188, 192
monocyte chemoattractant protein, 81, 96, 230
monocyte chemotactic protein, 40, 237
monocytes, 41, 231, 232, 233, 235
mononuclear cells, 34, 63, 83, 97, 233
monotherapy, 58, 240
mood, x, 155, 156, 162, 172, 194
mood disorder, x, 155, 156, 162, 172, 194
morbidity, vii, viii, xi, 30, 65, 78, 79, 89, 91, 92, 93, 102, 189, 194, 211, 212, 232
morphology, 44, 96, 231
mortality, vii, viii, xi, xii, 5, 7, 11, 29, 30, 37, 42, 44, 49, 51, 55, 65, 67, 69, 78, 79, 82, 83, 85, 89, 91, 92, 96, 99, 109, 138, 178, 184, 186, 187, 188, 189, 191, 194, 211, 212, 214, 220, 221, 227, 228, 232, 233, 236
mortality rate, 78, 85, 187, 214
mothers, 11, 64, 65
motion, 24, 34, 46, 199, 203
mouse model, 126, 128, 161, 164, 174, 205
movement, 159, 194, 205
MRI, xi, 35, 66, 174, 193, 194, 196, 202, 203, 205, 206, 207, 209
mRNA, ix, 106, 118, 127
MTI, 195
multiple sclerosis, 137, 149, 158
multiplicity, 48
murmur, 33, 64
muscle cells, 37
muscle mass, 57
muscle strength, 24
muscles, 2
musculoskeletal pain, 106
musculoskeletal system, 79
mutant, 226
mutations, 52, 91, 216, 105, 107, 217, 218, 224
myasthenia gravis, 136, 138, 147, 148, 150, 191, 194
mycobacterial infection, 157
mycophenolate mofetil, xi, 133, 138, 211, 215, 218, 223
myelin, 135, 137, 147, 203, 205
myelin basic protein, 135, 137, 147
myocardial infarction, 35, 37, 41, 43, 44, 47, 48, 49, 66, 69, 72, 79, 80, 93, 94, 228, 232, 236, 237, 239
myocarditis, 31, 33, 34, 35, 36, 64, 66, 67
myocardium, 30, 33, 36, 62
myocyte, 34, 35, 241
myosin, 34, 234, 241

N

NAD, 234
National Institutes of Health, 146
National Research Council, 124
natural killer cell, 90
necrosis, 26, 33, 34, 63, 67, 95, 102, 111, 113, 119, 158, 198, 239
neovascularization, 38
nephritis, x, xii, 1, 2, 4, 5, 6, 7, 8, 10, 11, 15, 82, 89, 95, 102, 127, 128, 138, 141, 142, 144, 146, 147, 149, 150, 161, 162, 170, 172, 177, 183, 184, 185, 186, 190, 218, 223, 227
nephrologist, 15
nephropathy, 33, 228, 234
nephrotic syndrome, x, 8, 177, 184
nervous system, vii, 25, 102, 163, 164, 166, 167, 168, 189, 192, 206
Netherlands, 77
network, 132, 159, 178, 238
networking, xi, 212
neuroblastoma, 167
neurofibrillary tangles, 163, 173
neurofilament, 158
neuroimaging, 157, 194
neuroimaging techniques, 157
neurological deficit, 202
neurological disease, 163
neuronal apoptosis, 160, 161
neuronal cells, 167
neuronal death, 165
neurons, 157, 160, 161, 166, 197, 205
neuropathy, 158, 164, 194
neuroscience, 208
neurotransmission, 165
neurotransmitter(s), 160, 165, 173, 197
neutropenia, 187

neutrophils, 122
New York, iii, iv, 56
New Zealand, 129, 152
nicotine, 161
nitrates, 59
nitric oxide, viii, 39, 40, 52, 77, 82, 127, 230, 237, 241
nitric oxide synthase, 40, 127, 230, 237, 241
nitrogen, 4, 127
NK cells, 122
NMDA receptors, 160, 161, 170
NMR, 209
nodes, 109, 115
nodules, viii, 30, 63
noninvasive tests, 70
normal development, 173
NSAIDs, 2, 49
nucleosome, 141, 151
nucleosomes, 139, 141, 151, 162
nucleus, 162
nutrition, 222

O

obese patients, 225
obesity, 47, 50, 80, 83
observations, 5, 39, 158, 228
obstruction, 43, 44
occlusion, 44, 80
oedema, 33, 51, 58
optic neuritis, 164, 189
orbitofrontal cortex, 204, 205
organ, viii, ix, x, 2, 5, 10, 33, 77, 78, 79, 85, 86, 97, 99, 105, 106, 107, 108, 126, 131, 132, 133, 138, 181, 183, 187, 188, 189, 212, 214, 219, 223
organization, 214
orientation, 209
orthopnea, 33
ossification, 101
osteoarthritis, ix, 61, 105, 106
osteoporosis, viii, ix, 18, 77, 78, 79, 85, 86, 87, 88, 92, 99, 101, 105, 106
outpatients, 18, 51, 101
overload, 54, 163
overproduction, 234
ovulation, 12
oxidation, 41, 86, 232, 240
oxidative stress, 38, 82, 96

P

pain, 2, 19, 24, 26, 31, 33, 51, 109, 167
palpitations, 33
paralysis, 242
parameter, 116, 183, 198
parenchyma, 203, 205
parents, 184
paresis, 19
paroxysmal nocturnal dyspnea, 33
particles, 41, 151, 160, 173
PAS stain, 117
pathogenesis, viii, ix, x, xi, 38, 40, 52, 53, 66, 68, 77, 78, 79, 80, 81, 86, 89, 90, 91, 97, 105, 108, 125, 127, 132, 136, 139, 148, 152, 155, 157, 158, 162, 163, 165, 193, 196, 205, 229, 232, 237, 238, 240
pathogens, 90, 132
pathologist, 51
pathology, 66, 109, 123, 134, 137, 160, 206
pathophysiology, 202
pathways, 127, 133, 134, 213, 240, 241
PCR, 108, 112, 126
pediatric patients, 43, 171
peptides, x, 38, 131, 133, 134, 135, 136, 137, 138, 139, 140, 141, 143, 145, 146, 147, 148, 150, 151, 152, 153
perception, 213
perfusion, 66, 70, 79, 207
pericardial effusion, 31
pericardial rub, 31
pericarditis, 31, 32, 64, 184
pericardium, 30, 31, 62
peripheral blood, x, 18, 26, 139, 141, 144, 152, 177, 181, 183, 190, 191, 226
peripheral blood mononuclear cell, 139
peripheral nervous system, 156, 194
peripheral neuropathy, 2, 158, 189
peripheral vascular disease, viii, 77, 79, 172
permeability, 166, 232
Persian Gulf, 125
Persian Gulf War, 125
pertussis, 127
PET, 45, 195
PGE, 120, 230
pH, 108, 112
phage, 160
phagocytosis, 123, 128, 129
pharmaceuticals, 213
pharmacogenetics, 213, 214, 223

pharmacogenomics, xi, 211, 213, 214, 219, 220, 222, 223, 226
pharmacokinetics, 212, 215, 216, 218, 222, 223, 224, 225
pharmacological treatment, 2, 4, 5
pharmacotherapy, 212, 213
phenotype(s), 70, 113, 123, 126, 128, 133, 172, 213, 219, 230, 235, 242
phosphocreatine, 196
phosphodiesterase inhibitors, viii, 30
phospholipids, 163
phosphorylation, 234
photomicrographs, 117, 119
photosensitivity, 184
physical activity, 84, 86, 88
physical exercise, 27
pilot study, 26, 95, 164
pituitary gland, 26
placebo, 48, 57, 74, 235, 239, 242
placenta, 11, 12, 13
planning, 88
plaque, 38, 40, 42, 44, 45, 68, 70, 84, 94, 96, 230, 232, 238, 240
plasma, 1, 3, 4, 5, 7, 8, 14, 27, 33, 57, 62, 71, 82, 83, 86, 96, 97, 158, 239
plasma cells, 33
plasma levels, 14, 82, 86, 96, 97
plasma membrane, 62, 158
plasmapheresis, 1, 3, 4, 5, 6, 7, 8
plasmid, 138
plasminogen, 40
platelet activating factor, 163
platelet aggregation, 63, 107, 232, 240
platelet count, x, 178, 182, 183, 186
platelets, 11, 107, 182, 185, 232, 233
plexus, 158
PM, 70, 71, 95, 237
pneumococcus, 92
pneumonia, 103, 184, 185, 187
pneumonitis, 183, 185
pneumothorax, 186
Poland, 227
polycarbonate, 108
polymer, 111
polymerase, 112, 127, 185
polymerase chain reaction, 112, 127, 185
polymerization, 107
polymorphism, 97, 102, 103, 134, 215, 217, 218, 224, 225
polymorphisms, 52, 60, 75, 91, 103, 213, 215, 217, 218, 219, 223, 224, 225, 226
polypeptide(s), 60, 159, 160
poor, 1, 4, 6, 54, 189, 201
population, viii, xi, 2, 43, 46, 48, 51, 63, 74, 78, 79, 80, 81, 82, 83, 85, 87, 88, 92, 99, 101, 102, 103, 106, 134, 148, 165, 167, 206, 211, 212, 214, 216, 218, 219, 224, 228, 235, 236
positive correlation, 41, 231
positive relation, 87
positive relationship, 87
positron, 70, 195, 207
positron emission tomography, 70, 195, 207
postmenopausal women, 48, 88, 99
precipitation, 3
prediction, 95, 231
predictors, 10, 39, 40, 45, 68, 95, 99, 101, 147
prednisolone, x, 177, 182, 183, 184, 185, 186
prednisone, 5, 10, 31, 36, 39, 43, 47, 64, 98, 102
preeclampsia, 11
pregnancy, 7, 8, 9, 10, 11, 12, 13, 14, 15, 88, 189, 192
premature death, ix, 106, 115
prematurity, 10
premenopausal, 87, 88, 98, 99, 100
premenopausal women, 98, 99, 100
pressure, viii, 17, 18, 19, 25, 30, 31, 33, 50, 51, 53, 54, 55, 57
preterm delivery, 10
prevention, 18, 45, 46, 47, 48, 49, 70, 71, 84, 88, 98, 123, 141, 182, 192, 231, 232, 233, 235, 240, 241, 242
privacy, 213
private practice, 38
probability, 41, 185, 218
probe, 112
processing pathways, 173
production, vii, ix, x, xii, 3, 5, 39, 40, 52, 82, 86, 101, 105, 107, 116, 118, 121, 122, 126, 128, 129, 131, 132, 133, 135, 137, 138, 141, 143, 144, 147, 149, 150, 152, 158, 162, 228, 230, 231, 233, 235, 237, 242
profit, 214
progenitor cells, 128, 181, 191
prognosis, xii, 1, 54, 65, 79, 92, 102, 191, 201, 206, 214, 218, 227, 228
prognostic value, 93
program, 27, 98
programming, 241

pro-inflammatory, xii, 86, 132, 133, 162, 166, 172, 228, 235
proliferation, 38, 40, 41, 52, 57, 68, 69, 113, 119, 121, 128, 140, 141, 142, 145, 165, 174, 231, 232, 234, 241, 242
promoter, 91, 224, 225
prophylactic, 91, 142
prophylaxis, 64, 91, 182, 188
prostanoids, viii, 30, 55, 56, 58
proteases, 90, 125
protective factors, 40, 95
protective mechanisms, 135
protective role, 80, 159, 229, 231
protein(s), x, 3, 4, 41, 42, 52, 60, 62, 69, 70, 82, 90, 91, 97, 102, 107, 113, 122, 126, 138, 140, 141, 142, 149, 150, 151, 155, 157, 158, 159, 160, 161, 162, 163, 165, 167, 168, 170, 171, 172, 173, 174, 183, 213, 216, 217, 224, 233, 234, 238, 241
protein structure, 90
protein synthesis, 162
proteinase, 165
proteinuria, ix, 4, 11, 43, 48, 81, 106, 108, 109, 113, 114, 115, 121, 140, 144, 184, 186
proteomics, 213
prothrombin, 233
pro-thrombotic, 230
protocol(s), 51, 108, 109, 137, 138, 144, 181, 182, 184, 186, 188
protons, 196
prototype, 228
psychiatric disorders, x, 155, 156, 162
psychiatric morbidity, 159
psychopathology, 162
psychoses, 167
psychosis, x, 155, 157, 161, 162, 164, 170, 171, 172, 186, 189, 194, 201
public health, 219, 220
public opinion, 220
public policy, 214
puerperium, 10, 12
Puerto Rico, 211
pulmonary arteries, 51, 53, 54
pulmonary artery pressure, 50, 51, 54, 56, 186
pulmonary circulation, 73
pulmonary function test, 183
pulmonary hypertension, vii, viii, 27, 29, 30, 50, 51, 52, 53, 56, 57, 63, 72, 73, 74, 186
pulmonary vascular resistance, 56
pulse(s), x, 17, 18, 21, 25, 26, 33, 72, 177, 179, 180, 181, 183, 184, 185, 186, 190, 223
P-value, 113
pyelonephritis, 184

Q

QT interval, 65
QT prolongation, 65
quality improvement, 71, 84, 98
quality of life, viii, xi, 18, 27, 78, 79, 85, 99, 212, 219, 221
questionnaires, 19

R

race, 85, 221
racial differences, 223
range, 2, 5, 24, 25, 62, 183, 194, 220
rash, 10, 11, 35, 184, 185
Raynaud's phenomenon, 25, 27, 63
reactive oxygen, xii, 228
reactivity, ix, 4, 48, 60, 61, 106, 107, 123, 131, 132, 150, 151, 159, 162, 187
reality, xi, 69, 170, 178
receptors, 41, 53, 56, 63, 72, 73, 123, 133, 145, 147, 160, 165, 215, 233
recognition, 47, 90, 97, 122, 123, 148, 151, 229
recovery, 121, 148, 184, 187, 188
recurrence, 4
red blood cell(s), 182
redistribution, 39, 41, 163, 178
reduction, 4, 5, 43, 49, 87, 147, 189, 201, 202, 232, 240, 241
refractory, x, xi, 6, 35, 177, 178, 181, 187, 189, 190, 192, 234, 235, 242
regeneration, 123, 125, 128
regression, 59, 61, 124, 231
regression analysis, 124
regulation, 52, 67, 95, 126, 128, 129, 145, 149, 162, 230, 233, 234, 237, 238, 239
rehydration, 108
rejection, 113, 120, 123, 224, 226, 230
relapses, 127, 159
relationship, 9, 38, 60, 61, 62, 80, 86, 87, 93, 123, 159, 161, 164, 167, 173, 174, 202, 212, 214, 215, 218, 225, 226
relaxation, 18, 35, 41, 58, 59, 197
relaxation times, 35, 197
relevance, x, 61, 145, 155, 171, 215, 219, 224
reliability, 45, 57

remission, 2, 4, 5, 170, 179, 180, 183, 184, 185, 186, 187, 190, 191, 206, 217
renal dysfunction, 106, 189
renal failure, 10, 81, 82, 86, 88, 186, 189, 221
renal function, 2, 4, 5, 12, 13, 86, 89, 186
repair, ix, 64, 105, 107, 123
reproduction, 15, 109
residues, 82, 136, 140, 160
resistance, 36, 83, 126, 144, 217, 219, 224, 225
resolution, vii, 30, 196, 203
respiratory, 186
responsiveness, 135, 148
restenosis, 47, 50
retinitis, 224
retinitis pigmentosa, 224
reverse transcriptase, 112
rheumatic diseases, xii, 3, 100, 101, 149, 215, 228, 242
rheumatoid arthritis, ix, 25, 60, 61, 98, 100, 105, 106, 124, 138, 150, 235, 242
rheumatologist, 219
rhythm, 33, 64
ribosomal RNA, 112
right atrium, 31
right hemisphere, 195
right ventricle, 32
risk, vii, viii, xii, 3, 5, 9, 11, 12, 14, 15, 26, 29, 30, 37, 38, 39, 41, 42, 43, 45, 46, 47, 48, 49, 50, 61, 62, 64, 65, 67, 68, 69, 70, 71, 72, 77, 78, 79, 80, 81, 82, 83, 84, 85, 86, 87, 88, 89, 90, 92, 93, 94, 95, 96, 97, 98, 99, 101, 102, 103, 106, 125, 126, 132, 133, 163, 187, 188, 189, 190, 192, 218, 221, 223, 227, 228, 229, 233, 235, 236, 241, 242
risk factors, viii, 26, 37, 38, 39, 41, 42, 43, 45, 47, 50, 65, 67, 68, 69, 70, 71, 77, 79, 80, 81, 82, 84, 85, 87, 92, 93, 94, 95, 97, 98, 102, 126, 192, 221, 229, 233, 235, 236, 241
rituximab, 188, 192
RNA, 97, 106, 111, 140
RNA splicing, 140
ROI, 203
room temperature, 109, 110, 111
Russia, 177

S

sacrifice, 119
safety, 8, 12, 24, 88, 145, 213, 215, 219, 220
sample, 2, 48, 112
scar tissue, 107
scleroderma, 25, 27, 53
sclerosis, 137
scores, 45, 70, 113, 116
SCT, x, 177, 178, 179, 181, 182, 183, 184, 185, 186, 187, 188, 189
search, 213
secretion, 26, 40, 128, 142, 147
sediment, 11
seizure(s), 11, 106, 157, 163, 164, 167, 194
selecting, 189
selectivity, 7
sensation, 19, 24
sensing, 73
sensitivity, 34, 40, 196, 220, 225
sensitization, 135, 199
sepsis, 107, 125, 179, 184, 185
septum, 54
sequencing, 215
series, vii, viii, ix, 6, 10, 11, 12, 30, 33, 34, 35, 36, 46, 55, 56, 57, 58, 66, 78, 89, 109, 110, 139, 189, 228, 229
serine, 90, 163, 165
serology, 183, 185, 186
serum, x, 4, 5, 7, 11, 38, 43, 60, 61, 69, 72, 81, 86, 87, 90, 91, 96, 101, 103, 108, 110, 111, 116, 118, 122, 123, 126, 155, 158, 159, 161, 163, 164, 165, 167, 174, 183, 231, 233
serum albumin, 110
severity, xi, 5, 27, 31, 43, 45, 49, 55, 85, 103, 113, 122, 123, 135, 161, 189, 194, 201, 202, 211, 212
sex, 2, 79, 215
shares, 90
shock, 31, 42, 69, 70, 107, 138, 150
sialic acid, 158
side effects, 3, 5, 133, 134, 138, 184, 222
signal transduction, 158, 234
signals, 122, 132
sign(s), ix, 31, 33, 59, 91, 106, 115, 185, 198, 200
similarity, 143
single photon emission computerized tomography, 207
single-nucleotide polymorphism, 215, 224
skin, vii, ix, 2, 5, 10, 17, 18, 21, 22, 23, 24, 25, 26, 91, 92, 105, 106, 107, 108, 109, 111, 112, 113, 114, 115, 119, 120, 121, 123, 125, 187
skin diseases, 125
smokers, 38
smoking, viii, 38, 43, 47, 50, 77, 84, 85, 88
smooth muscle, 37, 38, 40, 41, 42, 44, 52, 56, 57, 69, 81, 230, 233, 234, 241

smooth muscle cells, 37, 38, 42, 44, 57, 69, 81, 230, 233
SNP, 216, 217
sodium, 36, 133
solubility, 135
somatic mutations, 213
sounds, 213
species, xii, 139, 228, 234
specificity, 35, 46, 51, 60, 133, 134, 144, 146, 156, 158, 161, 165, 170, 194
spectroscopy, xi, 193, 195, 196, 197, 200, 202, 206, 207, 208
spectrum, 89, 92, 156, 196, 197, 198
speed, 213
sperm, 13
sphygmomanometer, 19
spinal cord, 192
spine, 88
spleen, 115, 141
splenomegaly, ix, 106, 108, 115
spontaneous abortion, 10
sprouting, 173
St. Petersburg, 109
stability, 139
stabilization, 232, 240
stages, 40, 51, 70, 142, 145, 150
standard deviation, 111
standards, 110
statin, 48, 71, 232, 233, 234
statistical analysis, 19
stem cells, x, 177, 178, 181, 185, 187, 191
stenosis, 43, 44, 46
stent, 50
sterile, 109
steroids, 5, 98, 99, 188
stillbirth, 10
strain, 122, 123, 129, 160
strategies, x, 40, 42, 43, 46, 48, 55, 59, 66, 78, 87, 88, 123, 131, 137, 138, 165, 219
strength, 25, 88, 107
stress, 27, 96, 106, 124, 126, 161, 163, 235
stress factors, 235
stretching, 17, 18
stroke, 39, 41, 43, 47, 49, 64, 79, 83, 94, 163, 189, 199, 201, 202, 240
structural changes, 208
structural characteristics, 135
subacute, 35, 189
subcutaneous injection, 138
subgroups, 84, 231, 241
substitution, 1, 3, 36, 149
suffering, 62, 232
sugar, 158
suicide, 159
suicide attempts, 159
sulfate, 2, 3, 6, 7, 8
sulfur, 39
sulfuric acid, 110
superiority, 137
supervision, 14
suppression, 13, 127, 132, 134, 135, 137, 138, 139, 144, 145, 147, 148, 150, 151, 152, 232, 234, 235
surface area, ix, 105
surface structure, 163
surveillance, 64, 132, 188
survival, viii, ix, 55, 77, 78, 79, 106, 108, 113, 114, 115, 120, 121, 122, 138, 140, 141, 142, 189, 219, 222, 226
survival rate, ix, 106, 108, 114, 115
susceptibility, 90, 91, 103, 169, 196, 225
swelling, 33, 35
switching, 122
symptom(s), ix, x, 2, 4, 5, 19, 24, 26, 31, 33, 35, 51, 58, 59, 91, 105, 107, 114, 155, 158, 161, 162, 184, 185, 186, 189, 200, 201, 202, 203, 205, 210
syndrome, 11, 48, 59, 60, 62, 80, 81, 83, 96, 102, 107, 114, 117, 125, 127, 159, 184, 192, 194, 201, 225, 235, 236
synthesis, ix, xii, 5, 36, 40, 99, 106, 122, 127, 136, 138, 164, 166, 169, 227, 230, 231, 233, 235, 240
syphilis, 91
systemic circulation, 58, 160, 164
systemic lupus erythematosus, iv, vii, viii, ix, xii, 6, 7, 8, 14, 18, 27, 29, 30, 44, 53, 60, 61, 62, 66, 67, 68, 69, 70, 71, 72, 73, 74, 75, 77, 92, 93, 94, 95, 96, 97, 98, 99, 100, 101, 102, 103, 123, 124, 125, 126, 127, 128, 129, 131, 146, 147, 148, 149, 150, 151, 152, 167, 168, 169, 170, 171, 172, 173, 174, 175, 178, 189, 190, 191, 192, 194, 206, 207, 208, 209, 210, 221, 222, 223, 226, 228, 229, 236, 237, 239, 242
systemic sclerosis, 17, 18, 27, 73
systems, xi, 2, 5, 78, 183, 187, 211, 213, 215, 226
systolic blood pressure, 19
systolic pressure, 19, 55, 57

T

T cell, ix, 40, 44, 90, 107, 123, 126, 127, 129, 131, 132, 133, 134, 135, 136, 137, 138, 139, 140, 141,

142, 143, 144, 146, 147, 148, 149, 150, 151, 152, 153, 186, 226, 230, 231, 234, 237, 238
T lymphocyte(s), 107, 132, 145, 149, 229
tachycardia, 33, 59, 64
target population, 228
targets, vii, 30, 50, 59, 84, 133, 162, 163, 165, 188, 215
T-cell(s), 68, 120, 123, 126, 133, 134, 136, 138, 141, 142, 145, 147, 148, 186, 188, 236
TCR, 146
technetium, 46
technology, 5, 51, 213
temperature, 17, 18, 21, 22, 23, 24, 25, 26, 110, 111
territory, 194
testosterone, 86
Texas, 241
TGF, 52, 122, 129, 141, 144, 145, 152, 153
thalamus, 204, 205
T-helper cell, 126
theory, 201, 202
therapeutic agents, 138, 145, 146
therapeutic approaches, 1
therapeutic targets, 133, 241
therapeutics, xi, 211, 212, 213, 222
therapy, viii, x, xii, 1, 5, 6, 7, 8, 12, 13, 30, 32, 34, 35, 43, 46, 55, 56, 58, 69, 70, 71, 73, 74, 84, 88, 89, 98, 100, 101, 126, 131, 132, 134, 135, 137, 138, 139, 141, 142, 144, 147, 149, 159, 177, 178, 181, 182, 183, 184, 186, 187, 188, 189, 191, 192, 194, 213, 219, 222, 223, 225, 227, 228, 231, 234
threshold, 26, 112, 133
thrombin, 232, 233, 240, 241
thrombocytopenia, 11, 33, 189
thrombosis, 11, 39, 43, 53, 61, 62, 68, 69, 71, 80, 83, 88, 94, 156, 205, 232
thrombus, 38, 62, 63, 164, 230, 232
thymus, 118, 132, 135, 148
thyroglobulin, 136
thyroid, 64, 136, 148
time, x, 5, 18, 33, 43, 64, 78, 79, 86, 88, 99, 107, 108, 109, 110, 112, 113, 114, 115, 116, 117, 118, 119, 120, 121, 123, 126, 134, 138, 139, 178, 183, 185, 186, 196, 200, 201, 202, 203, 205, 213, 220, 221, 228
tin, 1
tissue, ix, x, 27, 30, 34, 35, 38, 40, 55, 62, 65, 73, 90, 105, 106, 107, 111, 113, 120, 122, 123, 131, 132, 133, 148, 160, 163, 174, 196, 199, 203, 230, 233, 235, 240, 242
TNF, ix, 40, 48, 53, 63, 69, 81, 86, 97, 106, 107, 119, 120, 122, 138, 144, 230, 231, 234, 235, 239, 242
TNF-alpha, 69, 97, 231, 239
TNF-α, 40, 48, 53, 81, 86, 107, 119, 120
total cholesterol, 48
toxic effect, 166
toxicity, 186, 188, 191, 214, 216, 217, 218, 220, 223
toxin, 127
toxoplasmosis, 91
TPI, 158
training, 27, 51, 220
traits, 215
transcription, 112
transcripts, 108, 119, 120, 122
transduction, 241
transforming growth factor, 52, 141
transfusion, 181, 182
translation, 219
transmission, 3, 26, 234
transplant recipients, 192, 224, 226
transplantation, ix, x, 106, 112, 120, 121, 126, 177, 178, 181, 182, 183, 186, 188, 190, 191, 215, 223, 237
transport, 173, 197
transthoracic echocardiography, 63, 75
trauma, 106, 107, 113, 114, 116, 118, 119, 120, 121, 123, 124, 125, 126
trend, 57, 187
trial, 5, 6, 15, 48, 57, 71, 101, 102, 138, 150, 190, 226, 239, 242
triggers, 106, 126, 136
triglycerides, 38, 39, 40, 43, 64, 67, 81, 95, 231, 239
tuberculosis, 89
tumor, ix, 53, 63, 67, 81, 95, 106, 127, 138, 147, 148, 158, 235, 239, 242
tumor growth, 158
tumor necrosis factor, ix, 53, 63, 67, 81, 95, 106, 127, 138, 147, 148, 235, 239
turnover, 25, 100, 126, 197, 200
twins, 65
type 1 diabetes, 150
type 2 diabetes, 97

U

UK, 103
ultrasonography, vii, 30
ultrasound, 43, 45, 46, 47, 55
United Kingdom, 83, 214

United States, 39, 43, 83, 101, 106, 124, 191, 222
universe, 126
unplanned pregnancies, 10
unstable angina, 236
urine, 108, 109, 113, 183
UV, 106
UV radiation, 106

V

vaccinations, 92
vaccine, 125
Valencia, 111
validation, 93, 139, 168
validity, 51, 139, 164, 220, 226
values, 4, 46, 55, 87, 112, 118, 164, 203, 204, 205, 208, 210
variability, viii, 27, 30, 165, 213, 215, 219
variable(s), xi, 45, 212, 218, 219
variation, 22, 23, 103, 156, 223
vascular endothelial growth factor (VEGF), 52
vascular wall, 239
vasculitis, ix, x, xii, 1, 2, 5, 46, 81, 95, 105, 113, 121, 156, 161, 162, 172, 177, 181, 183, 185, 186, 202, 205, 227
vasoconstriction, 25, 234
vasoconstrictor, 232
vasodilation, 25, 56
vasodilator, 57
vaso-occlusion, 205
vasospasm, 25
VCAM, 230, 237
vector, 149
velocity, 34, 46, 54, 58
ventricle, 32, 58
ventricular arrhythmias, 36
ventricular tachycardia, 35
vessels, 18, 25, 43, 52, 164, 196, 205, 232
veterans, 124, 125
viral infection, 91
virus infection, 184
viruses, 90
visualization, 46, 111
vitamin B1, 84
vitamin B12, 84
vitamin D, 86, 88
vitamin D deficiency, 86
VLDL, 81, 82
vulnerability, 44

W

water diffusion, 199
weight reduction, 84
welfare, 124
western blot, 158
Western Europe, 90
white blood cells, 181
white matter, xi, 193, 194, 195, 200, 201, 202, 203, 204, 205, 209, 210
WHO, 57, 181, 184
wild type, ix, 105, 107
withdrawal, 189
women, vii, 9, 10, 11, 12, 13, 18, 29, 41, 45, 68, 70, 71, 83, 87, 88, 93, 94, 95, 96, 97, 98, 99, 100, 101, 107, 228, 229, 236, 239, 241
World Health Organization, 181
wound healing, ix, 105, 107, 123, 125, 127, 128
wound repair, ix, 106, 107, 108, 119, 128
writing, 139

Y

yang, 240
yeast, 163
yield, 111, 119, 136, 213
yin, 240
young women, 218, 229